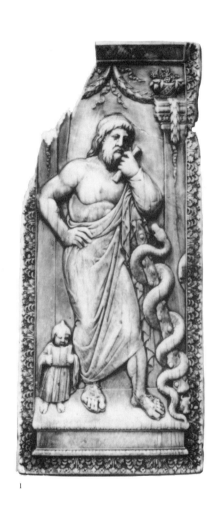

1

1 Asclepius, the god of
healing, with the sacred snake
coiled round his staff, in an
ivory panel from the Diptych of
Asclepius and Hgieia, made in
Rome about 400 AD.

For endpaper key see opposite p. 192

Triumphs

Introduction by

Sir Derrick Dunlop MD FRCP

Professor Emeritus of Therapeutics and
Clinical Medicine, University of Edinburgh;
Extra Physician to The Queen in Scotland;
former Chairman, Committee on Safety of Drugs
and Medicines Commission

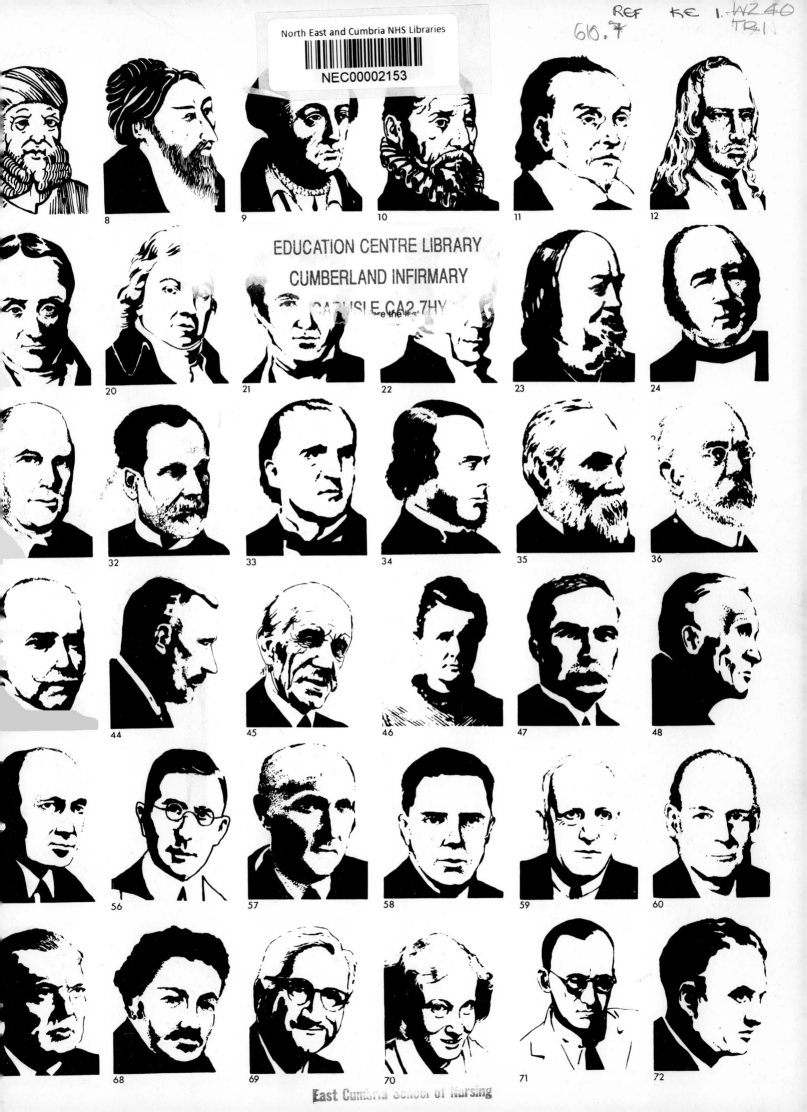

REF KE 1. WZ46
610.7 TRIN

# of Medicine

Edited by

Harry Keen MD FRCP
Professor of Human Metabolism, Guy's Hospital, London

John Jarrett MD MFCM
Senior Lecturer, Department of Community Medicine, Guy's Hospital, London

US Advisory Editor

Arthur M Levy MD
Professor of Medicine and Pediatrics, University of Vermont
College of Medicine, Burlington, Vermont, USA

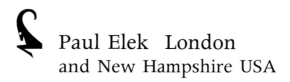

Paul Elek London
and New Hampshire USA

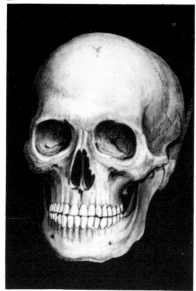
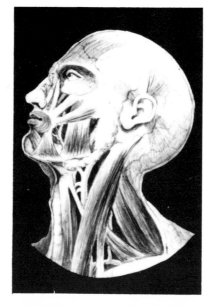
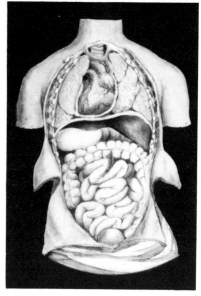
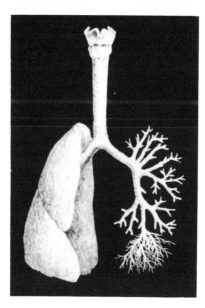
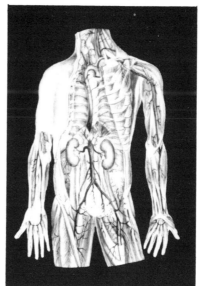
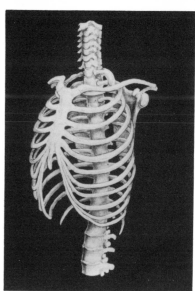

2 Hand-painted Victorian lantern slides probably used for teaching medical students. They show (top left to bottom right) the skull; the muscles of the head and neck; the lungs, heart, stomach and intestines; trachea, lung and bronchioles; the aorta and its branches and the kidneys; and the thoracic cage formed by the ribs and spine.

First published 1976 by
Paul Elek Ltd
54-58 Caledonian Road
London N1 9RN

and Paul Elek Inc.
10 South Broadway
Salem New Hampshire 03079 USA

ISBN 0 236 30925 0

Produced by Paul Elek Ltd
Picture Adviser:
J. Rytina MBKS AIIP AIMBI
Director, Department of Medical Illustration and Photography, Guy's Hospital, London

Filmset in Great Britain by Photocomp Ltd, Birmingham
Printed in Great Britain by The Garden City Press Ltd,
Letchworth, Hertfordshire SG6 1JS

Contents

List of Plates

Acknowledgments

The Editors and publisher wish to acknowledge specially the help given to them in the preparation of this book and the collection of illustrations by the following: Dr J. M. Annear, St Olave's Hospital, London; Professor C. R. Austin, Physiological Laboratory, Cambridge; Dr L. H. Bannister, Molteno Institute, University of Cambridge; Mr Michael Bewick, Guy's Hospital, London; Dr E. Bird, EM Unit, London School of Hygiene and Tropical Medicine; Dr Colin Blakemore, Physiological Laboratory, Cambridge; Professor Bryan Brooke, St George's Hospital, London; Professor Stewart Cameron, Guy's Hospital, London; Mr Stuart Campbell, Queen Charlotte's Hospital, London; Dr P. N. Cardew, Department of Audio-Visual Communication, St Mary's Hospital Medical School, London; J. S. Collins, Royal National Orthopaedic Hospital, Stanmore, Middlesex; Mr F. A. L. da Cunha, Oldham & District General Hospital; Dr D. L. Davies, Institute of Psychiatry, London; Dr T. Gibson, Guy's Hospital, London; Dr R. D. Hoare, Guy's/Maudsley Neuro-Surgical Unit, London; Dr J. Irving, Lewisham Hospital, London; D. Jackson-Feilden, Ferraris Development and Engineering Company Limited, London; Mr A. N. Johns, Guy's Hospital, London; Dr Brian Kaufman, Watford Hospital, Middlesex; Mr Hugh Kinder, Guy's Hospital, London; Dr P. J. Lawther, MRC Air Pollution Research Unit, St Bartholomew's Hospital Medical College, London; Dr Raymond Levy, Institute of Psychiatry, London; Dr John Lythgoe, MRC Vision Unit, University of Sussex; Dr Michael Maisey, Guy's Hospital, London; Dr I. F. Moseley, The National Hospital, London; Rosemary Nicholson, Westminster Hospital, London; Dr Julia M. Polak, Royal Postgraduate Medical School, London; Dr M. E. A. Powell, Kingston Group of Hospitals; Dr A. J. Salisbury, Cardiothoracic Institute, London; Mr L. F. W. Salmon, Guy's Hospital, London; Dr P. R. Salmon, University of Bristol; Dr Hugh Saxton, Guy's Hospital, London; John Smith; Professor Paul Talalay, Department of Pharmacology and Experimental Therapeutics, Johns Hopkins University School of Medicine; T. Tarrant, Institute of Ophthalmology, London; Professor J. R. Trounce, Guy's Hospital Medical School, London; Mrs Elizabeth Ward, The Silver Lining Appeal of the British Kidney Patient Association; Sidney Watkins, Wellcome Institute of the History of Medicine; Professor M. H. F. Wilkins, Biophysics Department, King's College, London; Dr Roger Williams, Liver Unit, King's College Hospital, London.

Individual authors have also taken particular trouble in supplying pictures for the book.

Thanks are also due to Faber and Faber Ltd and Harcourt Brace Jovanovich, Inc., for permission to quote four lines from *The Love Song of J. Alfred Prufrock* from *Collected Poems 1909–1962* by T. S. Eliot.

Editors' Preface

Medicine has been caught up like all other human activities in the technological revolution of the last hundred years. Traditionally it was a dormant profession in which the greatest virtue was the transmission of a system of ancient ideas from one generation to the next (although, of course, individual doctors had displayed a notable scientific curiosity). Now it has become a restless, critical discipline, trying desperately to encompass an explosive increase in knowledge in the biological sciences.

It is our purpose in this book to direct the attention of the reader to what we consider to be the major achievements in medical science, while attempting to avoid being blinded by the most recent or by the most spectacular. These achievements are not, in our view, limited to advances in the *treatment* of disease, impressive though these are. We have also focused upon some areas where the advance is in the *understanding* of diseases which we are, as yet, unable to treat with great success—for example the so-called inborn errors of metabolism which are examples of an almost fundamental explanation of disease, at a molecular level. The achievements are also impressive in the field of diagnosis. Radiography, the use of radio-isotopes, the measurement of complex substances, some at vanishingly low concentrations in blood and tissue fluids, all have illuminated the disturbances of structure and function which underlie the manifestations of human disease. And we have felt it right to point to the greatest triumph of all at the beginning of the book, the triumph which receives far less than its due recognition and that rejoices not in the dramatic cure but in the much less dramatic expectation of normality. We refer, of course, to the extraordinary achievements of preventive medicine and notably to the control of the infectious diseases. Much of the honor must go to the pioneers of the 19th century, Pasteur, Koch, Semmelweiss and others who brought the cause of the fearful contagions that beset mankind under the microscope and into the laboratory, so setting the scene for man's most dramatic conquest of disease. Credit must go too to the unsung battalions who protect the public health, day by day, year in year out. For all the miracles of antibiotics, our secure western societies would soon be ravaged by disease again were our carefully constructed and almost invisible defences to be seriously weakened. The absence of epidemic disease is now taken for granted; but not far separated from us in space or time cholera, typhoid, plague, malaria, smallpox and consumption wreak or have wreaked a terrible toll.

It will help the reader, as he tries to appraise modern medicine, to distinguish between the achievements of medicine at communal level, and those at personal level, though the distinction is, of course, neither sharp nor absolute. The surgeon's intricate operation on a diseased heart valve—supported by a team of bioengineers, who maintain the patient's circulation as he lies with his heart stopped in the surgeon's hand, following a period of intensive investigation with X-ray pictures of the chambers of the heart, records of the electrical activity of the contracting heart muscle, measurement of pressures and oxygen content in the circulating blood—will all be rendered unnecessary by the *prevention* of the streptococcal infection which led to the rheumatic fever that damaged the heart valve in the first place. A whole generation of chest physicians and surgeons who struggled to treat the depredations of pulmonary tuberculosis are now redeployed, working in other fields since the disease was brought under preventive control. Likewise, much of the machinery for finding and

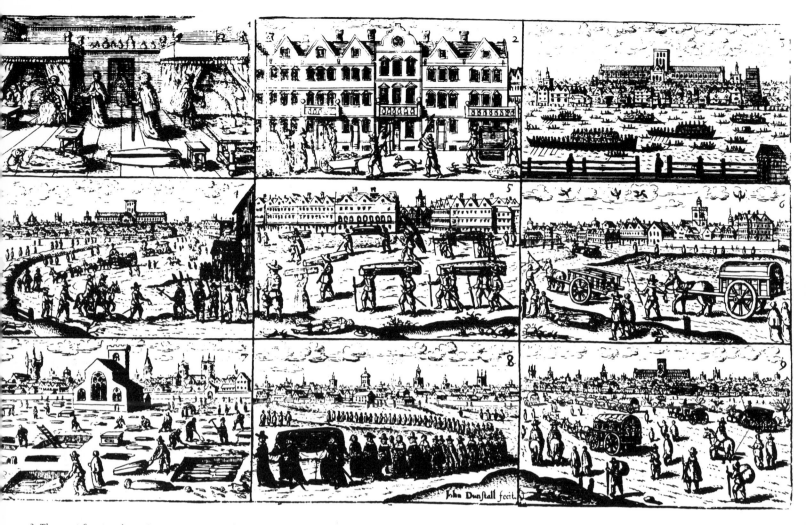

3 The most famous plague in history, the Great Plague of London of 1665. This late 17th century print shows typical scenes of death, flight by land and water, and the disposal of bodies, against the medieval backdrop of the City of London, about to be swept away in the Fire of the following year. Old St Paul's Cathedral can be distinguished in some of the pictures. It is difficult to conceive of the ever-present threat of death that hovered over existence a century or two ago. Great plagues would sweep across human communities. Hardly a family would escape; sometimes all would die. It is against this sort of grisly background that one should view the extraordinary security of life which we take for granted today.

4 The first of the non-invasive techniques which enabled the doctor to see below skin surface was the exploitation of the penetrating properties of the X-ray, discovered by Röntgen in 1895 (see illustrations 114 and 115). This early radiograph is a curious relic more of entertainment than instructive or diagnostic value. A composite of nine separate X-ray plates, it has been incorrectly assembled with the heart shown as lying in the right side of the chest. Apart from the development of X-ray techniques, many shown

treating lung cancer could be swept away by the cessation of cigarette smoking.

Like music and mathematics, medicine is a universal language, drawing contributions to knowledge from many countries and, theoretically at least, making discoveries available to the whole of mankind. Every country of the civilized world contributes to the body of medical knowledge. From barely recorded beginnings in Persia, India, North Africa and China through the great scientific culture of post-Renaissance Europe, the age of enlightenment has spread across the globe. There is no room for chauvinism in regarding these triumphs. Every country can look with pride to some contribution. The *delivery* of medical care is now becoming a main area of concern (what use is the most fascinating and life-saving discovery if it cannot be brought to those in need of it?): a separate book could be written on this subject.

Mankind cannot reasonably expect unmixed blessings, and we would not claim that modern medicine is such. What might at first sight seem to be an undiminished triumph proves on closer examination to exact its own considerable price from society. The great decline in infant mortality has led to a huge increase in population and, in western societies, the aged have become an increasing proportion of the whole. This,

together with the survival of sick and handicapped individuals, has contributed to the ever increasing total costs of medical care. The development of powerful drugs has not only cured or mitigated the effects of old diseases, but has also created new hazards to health. The massive machinery of diagnosis and treatment threatens to displace the dedicated nurse with the desiccated technician, to dehumanize the course of disease and almost to deny the inevitability of death. Because costs have risen faster than resources decisions have to be made—by the individual and by the community—as to how limited resources must be assigned. The doctor is now far less a priest, much more a super technologist relinquishing—sometimes with regret—his ancient authoritarian role in today's anti-authoritarian society and frequently seeking refuge in the perfection of machines. Medical research grows increasingly complex, reaching into hitherto undreamed of regions of molecular biology and biophysics and concerning itself almost exclusively with quantities, hardly at all with qualities. Yet despite—perhaps because of— the increasing intrusion of technology into medicine, the expectations of the public concerning its powers have never been greater. To the extent that the Biblical lifespan of three score and ten years is now the statistical norm for

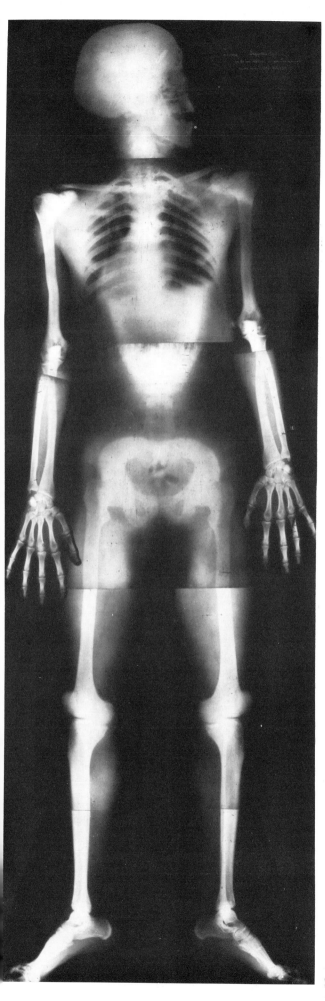

the average new-born baby, and that alleviation, if not cure, is available for most physical illness, these expectations might seem justified. However, when the expectations are not fulfilled the other side of the coin is disappointment and disenchantment. Never has public awe at the power of medicine been so intense; never have suspicions of it run so deep. At the same time doctors are accorded the highest honors in the land and submitted to the most punitive of malpractice suits.

The negative aspects of the triumphs are dealt with in each chapter as appropriate. But the book involves the *triumphs* of medicine and we make no apology for the generally optimistic tone. We hope that our readers will be entertained and informed by the contents of the book, and above all that it will help them to understand what medicine is, how it got there and, perhaps, where it is going.

in this book, other physical phenomena have been turned to non-invasive diagnostic use. Diagnostic ultra-sound is used to produce reflected images of the cavities of the heart, to outline the fetus still protected within the uterus (see illustration 204), and for the diagnosis of cysts and tumors deep within the body. The pattern of heat production from the skin surface may betray an underlying tumor or inflammatory disorder. Nuclear medicine, a new branch of diagnostics, makes use of the selective uptake by certain tissues of radioactive isotopes, the location of which then gives important information on functional or structural abnormalities (see illustrations 58 and 59). Most exciting perhaps is the EMI scanner which, by the combined use of radiology and computer analysis, builds up an image of an imaginary section cut across the body (see illustrations 33 and 145-7).

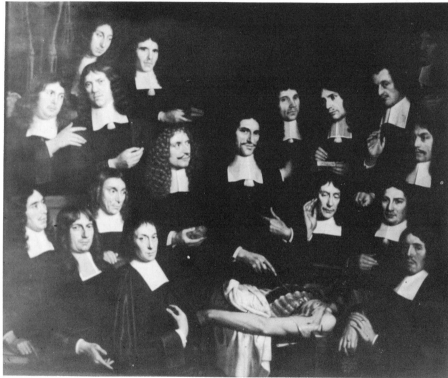

5

5 For centuries, the art of medicine was handed on as a set of inviolable rules and aphorisms which the practitioner disregarded only at the risk of being hounded as a charlatan and heretic. The age of enlightenment penetrated medicine late, and was ushered in by the careful and critical examination of the dead. The study of the normal structures of the human body, still a basic part of the education of the student of medicine, is portrayed above in 'The Anatomy Lesson' by Cornelis de Man, dated 1681. (Antony van Leeuwenhoek, the inventor of the microscope (see illustration 14), is the figure in the lighter colored wig, holding a sponge.) The painstaking correlation of disease in life with disordered structure after death laid the foundation of the modern development of scientific medicine. No longer is the anatomy lesson restricted to the naked-eye examination of the whole body. The powerful techniques of magnification and biochemistry have extended the understanding of structure and function in health and disease down to and beyond the level of the minuscule structures within the individual cells of the tissues of the body. Even the molecular mechanics of the genetic control mechanisms of living cells has been penetrated and described in detail. The chromosomes, species-characteristic rods exercising genetic control over the characteristics of every cell, have been shown to be composed of orderly sequences of nucleotides, the order of which conveys specific instructions to the protein-synthesizing apparatus of the cell, much as the sequence of holes on a pianola roll determines the complex melody which the player piano plays (see illustrations 51 and 52).

Introduction

Everywhere nowadays there is an increasing demand for more information about health, disease, prognosis and treatment. This is partly due to the wider discussion of medical matters on radio and television and in the press, books and magazines. The medical profession is unanimous as to the need for positive health education but is still divided on the desirability of educating the *healthy* public about disease. There are those who believe that the less the laity know and think about disease the better; that reading and talking about it only breeds neurosis and hypochondriasis and that television programs and articles on disease in the press are popular not so much for their educational value as for their sensational appeal. Others, including the writer, believe that the days of medical obscurantism are over, that fear arises from ignorance and that diseases lose half their awe-inspiring qualities if they are rationally and judiciously explained by competent, responsible authorities.

In the early civilizations medicine grew from the ribs of the priestcraft and treatment was mostly dispensed by spells, invocations and amulets. Priestcraft medicine survived into the Middle Ages and is not without its devotees today. Perhaps the cynic might say that the use of placebos which play a not unimportant role in the modern practice of medicine is not far removed from the practice of magic long ago.

In the golden age of Athenian civilization Hippocrates taught under his plane tree in Cos that a logical materialism and the application of natural methods were more important in medicine than superstition and magic. Nevertheless, about 300 years later the door which he had opened a little to rational medicine and therapeutics was effectually shut again for centuries by Galen, the personal physician to Marcus Aurelius. He believed disease to be due to changes in the humors of the body and classified medicaments into innumerable groups of herbal remedies which he claimed to have an effect on these humors. Galen must have been a remarkable man for in the long history of medicine there has been no one else whose authority brooded over its practice for so long and whose views were so universally held that it was heresy to challenge them.

The accurate description of the structure of the human body by Vesalius in the 16th century set the stage for the renaissance of science. Thus, the 17th century was notable for great advances in experimental physiology by William Harvey, in analytical chemistry by Robert Boyle and in physics and mathematics by Galileo. Advances in medical treatment during the century were not, however, comparable. Indeed Voltaire who was born only 52 years after the death of Galileo and 37 years after the death of Harvey defined medical treatment as 'the art of pouring drugs of which one knew nothing into a patient of whom one knew less'.

In the 18th century, though Galenism had been overthrown, no scientific therapeutics had emerged: just a fierce allopathy of bleedings, sweatings, vomitings and purgings. The natural revulsion to all this doubtless resulted in Hahnemann's popularity, for homeopathy at least did no harm. It also contributed to the therapeutic nihilism of most scientific physicians in the 19th and early 20th centuries.

Anatomy, physiology, pathology, bacteriology and diagnostic medicine had usually to blaze the trail along which scientific therapeutics could advance. Thus at much the same time as Boerhaave in Leyden was introducing clinical observation as we understand it today, and René Laennec, the inventor of the stethoscope, was beginning to put diagnosis on a firmer

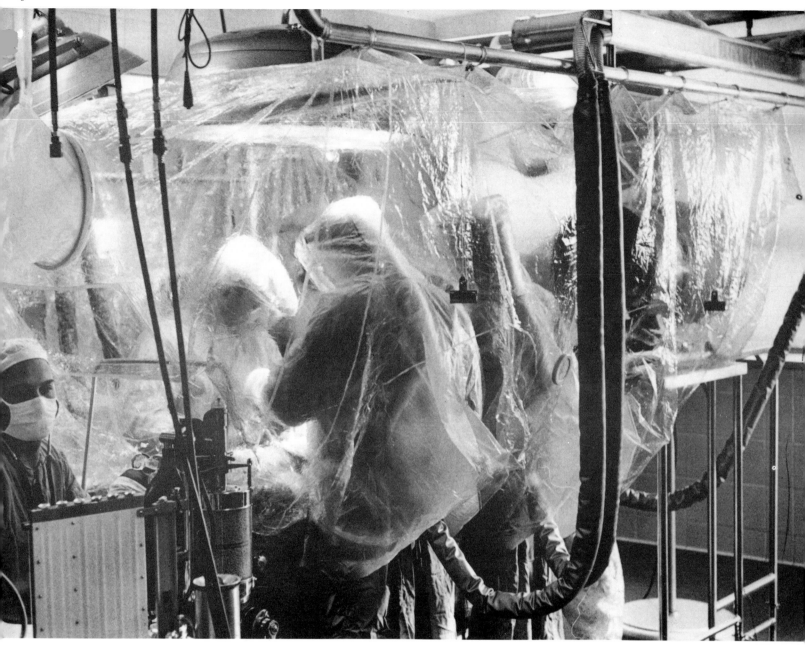

foundation, some 30 million leeches a year were being used in France in treatment. When the great German pathologist Virchow was revolutionizing pathology and altering our whole concept of disease, the pharmacopoeias then in use still included a mass of rubbish, the relics of medieval folklore. For years after Robert Koch had made his monumental discovery of the tubercle bacillus, tuberculous patients suffered from his disastrous recommendation that they should be treated with tuberculin. When Sir William Osler published his classical *Textbook of Medicine* about the turn of this century, therapeutic nihilism was still so rife that less than 10 per cent of the space in the first edition was devoted to treatment and much of that consisted of pious hopes and vague generalities: 'arsenic might prove useful'; 'the general health should receive attention'. He still had to rely for treatment very largely on bottles of medicine elaborately compounded, delicately flavored, meticulously bottled and exquisitely

labelled but, as Oliver Wendell Holmes said, 'if the whole materia medica, as now used, could be sunk to the bottom of the sea, it would be all the better for mankind and all the worse for the fishes'.

This was of course a considerable exaggeration for during the early part of the 19th century pharmacology became a science seeking to identify the active substances in the crude drugs which, so to speak, had been culled from the hedgerows, and to determine their actions in the body. Atropine, bromine, caffeine, codeine, emetine, iodine, morphine, nicotine, physostigmine, pilocarpine, quinine and strychnine were all isolated; and ether, nitrous oxide, chloral and chloroform synthesized. In 1860 coal tar was used to synthesize salicylic acid, the first product resulting from research on dyes, and the synthesis of that remarkable drug, aspirin, followed in 1899. A few years later the German pharmaceutical industry produced barbitone (Veronal),

6 Safe surgery owed much to the introduction of anesthesia, but the greatest hazard of all, infection, requires constant vigilance and ingenuity. Perhaps the ultimate in germfree surgery is shown here where, within the operating theater, the patient and surgeon are effectively confined within a plastic capsule, to which only highly purified air, free of microorganisms, is admitted. This scrupulous avoidance of infection is particularly important in transplantation surgery where the patient's immune responses, which normally guard against infection, have been suppressed with drugs to prevent the rejection of the foreign organ which the surgeon is implanting.

Cinchona bark

⬇

Quinine (antimalarial)

⬋ ⬊

Stomachics (bitters)   Quinidine (antiarrhythmic)

⬇

Synthetic antimalarials (Chloroquine, Proguanil, Pyrimethamine)

⬇

Antihistamines

⬋ ⬊

Phenothiazine tranquilizers   Antiemetics

7 Pharmacological advances originally stemmed from the discovery of the biodynamic agents in naturally-occurring substances, culled from the hedgerows so to speak: the poppy, the foxglove, the cinchona bark, rauwolfia, the coca leaf, the rye fungus, and so forth. Then through ingenious chemical juggling with the basic molecule, new substances often evolved. Thus, attempts to simplify the complex molecule of quinine, which had eventually been isolated as the active principle of the cinchona bark, led to the synthetic antimalarials. A study of their pharmacological properties revealed, quite unexpectedly, that they were antagonistic to histamine and so the antihistamines developed. The original ones were noted to be markedly soporific and to prevent travel sickness: hence the phenothiazine tranquilizers and modern anti-emetics. Thus all these drugs stem from the 17th century remedy, Jesuit's bark. There are many other examples of this pharmacological House that Jack Built.

the first of this well-known series of hypnotics. Thus, the modern tendency to regard the history of drug therapy prior to our chemotherapeutic and antibiotic era as a sort of prolongation of the Dark Ages is a little inappropriate.

The greatest discovery of the 19th century was that of Pasteur who established that infections were caused by germs and that it was possible to produce immunity against them by vaccines. His work led Lister to introduce antiseptic surgery which in combination with anesthesia made the century remarkable for its surgical progress.

In the closing decades of the last century and the first decade of this one the great pharmacologist Paul Ehrlich, inspired by the work of Robert Koch in the staining of histological specimens with dyes, explored the relationship between dyes and the living cells of the body; in the process he produced Atoxyl, the first effective drug against trypanosomiasis, and Salvarsan against the spirochete of syphilis.

The most exciting advance in the early part of the present century was the isolation of hormones from the endocrine glands. Starting with the use of thyroid extract in thyroid deficiency at the end of the last century, it continued with the isolation of adrenaline. When in 1889 Von Mering and Minkowski showed that diabetes could be produced by experimental removal of the pancreas of animals the idea was born of preparing a pancreatic extract which would replace the substance missing in human diabetics, and in 1921 Banting and Best eventually succeeded in extracting insulin from the pancreas of a calf. It is doubtful if there has ever been a medical discovery comparable in drama to the effect of the administration of these precious vials of insulin when they became available a few years later.

My generation of physicians who qualified shortly after the First World War have witnessed greater advances in treatment in their life span than have occurred in all the previous eons of time and there is no saying what the majesty and splendor of progress will be in the quarter of the century which remains; we may even be able to prevent the common cold! Young physicians

nowadays, armed with the therapeutic thunderbolts of Jove which the synthetic chemist has put into their often very ungodlike hands, must find it hard to imagine, just as we are beginning to find it hard to remember, what it was like to practise medicine when there was no insulin, vitamin B_{12}, sulfonamides, antibiotics, hypotensives, anticoagulants, specifics for tropical diseases, and potent diuretics, hormones and anticonvulsants.

As a result the pattern of disease is quite different today from that obtaining when I was a young doctor. Most hospitals for tuberculosis and many wards for the treatment of infectious diseases have been closed or given over to the care of old people or chronic bronchitics. Young people between the ages of 15 and 30 relatively seldom die from disease nowadays: the chief cause of death among them is accident, mostly on the roads; the next most common cause is suicide; and the third, a long way behind these, is the comparatively rare groups of blood diseases, the acute reticuloses, including acute leukemia. The atmosphere and length of stay in our mental hospitals has changed out of recognition as the result of the use of modern psychotropic drugs; and our general hospitals are mostly filled with patients suffering from the natural processes of ageing, from the various forms of atherosclerosis, and from a variety of types of new growth.

The chapters in this book, written by distinguished American and British authorities for intelligent, educated laymen, identify and describe the fundamental essence of the most important specialties, their history, their triumphs and the services they offer. The demand for medical services seems insatiable but unlimited demand is self-defeating and priorities must be determined. Such priorities must ultimately depend on an informed public opinion on medical matters. At present where such opinion exists it is often determined by small, ignorant and prejudiced but vocal pressure groups. Doctors should play a more active part than they do in presenting important medical issues to the public. This volume is a pioneer in this respect.

1 The Conquest of Infection

Infectious disease has always been the most feared of all the afflictions of mankind, particularly in the anxious centuries before bacteria and viruses were discovered, when the spread of illness from the stricken to the hearty appeared almost supernatural.

During the fearful cycle of epidemics which ravaged Europe during the 14th century, about 25 million people perished—one quarter of the population. No city or village knew when the arrival of a sickly traveller would herald yet another devastation. Plague itself, imported from the Far East, often through Marseilles, accounted for most deaths, and in later centuries smallpox assumed the grim mantle shed by plague. In the early years of the 19th century cholera and typhus fever added their terrors to community life, at the very time when rural populations were crowding into the busy industrial centers of both the Old and New Worlds.

In these early days the physicians, however devoted, were virtually powerless in the face of illness, particularly epidemic disease. The theories elaborated to account for the steady march of death through a healthy society were numerous. They ranged from divine anger to belief in noxious mists and vapors, the latter view containing a glimmering of the truth to come. Empirically, it was recognized that strangers, particularly those coming from distant parts, were dangerous and should be isolated, or quarantined. The need to isolate the sick, when epidemic disease was suspected, was also recognized, and in 1666 the whole population of the township of Eyam in Derbyshire most heroically cut themselves off from all contact with the adjacent countryside when a villager was stricken with plague: 259 of the 350 inhabitants died, but the disease spread no further.

Edward Jenner and smallpox. The irresistible rise of scientific enlightenment made no advance against infectious disease until the end of the 19th century, with one outstanding exception. The keen eye and vigilant mind of Edward Jenner, an English country doctor and naturalist, had determined the mastery of smallpox by the end of the 18th century, half a century before John Snow realized the source of cholera and a full 100 years before any other form of artificial immunity against epidemic disease was made

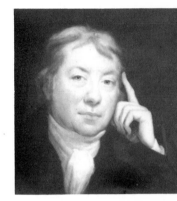

8 Edward Jenner (1749-1823), whose observations on the immunity to smallpox enjoyed by milkmaids with cowpox (vaccinia) led to the widespread application of vaccination against smallpox and opened the era of protective immunization against many other infections.

9 An illustration from Edward Jenner's *An Inquiry into the Causes and Effects of the Variolae Vaccinae*, published in 1798, showing the cowpox-infected hand of a milkmaid named Sarah Nelmes. Putting to the test the country observation that people with cowpox appeared never to contract smallpox, Jenner infected an 8-year-old boy called James Phipps with material from one of the sores on Sarah Nelmes' hand, and six weeks later inoculated him with material from a smallpox pustule. This historic—and, in view of the lack of any real knowledge about the processes of infection and immunity at the time, highly dangerous—experiment was the first great step in the history of the conquest of the scourges of infection.

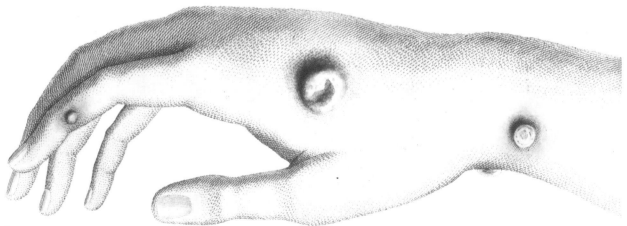

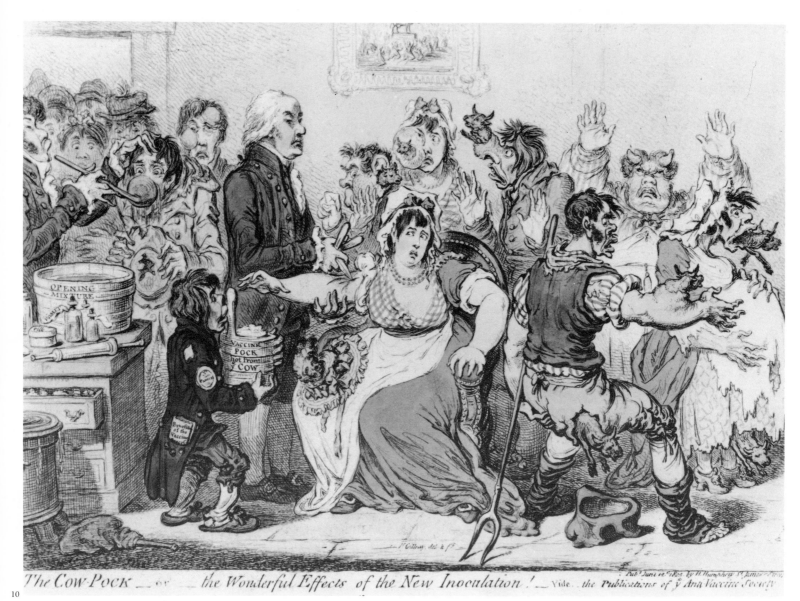

The Cow-Pock — or — the Wonderful Effects of the New Inoculation! — Vide. the Publications of y Anti Vaccine Society

10

10 The Cow-Pock, or the Wonderful Effects of the new Inoculation! A caricature by James Gillray published in 1802, eight years after Jenner's introduction of vaccination. The blessings of inoculation were not immediately appreciated by society. The concern and anxiety of much of the population is represented in the rather florid fantasies of bovine transformations which it is suggested the vaccine might induce.

11 Although John Snow showed that cholera was transmitted by water in his famous experiment with the public pumps in Soho in London in 1848, it was not until 1883 that Robert Koch (1843-1910) observed the cholera organisms themselves through the microscope. His drawing of the comma-shaped vibrios is reproduced here. Although Snow's observations laid the basis for preventive public health measures, it was microscopic observation of the organisms themselves that opened the way to the full understanding of the nature of infective processes.

available. Jenner was the empiricist *par excellence*: from the observation in 1796 that dairymaids were spared smallpox, he deduced that they contracted a 'protecting' disease from contact with cows, which he called cowpox. This 'protecting disease' took the form of a sore on the milkmaid's finger, contracted from the cow and conferring immunity against smallpox. By this brilliant inspiration Jenner anticipated much of the painstaking and laborious work a century ahead. He infected purposely the arms of his patients by contact with the milkmaids' sores, thus transferring future immunity to them also. It should be remembered that not only were the principles of immunity unknown, but the world was many decades away from knowledge of bacteria and viruses. Yet the foresight and persistence of this rural practitioner decided forever the only effective protection against smallpox. President Jefferson told Edward Jenner in a famous letter: 'Future nations will know by history only that the loathsome smallpox has existed and by you has been extirpated'.

The relatively late colonization of the New

World had spared its native population the ravages of plague. By the 19th century, however, maritime trade routes were open and busy between the Old and New Worlds, and the opportunities for the dissemination of the major infectious diseases were only too clear. Cholera, smallpox and typhus struck at Canada and the Americas, and the construction of the Panama Canal was all but halted by a mysterious and dangerous disease later recognized as yellow fever, which had struck as far north as Philadelphia in 1790 and was responsible, in that city alone, for over 10,000 deaths before the end of the 18th century.

The conquest of these fearful diseases was to be a difficult and perilous endeavor, dependent upon knowledge of the infecting agent, the cleansing of the environment and the production of vaccines.

John Snow and cholera. Many years before the deadly comma-shaped cholera germ was seen under the microscope John Snow, a London physician, had shown, by an ingenious epidemiological survey, that the disease was spread by water, and not by mists and fogs. This he demonstrated by noting the location of each case in his practice and marking it on a map of London. In 1854 he was able to show that the pattern of cholera corresponded to the distribution of water from a hand pump in Broad Street. He settled the controversy which this heretical notion aroused by removing the handle from the pump, and showing that the disease then diminished. Not only did Snow dispel the false notion of airborne spread of cholera, but he also most convincingly demonstrated the value of the 'spot map' which had already been tentatively used, though without great success, in the Philadelphia yellow fever epidemic of the late 18th century.

Cholera as an epidemic hazard was to receive further blows from antibiotic and vaccine research in the years ahead, but Snow convincingly revealed a method of control which was effective and was imitated in the

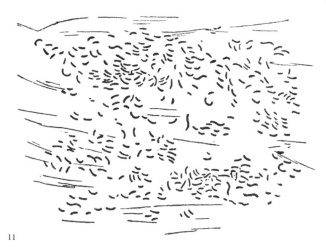

11

confrontations with other diseases, such as typhoid fever: find out the source, or vehicle, of the disease and reduce all chances of contamination. In fact Snow and William Budd, an epidemiologist from Bristol, laid down the principle that sewage and drinking water must be separated at all times unless the water was effectively sterilized—a difficult process in the last century.

Germs. While the civilized world enjoyed the benefits of Jenner's vital discovery of vaccination, and while the efforts and observations of Snow and Budd and others painfully strengthened defenses against the major diseases, scientists in all the countries of the world were reaching the brink of the most vital discovery of all, a discovery which was to transform defenses against infectious disease, and ultimately lead to the artificial creation of immunity against infectious disease.

In 1673 a Dutch draper, Antony van Leeuwenhoek, constructed a crude but effective microscope and was able to observe, and describe, protozoa and bacteria. He wrote to the newly-

formed Royal Society of London about his discoveries, and one letter, written in 1683, leaves little doubt that he had witnessed the movements of bacteria. Most unfortunately his descriptions, though leading to great scientific interest, were not linked in any way with disease, and he and his contemporaries failed to realize the tremendous capabilities, both for good and evil, possessed by microorganisms. It was nearly 200 years later that Louis Pasteur realized the true association between certain microbes and specific diseases, and his work was enhanced by a most fruitful partnership with Lister, a surgeon

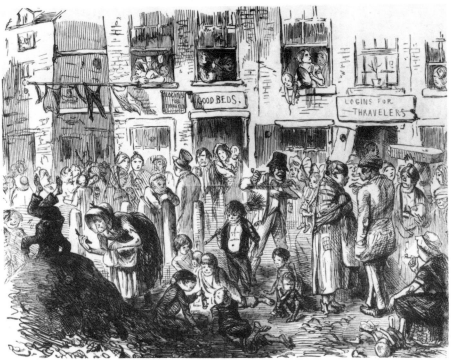

12

13

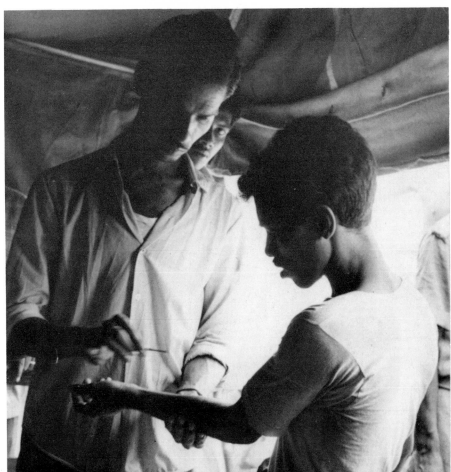

12 A Court for King Cholera: a cartoon by Leech in *Punch* for 25 September 1852. The invasion of Western Europe by cholera in the early 19th century was almost entirely attributable to conditions such as those depicted here.

13 While cholera is a part of history in the developed countries of the west, in many regions of the Third World the fight against this disease of overcrowding and poor sanitation continues. Here a youth is being vaccinated against cholera in a refugee camp near Calcutta, in India.

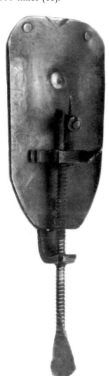

14

working in Glasgow.

Lister accepted Pasteur's opinions concerning bacteria and disease, and decided that the infection of surgical wounds, then exacting a fearful toll in the operating theater, might well be due to the invasive effects of microbes. Knowing the power of carbolic acid as a poison to living creatures, Lister decided to assay its effect against the invisible germs surrounding operation wounds, and used this disinfectant freely on the patient's skin, on his own hands and as an aerial spray. His results were outstanding. Through Lister and Pasteur, the great advance had been made. Germs caused infection, and could be mastered, even though only by crude methods.

The era of the bacteriologist had dawned, and scientists of great distinction such as Koch in Germany, Laennec in France, and Almroth Wright in England, were gradually identifying separate species of bacteria by the microscope, by biochemical tests, and by refined and sophisticated tests involving sera. Particular infectious diseases were firmly linked with particular germs to the extent that in the 1880s and 1890s environmental factors in the causation of disease tended to be unwisely neglected, such was the immense medical and scientific enthusiasm for the new discovery. Thus the physical basis for the transference of infection had at last been elucidated.

The exploitation of immunity. Centuries before the acceptance of the germ theory of disease, physicians had noted that the survivors of certain epidemics appeared to be entirely safe when the disease reappeared. John Hunter, who

in his day had taught Edward Jenner as a student, summed up this observation in the famous words: 'The body, once affected by some stimuli, never forgets, as it were, their action, and thereby is never again affected by that poison, as in the smallpox, measles, etc.' These words were pronounced in the mid-18th century, and described the state of immunity as then appreciated. Once the end of the 19th century had been reached, the scientists, now equipped with knowledge of the existence and structure of bacteria, were able to formulate more detailed views concerning immunity. They visualized the period of illness during infectious disease as a period of battle between the invading microorganisms and the defenses of the body, the contest ending either in death or recovery, recovery often being associated with future immunity. Thus, apart from the general defenses of the tissues, such as that provided by roving white cells capable of ingesting and destroying an invader, there must be some specific antidote prepared by the body as a special 'tailor-made' defense against the particular invader. Whether the patient lived or died would then depend upon the invasive qualities and speed of multiplication of the germs on the one hand; and the rapidity with which the body could produce its specially-prepared defenses on the other. This view of the dynamics of infectious disease permeated many of the scientific papers of the late 19th century. It could readily explain immunity, on the basis that the production of defensive material could never be exactly geared to the requirements. It was likely to be produced in excess, and for

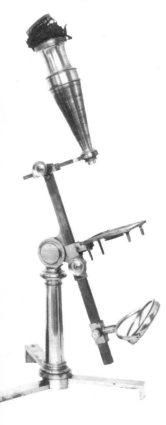

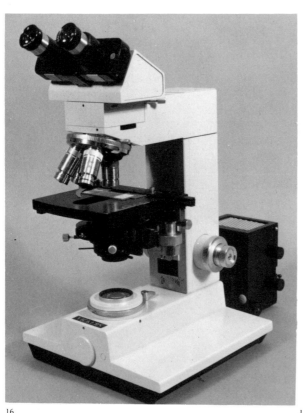

16

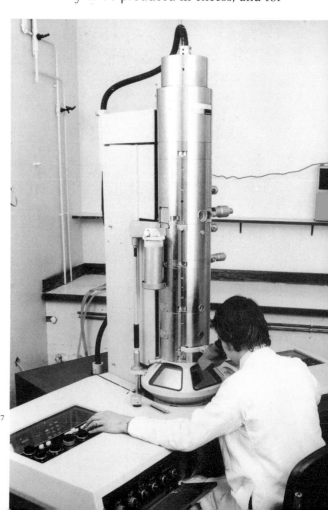

17

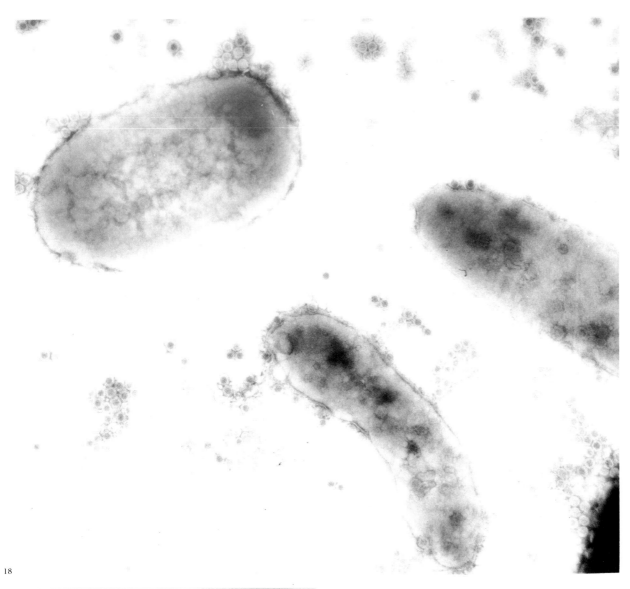

18

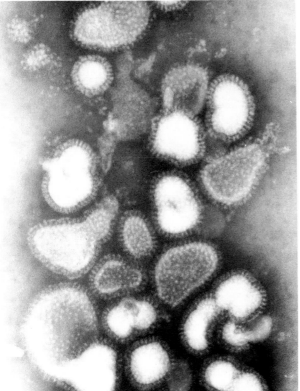

19

considerable periods after the actual infection had been defeated. Accordingly, it was argued, when the same invading germ reappeared months or years later, there would be no delay in producing the specific antidote. The invader would virtually fall into an ambush at whatever point it entered the tissues, and the individual would not suffer from the disease: he would be *immune*.

This theory of immunity, worked out by Pasteur, Koch, Almroth Wright and the other great medical scientists of that golden era, was originally based upon fundamental but brilliant reasoning, and it led to an immensely exciting and novel concept. Could Nature be imitated? Could the state of immunity, created by experience, possibly dangerous experience, of actual disease be mimicked by artificial means so that protection against various diseases could be created without illness?

The outstanding figure at this time was Almroth Wright, Professor of Pathology at the Army Medical School, Netley, England. The British Army had suffered greatly during the Crimean campaign of the 1850s from the effects

18, 19 The resolving power of the electron microscope is shown in this photomicrograph of a bacterium (*Escherichia coli*), revealing details of its internal structure (18). Also shown in this picture are small reovirus particles associated with gastro-enteritis in children and visible as wheel-like structures, for which reason they are known as rotaviruses. The influenza virus is shown under even greater magnification, revealing the high degree of organization within such extremely small particles (19). The magnifications are approximately 44,000 and 125,000 respectively.

21

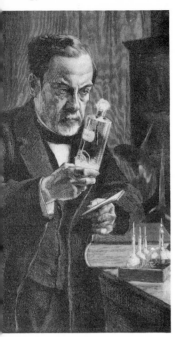

20 Louis Pasteur (1822-95), pictured at his laboratory bench holding the glass vessel in the like of which he conclusively disproved the theory of spontaneous generation of microbes in decaying matter, and opened the way to our modern understanding of bacterial infection as a cause of disease. It is interesting to note that his work was initiated by the French wine manufacturers' desire to control the disasters to wine production which threatened their industry. His studies of the activities of bacteria introduced the term 'enzyme', from the fact that he first described the chemical substances in yeast—*en zyme*.

21 Sir Almroth Wright (1861-1947), who introduced the widespread use of protection against typhoid and paratyphoid fever by the use of injection of the killed organisms of the disease, or immunization, shown in his primitive laboratory early in this century. It was mainly towards the British Army in the field that his researches were directed and his affiliations are apparent from his somewhat untidy military garb. The early microscope and hand-driven centrifuge were the rather primitive tools with which he achieved his considerable contribution to knowledge. It was he who was lampooned as Sir Colenso Ridgeon in Bernard Shaw's play *The Doctor's Dilemma*. Shaw was a violent opponent of the practice of compulsory vaccination and inoculation.

of disease, particularly typhoid fever. Indeed *Punch*, a London periodical, had made in 1861 an ironic suggestion that the Guards Memorial in Waterloo Place, London, should bear the names Fever, Dysentery and Cholera rather than Alma, Inkerman and Sebastopol. The development of any form of treatment which could protect soldiers in advance of infection would be a great advance in military medicine, particularly in the face of the Boer War of 1899-1902, which was likely to provide conditions comparable to the Crimea.

Wright had observed the work of Pasteur in the production of *living* but weakened cultures of organisms which, when injected, stimulated the body's defenses to create the specific antidote (now termed the antibody) able to protect against future invasions of the fully-virulent germ. Pasteur's experiments had been concerned with anthrax in cattle and rabies in humans. The rabies vaccine, while affording some protection, was extremely difficult and tedious to prepare and not without its own dangers.

Almroth Wright decided to attempt a new process of creating artificial immunity, likely to be quicker, safer, and more readily adaptable to mass production. He cultured living typhoid organisms by placing them in nutrient broth until they formed relatively large colonies, and then killed them by raising the temperature and adding a weak disinfectant. His aim, securely achieved, was to render the bacteria lifeless while causing the minimum destruction and distortion of their structure. The essence of the scheme was to deceive the body into thinking that the germs were alive and thus to set into train the production of antibodies.

This was a most crucial endeavor, and determined the attitude of doctors to killed vaccines for many decades to come. The first trials were conducted in 1898, upon Wright himself, doctors on probation at Netley and inmates of an asylum in Kent. Laboratory lists

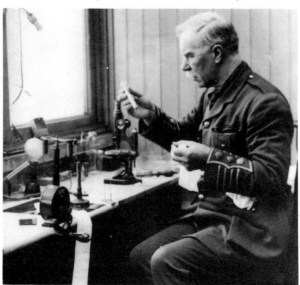

21

showed that, after an interval, the blood of the immunized volunteers contained substances able to disrupt the structure of living typhoid germs. Clearly the experiment had been successful and a means of protecting soldiers in the field had been produced.

Unfortunately Wright was unsuccessful in his attempts to persuade the War Office to make immunization against typhoid compulsory, and finally only about 14,000 men who enlisted for service in South Africa were protected, slightly more than four per cent. During the siege of Ladysmith it was noticed that typhoid assailed 14 per cent of the uninoculated, while only two per cent of those protected suffered an attack. In fact, these results led to considerable controversy as doubts were cast upon their statistical validity, but later and more carefully controlled trials in India vindicated Wright's claim.

The killed typhoid vaccine produced in 1894 was the precursor of a whole spectrum of immunizing agents whose efficacy depended upon the same reasoning.

The early attenuated vaccines. Louis Pasteur, some years before the very important work of Almroth Wright, had successfully experimented with living vaccines. Since injection of living organisms without any pre-treatment of the culture would provoke the disease, it was necessary to weaken, or attenuate, the bacteria before they were introduced into the body. Pasteur in 1880 had tried exposure to heat and to weak disinfectants to attain this end. His aim was to maintain the antibody-provoking qualities of the germ while diminishing its virulence to the point at which active disease could not be caused. Cholera, anthrax, swine erysipelas and rabies were diseases against which attenuated vaccines were prepared. These were in general successful, but there remained for many years a degree of prejudice against living vaccines, as the possibility of reversion to virulence was always in mind. Nevertheless, the new century dawned with the principle of attenuated living vaccines, as well as killed vaccines, firmly established as a form of protection against infectious disease.

Antibacterial and antitoxic sera. The consequences of many infections are due to destructive efforts by the bacteria themselves. In others the microorganisms are relatively harmless, but they produce a powerful chemical poison which can damage or destroy vital organs. Diphtheria is such a disease, and demonstrations in Paris by Emile Roux in 1858 showed that the diphtheria germs could create a poison, or toxin, which could be filtered through unglazed porcelain and, though sterile, could then, if injected, produce all the signs and symptoms of diphtheria. Later work by Behring in 1890 showed that animals which had been injected with this diphtheria toxin produced in their blood a defense substance which he termed an *antitoxin*. It was comparable to the antibodies which all species produced to confront bacterial invaders, but was capable of specifically opposing the chemical poison itself. Behring appreciated that human cases of diphtheria, then a deadly and common disease of childhood, could be assisted by an injection of blood serum from an animal which had received diphtheria toxin. This serum would contain the vital antitoxin which was perhaps being manufactured at too slow a rate in the patient's own tissues.

Tests proved his point. On Christmas night in 1891 the first patient, a little girl, was saved in Berlin and within three years over 20,000 children had received this treatment in Germany. The term 'passive' immunity was applied to this form of treatment, as the antitoxin had been made by other animals (sheep and goats) and not by the patient. No permanent immunity was conferred: the antitoxin remained viable long enough only to meet and destroy the circulating toxin.

In later years the use of antitoxic sera was to be extended, and antibacterial sera, produced on the same principle, added to the forms of treatment available.

Poised for progress. Progress from the recognition of germs as agents producing disease to the evolution of the science of immunology was extremely rapid and spanned less than half a century. By 1900 the three great growing points of immunological research and development had been established from the three archetypes of protective injections: killed vaccines, attenuated vaccines and antitoxic sera. From these grew all the vast armament possessed today against infectious disease. To these three styles of protection must be added the unique, solid and continuing contribution to the mastery of smallpox provided by Jennerian vaccination. There is no other example of one disease, voluntarily contracted, protecting against another.

Public health. Not only because of the established science of immunology were the early years of the 20th century the platform for the conquest of infectious disease. Two other significant trends were apparent. First, as the early impetus of the Industrial Revolution stabilized, the governments of both the U.S.A. and Britain had instituted programs of public works for the development of cleaner water supplies and efficient disposal of sewage, and had begun to exercise control over housing standards.

Secondly a new species of public health physician began to appear, with the task of applying national health legislation to local conditions, with the control of infectious disease a prime responsibility. The first 'Medical Officer of Health' had been appointed to Liverpool in 1847, and by the end of the century such appointments were obligatory in England. A major responsibility of the Medical Officer was the compilation of vital statistics for his area, such as the death rate, the infant mortality rate and the maternal mortality rate. Thus statistically-based comparisons could be made and conclusions drawn on which action could be based.

Thus there now arose, on both sides of the Atlantic, possibilities for co-operation between the emerging basic medical sciences and the new public health organizations which foreshadowed, though perhaps distantly, the removal of serious infectious disease as a health hazard.

The twentieth century
Yellow fever. In 1900 Major Walter Reed of the United States Army led a team of scientists who were sent to Cuba to investigate the cause of yellow fever, which had affected the American troops stationed there. Hitherto it had been considered that the disease could spread readily from man to man; Reed and his team demonstrated that a particular species of mosquito was necessary for the infection of man. James Carroll, a bacteriologist on the Commission, volunteered to be bitten by an infected mosquito to prove his point. He nearly died but the source of infection was then settled. After two further years of research it was conclusively proved that only a particular species of mosquito, *Aedes aegypti*, could transmit the disease. The actual germ is a virus, of a size not then visible in a microscope field and, though the steps taken by the Commission to reduce the breeding opportunities of the mosquito virtually eradicated the disease from Cuba, many years were to pass before the causative agent was identified and described.

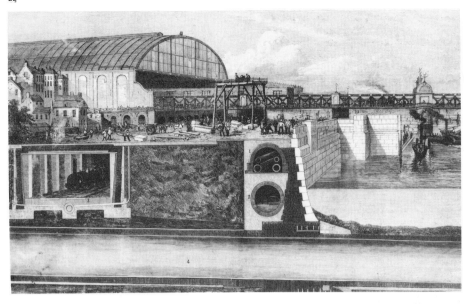

22 While we owe much of our present-day safety from infectious disease to the scientific understanding of infectious organisms and the practice of immunization, the heroic works of public health engineering which were a feature of the second half of the 19th century in London and other big cities in Europe and America continue to give us their benefits today. This picture from the *Illustrated London News* in June 1867 conveys graphically the scale of the works involved. It shows an imaginary section through the new embankment on the north shore of the Thames, then under construction in front of Charing Cross railway station and in part covering the area of old Hungerford Market next to which the young Charles Dickens worked in a factory making boot blacking. As well as the main sewer (marked '2') it shows gas and water pipes and the new underground railway.

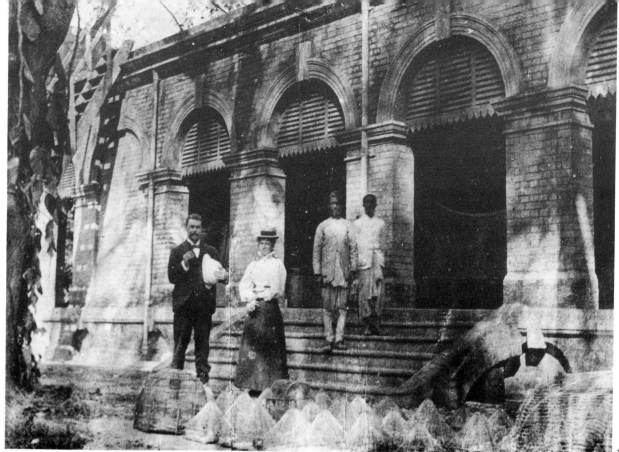

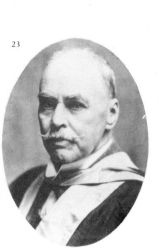

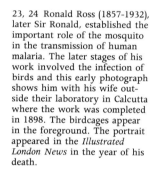

23, 24 Ronald Ross (1857-1932), later Sir Ronald, established the important role of the mosquito in the transmission of human malaria. The later stages of his work involved the infection of birds and this early photograph shows him with his wife outside their laboratory in Calcutta where the work was completed in 1898. The birdcages appear in the foreground. The portrait appeared in the *Illustrated London News* in the year of his death.

Yellow fever cases fell from 1,400 in Havana in 1900 to none in 1902, following an extremely vigorous anti-mosquito campaign. Nevertheless the final victory over this dreaded disease which had held up the completion of the Panama Canal for 20 years was not achieved until 1937, when, after eight years' patient work, an effective attenuated vaccine was produced which stimulated production of protective antibodies in human tissues. The vaccine was eventually prepared from virus grown on chick embryos, and the protection conferred is certain and lasts at least ten years.

An alarming incident in 1942 cast temporary doubts on the safety of the vaccine, when 28,000 American troops developed jaundice after mass immunization. Research eventually demonstrated that their illness was due to contamination of the vaccine with another virus, that causing serum hepatitis, and there was no reflection upon the safety of the now famous 17D yellow fever vaccine.

It is likely that the attenuated yellow fever vaccine is the best and most reliable of all the attenuated living virus preparations used for protection against disease, and no cases of yellow fever have ever been recorded in those immunized.

Malaria. Malaria, with yellow fever, had a disastrous effect upon exploration and commercial development during the 19th century, and accounted for the sombre title, attributed to West Africa, of the White Man's Grave. The disease, with its fever, delirium and high death rate, the classical disease of the tropics, was a mystery until 1880, when tiny objects, later to be

described as malarial parasites, were seen in the blood of a feverish patient by a French surgeon, Laveran, working in Algeria. These parasites were originally thought to be germs of the bacillus group. The great Italian pathologists of the late 19th century, following up Laveran's discovery, noted that different shapes of parasites appeared to be associated with different clinical forms of the disease. It was not until 1894, however, that Sir Patrick Manson suggested that these parasites were transferred from victim to victim by some type of suctorial insect, probably a mosquito. Eager research by Major Ronald Ross and others soon confirmed this view and a classical paper by Manson in 1900 established beyond doubt the role of the anophelene mosquito in the spread of the malaria parasite. Later work revealed the complicated life cycle of the parasite, termed the 'plasmodium', a cycle partly evolving within the mosquito and partly within the blood of man. Eventually, different parasites were identified, and firmly associated with the different forms of the disease. The stage was now set, in the early 1900s, for the slow but certain conquest of malaria.

Clearly there were two lines of approach to the problem. Firstly, to eradicate the mosquitoes; secondly, to produce a substance which would oppose the development of the plasmodium in human blood, should a mosquito bite inject it. To solve the first problem doctors, entomologists and engineers had to combine. The mosquito concerned has its own life cycle, including a larval stage. The larva must spend some time in water: accordingly, all free surfaces of fresh

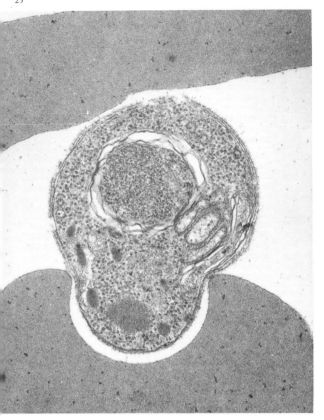

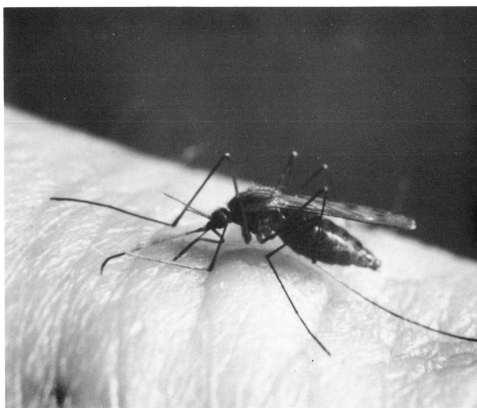

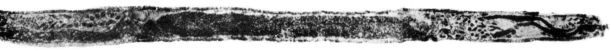

27

water must be removed or covered. Thus the larvae could not survive and the generation of mosquitoes would be lost. This attitude remains a fundamental element of malaria control, though protective clothing, chemical repellents for use on skin and, more recently the use of insecticides have heightened the war against the mosquito.

The first drug to be tried against the malaria parasite was quinine. It was soon realized that it was better to take this drug as a prophylactic, so that the plasmodium, if injected by a mosquito, found itself in an instantly hostile environment. Quinine was succeeded in the 1940s by mepacrine as a prophylactic. Other synthetic compounds followed rapidly, each with specific therapeutic powers in relation to particular forms of the plasmodium. The most effective general prophylactic, to be taken before exposure, is probably proguanil, though chloroquine may have to be used if an unusually resistant plasmodium is encountered. The drug to be used in actual treatment may be a matter of very careful selection, but the choice is wide.

Accordingly, malaria, once understood, failed to withstand the combined assault of the public health engineer and the clinical pharmacologist, and the W.H.O.'s progress to malaria eradication is interrupted only by the physical, financial and occasional diplomatic difficulties of mounting the campaign, simultaneously, in the developing areas of the world.

Leprosy. Leprosy, once a plague with over three million deformed and tortured victims, can now be controlled with certainty when the diagnosis is made and the patient treated. Centuries ago it was the world-wide disease, with colonies in Norway and Iceland. Although never acutely infectious it could spread insidiously through primitive communities, and the fear of disfigurement and crippling illness led to the segregation of sufferers. General advance in hygiene and the widespread adoption of isolation measures have now confined leprosy almost exclusively to tropical regions, where medical services are rudimentary. Nevertheless, great therapeutic advances during the last 40 years have changed the outlook from despair to hope, and it is only the difficulty of identifying cases and securing co-operation of governments and patients that hinders the eradication of this most feared of diseases.

The first effective treatment was hydnocarpus oil in the 1930s, now replaced by a synthetic preparation, di-amino, di-phenyl sulfone. Introduced by Lowe in 1950, this drug revolutionized the treatment of leprosy and was the first really effective measure of progress since the discovery of the hardy bacillus leprae by Hansen in 1880.

Since 1957, the sulfones have been supplemented by cortisone, and recent work from Indonesia suggests that massive doses of hydroxyprocaine-

25-9 Human malaria is an infection by a microscopic parasitic organism with a complicated life-cycle lived partly in mosquitos and partly in man. These photographs show something of the role of powerful modern techniques of microscopy in studying the disease, still a major killer in tropical parts of the world and the subject of large-scale control programs by international agencies such as the World Health Organization. Females of some species of the Anopheles mosquito (26)—the males are incapable of biting—take up the parasite when feeding on the blood of a person infected with malaria. The parasite penetrates into the mid-gut cell (28, p.26) and travels to its basement membrane (28a), where it becomes a spherical oocyst. Within the oocyst 'sporozoites' (27) are formed, and these travel through the mosquito's body to the saliva glands, from which they are injected into the next victim. A remarkable photograph (25) shows the entry of a further stage, a merozoite, into a red blood cell. The characteristic pattern of recurrent chills and fevers occurs when the merozoites, having multiplied, burst out of the red cells into the blood plasma. In some forms of malaria a latent infection is maintained for several years in the liver. Illustration 29 shows a schizont from which many new merozoites (visible as large, distinct, granular particles) would in due course discharge into a nearby blood vessel. The approximate magnifications are as follows: 25, 13,500; 27, 10,500; 28, 5,500; 29, 2,000.

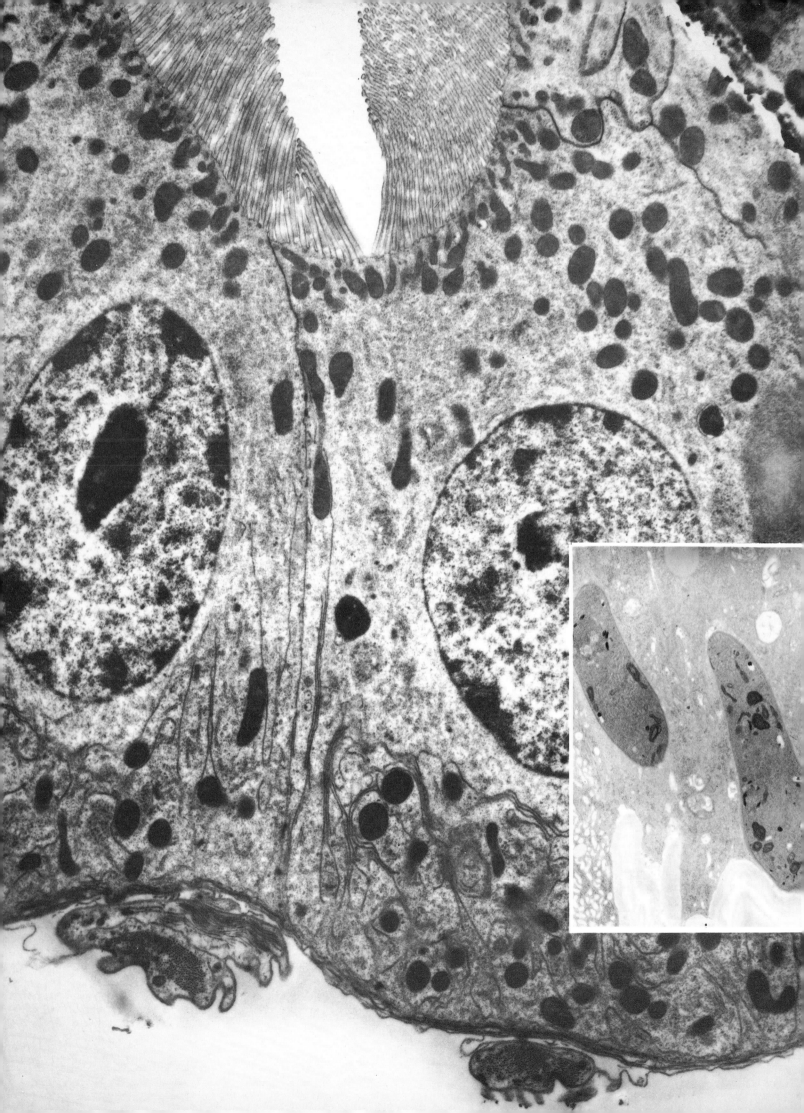

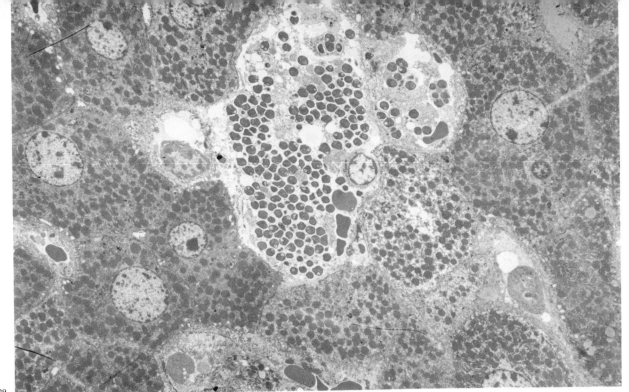

28-9 *See page 25.*

penicillin may complete the agents now available to master leprosy, which, though cured or controlled by drugs, has not yet yielded to the bacteriologists' weapon par excellence, a vaccine.

The battle against diphtheria. Diphtheria antitoxin, prepared from the blood of horses which had been injected with virulent diphtheria toxin, had been used in the treatment of established diphtheria since 1891. Though this development saved many thousands of lives it had a limited usefulness, as speed of diagnosis was essential: antitoxin was useless if administered late, and it did nothing to protect the healthy against future attacks of the disease. What was wanted was some type of safe provocation to the body's own defenses, so that antitoxins would be permanently available in the circulation for life-long protection. It is said that the discovery of how this could be done was entirely accidental.

Alexander Glenny, a London scientist, was concerned in 1904 with the immunization of horses with diphtheria toxin in order to prepare antitoxin from their blood later. He observed that certain batches of diphtheria toxin were equally efficient in inducing an antitoxin reaction even though they could be shown to be much less toxic themselves. Further investigation showed that the toxicity had been diminished by accidental contamination with formalin during laboratory procedures. This mixture of toxin and formalin created a species of 'tamed' toxin, still capable of producing the antitoxic response yet itself harmless. It was unfortunate that 20 years elapsed before the toxin-formalin (toxoid) mixture became the basis of immunization against diphtheria. Meanwhile, however, other attempts had been made to create a safe method of immunizing, and mixtures of antitoxin (produced from immunized animals) and toxin were tried, in the hope that the toxin would, by contact with antitoxin, be robbed of its capacity to damage tissues while still providing sufficient 'shock' to the body's receptors to produce permanent new antitoxin. This method was in fact tried by William Park, the Director of Hygiene Services for New York City in 1914, and in that year over 10,000 children were successfully immunized. By 1924, however, the simplicity and cheapness of the toxoid type of vaccine led to the discontinuance of toxin-antitoxin mixtures.

In Britain there were several clinical trials of diphtheria toxoid, during epidemic periods between 1924 and 1935. In 1940, when the overcrowding and disturbed social conditions of war made epidemics likely, the government sponsored a massive immunization campaign, and this illustrated beyond question the efficacy of anti-diphtheric immunization. In the decade preceding the Second World War there had been over 58,000 cases and 2,000 deaths per annum: during the decade 1956–65, when the procedure was established and widely accepted, cases averaged less than 50 per annum, and deaths less than four. In 1959 and 1964 there were no deaths. All the Western nations mounted similar campaigns and in 1933 William Park, by then Professor of Bacteriology in the University of New York, injected the millionth child in New York against diphtheria.

Since the spread of any infectious disease depends upon contact between cases and susceptible, or unprotected, persons, a high rate of immunization protects everyone. Diphtheria, once the most deadly scourge of childhood, has virtually disappeared from all advanced countries, but its occasional reappearance is a reminder of the absolute necessity to keep the 'immune rate'

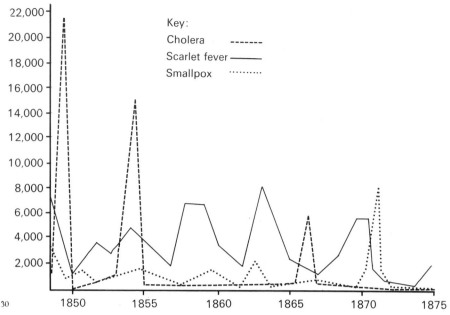

30 The waves of epidemic infections which swept across the crowded urban populations of Britain in the last century are represented vividly in the rise and fall of deaths attributed to cholera, scarlet fever and smallpox in mid 19th century London. Cholera and smallpox, now thought of as diseases of developing nations, scourged Europe until remarkably recent times and have been eradicated almost entirely as the result of the application of public health measures–sanitation and water supply in the case of cholera, vaccination and isolation in that of smallpox. The subsidence of scarlet fever, however, has probably in part been due to a change in the character of the streptococcus responsible for the disease. The severe and sometimes lethal infection, associated with intense reddening of the skin, is now rarely seen, though less virulent streptococcal infections continue to occur. They are now aborted early with antibiotic treatment.

very high if the disease is to be kept at bay.

Tetanus and whooping cough. One of the most feared diseases is tetanus, which may follow the soiling of an open wound with earth or other organic debris. The muscles of the body go into a form of agonizing spasm and the whole frame arches upwards. The illness is due to a toxin produced by the tetanus bacterium, and its effects may be opposed by the timely injection of anti-tetanus serum prepared from horses. However, as in the case of diphtheria it is much safer to accept immunization with a formal toxoid prepared by mixing tetanus toxin with formalin.

Whooping cough, or pertussis, was once a very common disease of young children, leading not infrequently to permanent respiratory disability. A killed vaccine was produced as early as 1923 by Thorvald Madsen of Copenhagen and results of the use of this vaccine in the Faroe Islands and elsewhere showed that it was effective. Dr Pearl Kendrick of Michigan was prominent in the refinement of the pertussis vaccine and between 1946 and 1959 the British Medical Research Council carried out controlled statistical trials to test the effect of immunization. Though not absolutely effective in all cases, it was shown that 87 per cent of house-contacts of established cases contracted whooping cough if not immunized, while only 14 per cent of the protected became victims.

The three diseases diphtheria, tetanus and whooping cough are considered together here, as routine protection against the three is offered in many countries of the world in the form of a single injection, containing diphtheria and tetanus toxoids and killed whooping cough germs. This type of 'package' immunization is greatly favored as it obviates the need for several injections and is economical in medical time and equipment.

Normally this 'triple-antigen' injection is given

on three occasions, with an interval of six weeks between doses one and two, and six months between doses two and three.

The conquest of poliomyelitis. Few diseases have struck such terror as poliomyelitis, or infantile paralysis. A virus disease, it attacks the cells in the spinal cord which control the voluntary movements of the muscles, and an attack can leave the victim a hopeless cripple, who may have to be kept alive by artificial breathing devices for the remainder of his life. In 1916 a major epidemic struck the U.S.A. and 27,000 persons were paralyzed and 6,000 died, 2,000 in New York City alone. Various experimental preparations, largely designed to create temporary passive immunization in epidemics, were tried during the next 20 years, but none was fully successful. In 1934 two vaccines were produced, each curiously prophetic of the more sophisticated varieties to come about 30 years later. The first was developed by John Kolmer of Philadelphia, who based his work upon the observations of Flexner that occasionally monkeys could be protected by injections of living virus which had been chemically attenuated. Meanwhile William Park of New York produced his own protective vaccine from the spinal cord of infected monkeys, the virus having been inactivated by direct contact with formaldehyde. Widespread immunization involving over 10,000 children was undertaken with these preparations and, most unfortunately, cases of paralytic polio occurred among those whom it was hoped to protect. In such large numbers it might well have been that polio was due to strike at those individuals in any event, but nevertheless the preparations were discredited.

By 1949 it was known that there were three strains of polio virus, and that protection against one strain did not necessarily produce protection against the others. This discovery, made by David Bodian of the Johns Hopkins University in Baltimore, explained many anomalous results in research, and stimulated Professor Jonas Salk of the University of Pittsburgh to produce a trivalent vaccine, designed to master the three known virulent strains. In 1954 the Salk vaccine (a 'killed' preparation) was tried upon 450,000 children. The results, carefully matched with a control group, showed that the incidence of polio among the vaccinated had fallen to one quarter. Then, in 1955, tragedy struck at the vaccines: living virus accidentally remained in two batches, and altogether 204 vaccinated children, and certain of their close contacts, were stricken with the very disease they sought to avoid. After several technical investigations the source of the disaster was identified and the vaccine was again the agent of a nationwide campaign.

From 1949, when John E. Enders succeeded in

growing polio virus in tissue culture, thought and talent had been devoted to the possibility of a safe living vaccine, which could be taken orally. Again, the path of progress was far from straightforward. Hilary Koprowski of the Lederle Laboratories, New York, produced a vaccine which appeared entirely safe until it was observed that when the living attenuated virus was excreted by experimental animals, it could apparently regain its original virulence and cause severe damage to the nervous tissues of other monkeys.

Perhaps the final triumph in the tortuous and at times heart-breaking battle against poliomyelitis was recorded by the efforts of Albert B. Sabin of the Children's Hospital in Cincinnati. By 1957 he had produced a living vaccine which could not be faulted, and which withstood every safety test.

Living vaccines had tremendous advantages over the killed version. Not only did they produce solid and totally effective immunity, but they inevitably multiplied in the gut and silently spread the protecting condition just as virulent polio would have spread in an epidemic. Thus the fearless were protected with the careful, and when mass campaigns were undertaken, it was likely that no one was spared contact with the living virus, able only to protect and never to injure. In the middle 1960s Sabin vaccine, now effective against the three paralytic strains, had

supplanted Salk (killed) vaccines and remains the permanent vehicle of immunity.

It is customary to begin immunization against polio at the age of three months, and to give two further doses, normally at the time the triple antigen is given against diphtheria, tetanus and whooping cough.

Tuberculosis. The combined onslaught of drugs, vaccine and X-ray investigations has led to the virtual disappearance of tuberculosis from Britain, most of Europe and the North American countries, and the story of its conquest is given in a later chapter.

Virus diseases. Soon after the discovery that bacteria were associated with disease, it became evident that an exceptionally small type of microorganism, termed a virus, could also produce illness, including some of the deadliest diseases known to man. Many years had to pass before virus particles could actually be seen through the microscope, and often the only form of identification depended upon the ability of suspected material from a known case to cause further cases, in man or animals.

Today viruses are known to have other potentially dangerous characteristics besides their submicroscopic size. They have the need to live within human or animal cells, and their presence inside the cell envelope may disrupt the whole structure and function of the host cell. When virus invasion is widespread and successful, death of the animal may occur rapidly. A further reason for fearing virus invasion is the inability, in general, of antibiotics to affect the invader. However (with notable exceptions such as influenza and the common cold) viruses induce immunity in the survivors, thus indicating that vaccine protection is possible.

Four significant virus diseases may be considered. Smallpox had been mentioned in association with Edward Jenner. Immunization by purposefully contracted vaccinia, or cowpox, provides complete and excellent protection. This is the standard procedure, and its efficacy has no doubt deflected interest from any other form of vaccine. In view of the very high mortality rate of smallpox in the unprotected, and the uncertainty of vaccination once exposure has occured, two further forms of treatment have been developed in recent years, though they are useful only during the incubation period and never once the disease is fully established. One form of protection is administered by injecting the anti-vaccinia antibodies from a recently vaccinated person into the potential victim, the other by giving a synthetic chemical known as methisazone.

Influenza is a disease of unpredictably fluctuating virulence. The great epidemic of influenza which swept the world in 1918 and 1919 killed at least 15 million people, more than

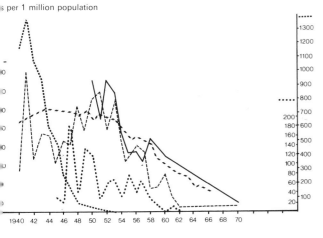

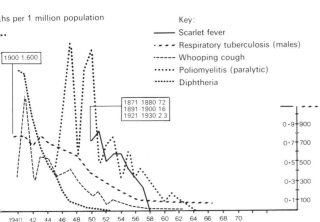

31 The diagrams here show graphically the final stages in the abolition of five serious and often lethal infections from the population of England and Wales. The upper graph shows notifications, and the lower, deaths attributed to each of these diseases per million of population since 1940. The scale against which each disease curve should be read is different and is indicated by the key lines at the head of the scales on each side of the diagrams. A further indication of the dramatic falls in mortality from tuberculosis and scarlet fever is given in the boxes. For tuberculosis, figures for males only have been given, for ease of tabulation. The considerable year to year variation in rates, notably for example in poliomyelitis, demonstrates the epidemic waves of the disease which used to sweep across unprotected populations, with intervening periods of comparative dormancy.

died from all effects of the Great War. Most unfortunately the influenza viruses mutate frequently and this makes the production of a reliable vaccine almost impossible and in any event, extremely expensive.

Measles, while in itself a relatively trifling disease, may cause complications in children, especially those who are debilitated for other reasons. One injection of a living attenuated vaccine confers complete protection and by the end of 1966 over 20 million doses had been given to children in the United States, and this vaccine is now standard procedure both in North America and Britain.

Rubella, or German measles, is a virus disease of very special interest because of its ability to damage the growing tissues of an unborn child and lead to congenital deformities. Though it is harmless and negligible itself as a disease, this feature of rubella has led to very strenuous attempts to produce a protective vaccine, particularly after events in 1964 when a rubella epidemic in the United States led to the birth of tens of thousands of deformed children in the U.S.A. and Britain.

Although it is difficult to envisage the control of influenza by vaccine, there are hopes not only that smallpox, measles and rubella will be effectively controlled, but also that perhaps immunization campaigns against these diseases could be spread widely enough for them to be indeed eliminated from the earth altogether: and as they depend upon human transmission their extinction would be permanent.

Chemotherapy and antibiotics. The major victories against infectious disease have been achieved through perfection of immunization techniques. However, a new generation of drugs has arisen in the last 40 years which, quite unlike the preparations available to the physicians of old, are specifically lethal to bacteria, though rarely effective against viruses. These substances have a limited use in the creation of immunity, in that curative doses, taken before exposure, will protect against a sensitive organism: but the protection is never more than temporary and cannot be compared in effectiveness with exposure to attenuated or dead microorganisms.

Antibiotics share with chemotherapy a limited role in the history of the mastery of infectious disease. The chief use of both chemotherapy and antibiotics is in the treatment of established cases. The great progress has been in the field of prevention rather than treatment, and particularly in the field of vaccines.

Some of the chief milestones in the history of chemotherapy and antibiotics are recounted in chapter 15.

Thus over a period of about 100 years, practically every infectious disease succumbed to the painstaking advances of medical scientists.

Different epidemiological techniques (and often a combination of techniques) have defeated different diseases. Plague recoiled from the discovery that cases originated from a microorganism carried on a particular flea harbored by a particular rat: and this victory was reinforced by the discovery of a vaccine, chemotherapy and antibiotics. Step by step and disease by disease the territories of infection were conquered by the medical scientists, their chief and principal weapon always being the protective vaccine. Problems of infection still remain, and the epidemiologist cannot sheath his sword until all known discoveries are accepted and utilized throughout the world— and until control has been established over the viruses, especially those likely to mutate, such as virulent influenza. Indeed the presence of atmospheric radiation enhances the possibility of mutation in microorganisms, and diseases entirely new to the human race may yet arise and challenge the ingenuity and persistence of a new generation of medical scientists.

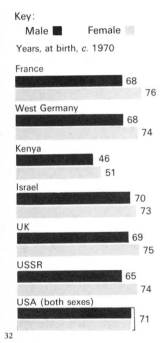

Key:
Male ■ Female ▨

Years, at birth, *c.* 1970

France
68
76

West Germany
68
74

Kenya
46
51

Israel
70
73

UK
69
75

USSR
65
74

USA (both sexes)
71

32

32 This diagram shows the average expectation of life at birth in seven different countries, for males and females respectively. (Figures by sex for the U.S.A. are not readily obtainable.) Except for Kenya, the countries shown are developed and industrialized, and there are only small differences in life expectation between them. In each, women have a substantially higher expectation than men. This principally reflects the different incidence of coronary heart disease after middle age. Kenya is shown as an example of a developing country. Here the much shorter life expectancy is mainly due to the much higher rate of mortality during the first few years of life.

2 Digestion and Absorption

Do I dare
Disturb the universe?
In a minute there is time
For decisions and revisions which
   a minute will reverse.

               T. S. ELIOT
The Love Song of J. Alfred Prufrock

Epidemiologists, scientists and alert clinicians, unlike J. Alfred Prufrock, have dared to disturb the universe, and the subsequent perturbations have been felt throughout human existence, not least in the concepts of gastro-intestinal function and disease. Decisions and revisions there have been in plenty, and indeed, the rapidity of change which mesmerized Prufrock has been a source of stimulus to the scientists. What follows is an attempt to show how the more important advances have influenced our understanding and treatment of several disorders, and to show where future advances can be expected.

The gut with its related organs the liver, gall bladder and pancreas provides the pathway for the processing and absorption of the foods and fluids necessary for life. The gut is a soft elastic tube of muscle and its internal lining of delicate membrane (the mucosa) works with extraordinary efficiency, absorbing virtually everything fed into it. Obesity, one of our modern epidemics, bears witness to this, and indicates that although our gut was evolved to eat for survival, it is capable of coping with eating for pleasure or indulgence. The mechanisms which regulate food intake are not yet understood. Swedish scientists have induced gluttony in sheep by stimulating nerve cells in the hypothalamus but there is no evidence that obese humans have hypothalamic dysfunction. It may be the bulk of food, not its nutritional content, which determines satiety. In this context, an operation in which 90 per cent of the small intestine is bypassed enhances weight loss not as one might expect by a decrease in the amount of food absorbed, but by a drop in the actual intake. Perhaps there is some reflex mechanism at work here which has yet to be discovered. In the meantime the problem of obesity is one whose solution is still to be sought, and it can only be said, as did Samuel Johnson, 'Sir if she is too fat, it is plain that she has eaten too much'.

Digestion. The complex molecules of food are broken down into simple units by an array of

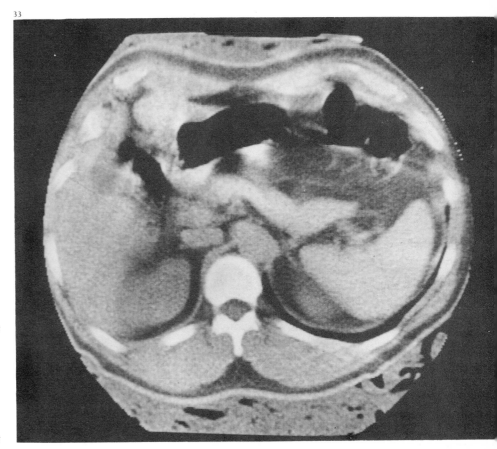

33 The extraordinary new EMI scanner 'cuts' an X-ray section through the body at a given level by linking the absorption of multiple X-ray beams with a computer—a technique known as computerized axial tomography. This section through the abdomen shows, as if viewed from below, the vertebral body and lower rib cage, appearing as the whitish structures in the lower part of the picture, protecting the liver, the solid organ lying to its left, and the spleen on the right.

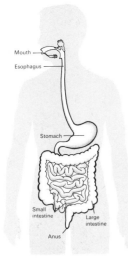

34

34 The gastro-intestinal tract. The selective and rejecting role of taste gives the mouth a most important protective function. The esophagus or gullet conducts food through the chest to the stomach by virtue of a complex and finely coordinated sequence of contraction waves. The stomach holds the ingested food, subjecting it to the primary physical and chemical breakdown processes, only passing its contents on to the adjacent small intestine when chemical messages signal completion of this process. The major function of the small intestinal transit is the final breakdown of complex molecules to those of smaller absorbable size, carried into the circulation at various levels, the residue being passed on for dehydration, temporary storage and final excretion to the large intestine.

35 The importance of the gastro-intestinal tract as an endocrine organ in its own right has only quite recently been fully appreciated. Many different cell types, each producing its own specific chemical messenger, are to be found running the length of the intestine. (Among these hormones some have known physiological functions, such as glucagon (A), insulin (B), secretin (S), and cholecystokimin (I). Others—enteroglucagon (L), somatostatin (D), pancreatic polypeptide (D₁)—do not have functions which are understood. The enterochromaffin cells (EC) are related to the sympathetic nervous system, while those marked ECL produce an unknown product.) The cell types are identifiable by highly specialized techniques which link a fluorescent dye to cells specifically recognized by antibodies artificially produced in experimental animals. This new technique of immunohistochemistry has opened the way to a much fuller understanding of the function as well as the structure of the cells of the body by the identification of the individual product of the cell.

gastro-intestinal enzymes, a process largely under hormonal control. These simple units are then absorbed through the mucosa of the small intestine. Any residual fluid is absorbed in the colon, and the resulting waste stored in the rectum prior to elimination in the feces. Coordinated movement of the food through the gastro-intestinal tract is achieved by a network of nerve fibers in the gut's muscle coat which, while having innate activity, also respond to hormonal levels and to stimuli from the higher nerve centers. The transit time from mouth to colon is about four hours, but imbalance of nervous control can cause major alterations in this, and give rise to either diarrhea (rapid transit) or constipation (slow transit).

Knowledge of the hormonal control of digestion has been gleaned over the past 70 years. That secretions from the intestines actually participated in digestion was first definitively demonstrated by the American army surgeon William Beaumont in the early 19th century. One of his patients was a young Canadian, Alexis St Martin, whose stomach had been exteriorized following a gun shot wound. Beaumont was thus able to describe the appearance and properties of the gastric juices. He showed they contained hydrochloric acid and demonstrated the profound influence of mental activity on the stomach secretions. By bathing various foods in gastric juices he showed their differing digestibilities, and in the course of these experiments first showed that bile was a useful adjunct in the digestion of fats. His book, *Experiments and Observations on the Gastric Juice and Physiology of Digestion,* is a classic in physiology.

Despite Beaumont, nobody knew what regulated the secretion of these juices, although the nervous system and particularly the vagus nerve was heavily implicated. That it was not nervous regulation alone was shown by the London doctors Starling and Bayliss in 1902. While investigating the flow of pancreatic juice into the duodenum, they showed that a chemical transmitter released from the small intestine into the blood stream stimulated pancreatic production of digestive juices. This was the first example of such a chemical transmitter, and Starling coined the word 'hormone' (from the Greek *hormeo,* to urge on). Starling realized that there were likely to be many hormones, and secretin was the specific name he gave to the first. Secretin's structure has now been established, and the upper gastro-intestinal cells which secrete it identified. It is also known that the stimulus for its release is acidity.

It was not until 1928 that Andrew Ivy in America identified another hormone working on the pancreas, pancreozymin. While secretin caused the flow of a large volume of alkaline

secretion, pancreozymin produced a highly concentrated enzyme-rich fluid containing trypsin, lipase and amylase, which help digest protein, fat and carbohydrate respectively. Speculation about hormones controlling the acid secretion of the stomach were first made in 1905. It was also suggested that such a hormone might be secreted from the antrum of the stomach. In 1955 the U.S. surgeon Lester Dragstedt finally discovered this hormone, gastrin, and shortly afterwards its chemical structure was determined and shown to be very similar to that of pancreozymin.

Pancreozymin, while triggering pancreatic secretion, also causes the gall bladder to contract. Bile salts which are stored in the gall bladder are then delivered to the gut. These salts enable fat to be digested by making an emulsion of it; unemulsified fat simply passes down the intestine.

Blood levels of these hormones can now be measured by radio immuno-assay techniques and this had led to an understanding of their roles in disease states. High gastrin levels are found in the rare Zollinger-Ellison syndrome in which multiple ulceration of the stomach and duodenum is often coupled with profuse diarrhea. For many years this disorder has been recognized by the very high acid secretion which accompanies it, but only by application of basic research was it possible to identify a gastrin-secreting tumor as the underlying cause.

35

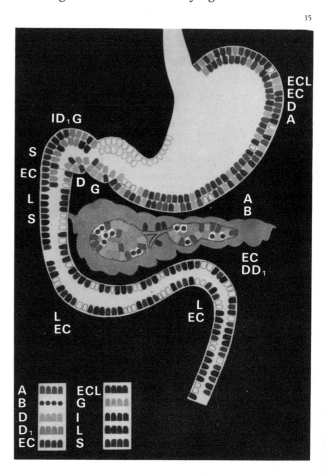

Undoubtedly similar pathological roles for secretin and pancreozymin await discovery.

Although secretin, pancreozymin (also called cholecystokinin) and gastrin are the big three, several other gastro-intestinal hormones have now been identified. These are (i) motilin, which increases motor activity of the stomach, (ii) vaso-active intestinal polypeptide (VIP), which inhibits acid secretion by the stomach as well as increasing the flow of fluid into the gut, (iii) gastric inhibitory polypeptide (GIP), which has a similar action to VIP as well as damping stomach mobility, (iv) enteroglucagon, which is secreted in response to sugary meals, and causes several metabolic reactions including increased fluid flow into the gut, and (v) enterogastrone, whose secretion is stimulated by the arrival of fat in the duodenum and which causes a fall in gastric acid secretion and gastric mobility.

The exact role of many of these hormones is uncertain, but they certainly act in concert. VIP and GIP have both been implicated in a rare but severe and potentially fatal disease in which the sufferer gets profuse and increasingly watery diarrhea, akin to cholera. Tumors excreting these two hormones have been found in association with the disease and their removal relieves the symptoms. The association of symptoms with abnormal levels of the hormones helps shed light on their action, and we can expect further syndromes to be delineated in the coming years.

All these gastro-intestinal hormones are secreted from similar cells, scattered throughout the epithelial lining of the gut and called generically 'clear cells'. These cells have characteristic pathways for handling amines, and have been dubbed APUD cells (an acronym of Amine, Precursor, Uptake and Decarboxylation). Precisely which hormones are produced where in the gut is under investigation, but the APUD series extends down into the colon, and release of hormones in constipation could account for the general symptoms sometimes attributed to constipation. It is appropriate that the gastro-intestinal tract, in which the first hormone, secretin, was discovered, now proves to be the biggest endocrine organ in the body, with an amazingly wide range of hormones acting in complex, and as yet undefined, ways.

Although not conventionally described as hormone, 5-hydroxy tryptamine (serotonin) is produced by the APUD cell series, and can, like a hormone, exert effects on dormant organs. Under normal circumstances, however, it is denatured by the liver, to which it is carried by the portal system. Occasionally, serotonin-producing tumors arise in the gut, and if these spread to the liver, active serotonin may be secreted directly into the systemic blood stream. Characteristic symptoms of flushing attacks, asthma, diarrhea and sometimes heart disease,

go to make up the disease, which is rather loosely called the carcinoid syndrome. Chemical antagonists to serotonin may be of some avail, but in view of the fact that the tumor is usually widespread by the time symptoms occur, radical cure is seldom possible.

Gastro-intestinal hormones are secreted by cells in contact with the gut lumen, which are thus ideally placed to sample the composition of ingested foods and react accordingly. But there is also a 'remote-control' nervous element, via the vagus nerve, so called because of its wandering, 'vagabond' course. The interrelationship of these two control mechanisms is under intensive investigation at present and is of particular importance in the medical and surgical treatment of peptic ulceration.

Peptic ulceration. Our knowledge of peptic ulceration is incomplete. That it is on the increase seems clear, and that ulceration of the mucosal lining of the esophagus, stomach or duodenum cannot occur in the absence of acid is a basic truth which has not been contested since the American physician Sippy's aphorism of 1912, 'No acid, no ulcer'. Under the influence of both the vagus nerve and gastrin, large quantities of concentrated hydrochloric acid are produced by the stomach. Our present view is that there is a mucous barrier which prevents this acid from attacking the mucosa, but which may be eroded by a variety of factors, and which will then permit ulceration. The mucous barrier concept is supported by investigations in which acidity is measured by electrodes placed in the cavity of the stomach and in its wall. Irritation of the wall causes an increase in acidity of the mucosal cells, which then die causing a mucosal break or ulceration. What factors cause this destructive irritation in the stomach? Increased acidity is indubitably one, and this may be mediated by increased vagus nerve stimulation caused by stress or, as we have seen, by gastrin-producing tumors which drive the acid-producing cells.

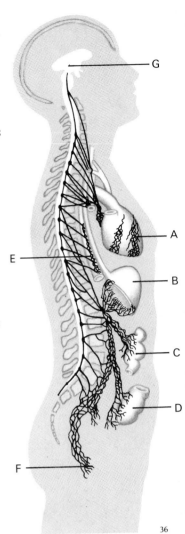

36

36 The gastro-intestinal tract, like the heart and blood vessels, is subject to the unconscious control of the autonomic nervous system. The functional control exercised by these nervous pathways is of great importance. The rate and force of the heart (A) and the state of contraction of the stomach and intestine (C and D) are both subject to autonomic nervous control. A plexus or sheath of fine nerve fibers accompanies the arterial supply (E) out to its final ramifications, supplying nervous impulses to the structures receiving the blood supply. The glandular function of the pancreas, the flow of blood to the intestines, the regulation of sexual function (F), particularly in the male, are all dependent on the integrity of the autonomic nerve supply. The central coordinatory role of the brain in much of this activity is indicated in the diagram which shows the origin of many pathways in the hypothalamus (G).

37 Optical fibers, used here in a table lamp, transmit a perfect image from end to end under almost any conditions of flexion and convolution. In the fiberoptic gastroscope one series of fibers transmits the light from a light source to the site to be viewed, and the desired image returns to the viewer along another.

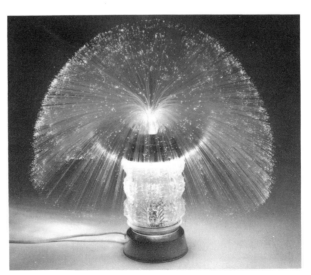

37

38 Almost every body cavity and vessel, duct or tube is now accessible to the radiologist. In this illustration the pancreatic duct has been outlined with radio-opaque 'dye' injected through a tube (a flexible gastroscope) maneuvered under visual control so that its tip has entered the ampulla of Vater in the duodenum, through which bile and the secretions of the pancreas are discharged. Obstruction of this duct, which may be shown up by procedures such as this, interferes with the discharge of the digestive enzymes, and partially digested food, in particular fats, pass through the bowel and are excreted, depriving the body of essential nutrients.

39 Here radiology has been used to identify the site of bleeding in a hemorrhage in the gut. A catheter has been introduced into the abdominal aorta from a leg artery and hooked over into the coeliac artery. A radio-opaque 'dye' has been injected and can be seen escaping from an artery as indicated by the diagram. This identifies the point of hemorrhage for later surgery.

40 In this picture a 'barium meal' has been used to show up the outline of the stomach in the search for a suspected ulcer. Barium sulfate is used to outline the stomach, since it is opaque to X-rays and its insolubility prevents its absorption. An ulcer crater is clearly visible in the picture. The barium mass may be followed during its passage through the remainder of the small intestine, where deformities of outline would reveal areas of ulceration, inflammation, or thickening of the bowel wall. A tumor within the abdominal cavity may distort the barium shape by pressure from without. The large intestine is more often outlined by the careful introduction of a similar barium mass from below in a 'barium enema'.

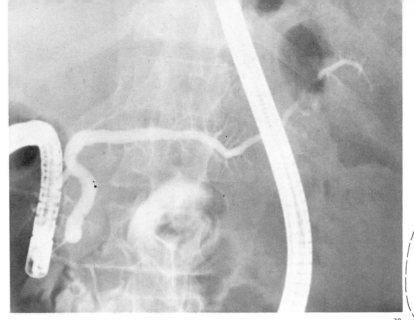

38

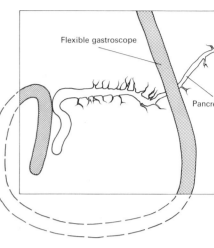

Flexible gastroscope

Pancr

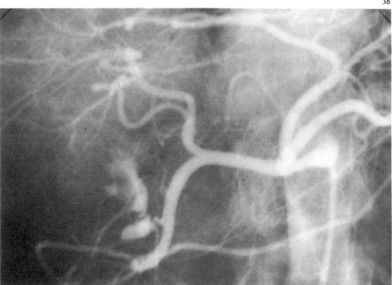

39

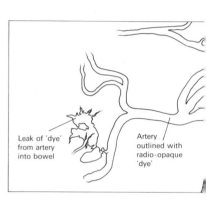

Leak of 'dye' from artery into bowel

Artery outlined with radio-opaque 'dye'

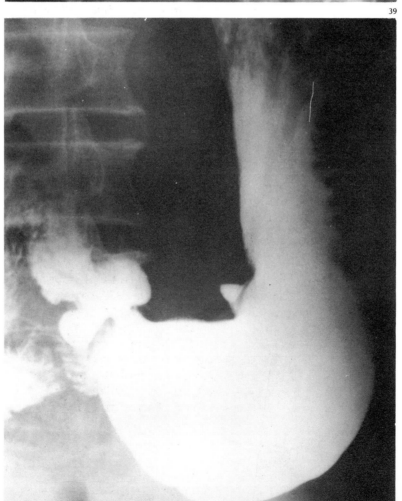

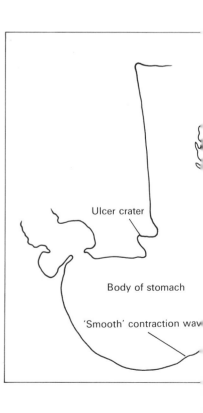

Ulcer crater

Body of stomach

'Smooth' contraction wav

40

Drugs such as steroids and salicylates can likewise cause damage, an effect that can be studied experimentally in animals. As far as gastric ulcers are concerned, reflux of bile salts from the duodenum may initiate damage. This was first demonstrated in the long-suffering stomach of Alexis St Martin, and has been confirmed in dogs by observing the effects of bile salts introduced into specially created stomach pouches.

The detection of gastric and duodenal ulceration has become progressively more accurate over the years. In 1868, twenty-seven years before Röntgen discovered X-rays, Kussmaul inserted a hollow lighted tube into the stomach of a friend, and through it made direct observations of the interior. The tube was rigid and his view was poor, a state of affairs which existed, despite modifications to the instrument, until the Japanese perfected a fiber-optic gastro-duodeno-scope in the early 1960s. This was flexible and maneuverable and by providing better illumination has given a near certain means of identifying and even photographing ulcers or other abnormalities of the upper gut. Removal of small pieces of tissue for microscopic or chemical examination is also possible with the gastroscope. Tissue samples obtained in this way have advanced the understanding of chronic gastritis, and can show very early whether there is any cancerous change in the lesion. In Japan stomach cancer is common and fatal if not diagnosed early. Early gastroscopic diagnosis is now a routine procedure, and fatality from gastric cancer correspondingly less.

In the West, gastroscopic diagnosis is a vital adjunct to barium meal X-ray diagnosis. Hammeter in Germany first displayed a gastric ulcer by barium meal X-ray in 1908. Since then it has been a standard diagnostic technique. Not all ulcers are demonstrable by X-rays but if the investigation also includes gastroscopy, a correct diagnosis is usually obtained.

With the serious and common problem of hemorrhage from the upper gastro-intestinal tract, usually from a peptic ulcer, informative barium meals are difficult and in the pre-gastroscope days an intelligent guess had to be made for the site of the hemorrhage. Now it is possible to observe the lesion directly, and to take measures appropriate to what is seen. Occasionally bleeding is so profuse that gastroscopy fails to reveal the source, and in these circumstances arteriography is used. A fine tube is inserted into one of the femoral arteries and guided first into the coeliac artery and then into the superior mesenteric artery, which supply blood to the stomach and duodenum. A dye injected through the fine tube enters the circulation and a rapid sequence of X-ray pictures traces the course of the dye and identifies the site of bleeding. Further, local infusion of drugs which constrict the relevant artery can be used as a method of treatment and is showing great promise. Treatment involves, in the first instance, support for the circulation by transfusion of the estimated volume of blood lost. If this fails, a direct surgical attack is made on the site of bleeding. Advances in surgical and anesthetic techniques have made surgery safer, but the risks remain. If this technique of arterial drug infusion proves itself, it will constitute a major therapeutic advance.

Hepatitis. Blood transfusions, often necessary in serious hemorrhage, have attendant risks, but a series of perceptive observations by Blumberg in the 1960s removed one of them. Before detailing his discoveries, we need to discuss the liver's structure and function. Because it synthesizes and secretes bile salts, the liver is intimately involved in fat absorption. It also plays a central role in the processing of carbohydrates, fats and proteins, the manufacture of blood clotting factors and the excretion of bilirubin, the breakdown product of worn-out red blood cells. It has two blood supplies, one a conventional supply from the hepatic artery and the second a flow of nutrient-rich blood directly from the stomach and intestine via the portal vein. The blood flows through the metabolically active liver cells and then returns to the heart via the hepatic vein. Bile made by the liver flows in a similar branching network to that of the blood, but of course in the opposite direction, from the liver through the bile duct system to the gall bladder and hence into the duodenum.

Hepatitis or inflammation of liver cells is a common disorder usually giving rise to jaundice—a yellow discoloration of the skin owing to retention of the pigment bilirubin, which a diseased liver cannot excrete properly. There are two common forms of hepatitis. One, serum hepatitis, is transmitted in blood transfusions, or by the use of one needle to inoculate a group of people. This latter mode of transmission had military significance during the Second World War when substantial numbers of troops contracted serum hepatitis following inoculation. Although a viral cause was suspected in serum hepatitis, no virus had been found. M. Blumberg, an American research scientist studying patterns of variations in blood proteins, observed what he took to be a new variant both in the blood of one of his subjects, and in that of an Australian aboriginal. He then noticed that certain individuals who were negative for this variant, became positive and at the same time developed serum hepatitis. He went on to comfirm that the Australia antigen, as he called the particle, was almost always associated with this disease. We now have reliable ways of detecting the Australia antigen in the blood of a potential donor, thus

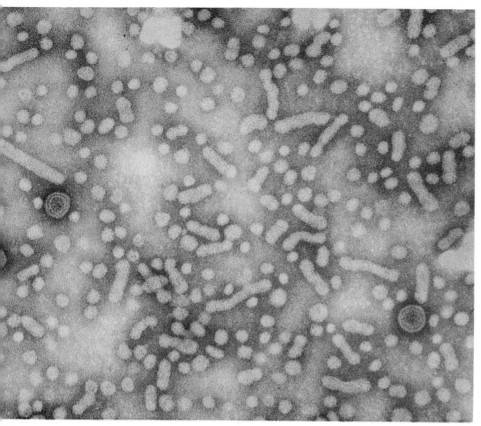

41 An electronmicrograph of approximately 151,200 times magnification of plasma from a patient with serum hepatitis. The picture shows three types of particle, a small round particle, short rods, and doughnut-like 'Dane' particles thought to be the complete viral bodies associated with the liver damage of hepatitis. It appears that the Hepatitis B associated antigen (Australia antigen), i.e. the small particles and short rods, is the same protein as constitutes the outer coat of the Dane particle. In viral infections the nucleic acid supplants some of the cell's own nucleic acid so as to replicate itself and make the cell embark upon abnormal production of the viral body's protein, a process which is likely to lead to the destruction of the cell or a chronic state of viral latency.

making blood transfusions much safer. Most people who get serum hepatitis eliminate the antigen during convalescence, but some, including patients on long-term renal dialysis, may harbor it for many years, thus acting as a reservoir for the disease. Although the great majority of people with acute hepatitis recover, a few go on from the acute illness to a chronic state of ill health, and ultimately to cirrhosis of the liver. These different responses to infection may be due to the particular genetic and immunological make-up of these individuals. Analysis of this problem will help to unravel the complicated inter-relationships between genetic make-up, immunological reactivity and liability to disease.

Until 1973 the actual nature of the Australia antigen was obscure. Was it really a virus, and if it was why could no one isolate nucleic acid, a *sine qua non* of viruses, from the particle? Although nucleic acid has still not been identified within the particle, experiments on animals have shown the antigen to fulfil the criteria classically associated with an infective agent. These were enumerated by Koch and are as follows:

1. The putative agent must be found in all cases of the disease.

2. It must be capable of being grown outside the body, in pure culture for a number of generations.

3. Introduction of the agent into a healthy organism must reproduce the disease.

4. It must be capable of being recovered from this organism and grown in pure culture.

The Australia antigen is thus the infective agent causing serum hepatitis and is almost certainly a virus.

Infectious hepatitis, a disease similar to but milder than serum hepatitis, has, despite intensive research, revealed no virus associated with it. Both diseases occasionally cause acute liver failure, usually fatal. The toxins which cause the liver failure have not been identified, but several ingenious methods have been used to try and cleanse the blood of them. These include perfusion of the affected blood through pigs' liver, baboons' liver, and even the livers of well disposed relatives—all, unhappily, with singularly little success. A new approach is to de-toxify the blood by running it through a charcoal column. Charcoal absorbs all manner of blood toxins, whilst not interfering too much with the normal blood constituents. The bond between charcoal and toxins is a physico-chemical one, and it is thanks to the close collaboration between doctors and physical chemists that this new technique is now being tried at King's College Hospital, London. First reports are encouraging, and as charcoal hemo-perfusion also has applications in the treatment of severe self-poisoning it is one area in which rapid and substantial advances can be expected. Failing any of these methods liver transplantation has been mooted as a treatment for acute hepatic failure, and this is discussed in chapter 11.

The bile salts. Bile was considered by Hippocrates and Galen and then, by virtue of the galenic tradition in medicine, by other scientists up till the seventeenth century, as an end product of liver metabolism, 'as a mere excrement, and of no other use than by its acrimony to promote the excretion of the gut'. It was not until researchers experimentally tied the bile duct of dogs, thus preventing bile from reaching the intestine, that its importance in fat digestion was realized. In these experiments the dogs although eating ravenously, lost weight and passed copious stools containing large quantities of fat. A few years later it was shown that bile salts were a major constituent of bile. Other researchers found that the bile salts were not all excreted in the feces but, after performing their digestive function, were reabsorbed back into the body, undergoing what is now called an entero-hepatic circulation. Reabsorption takes place exclusively in the terminal ileum, which is also the exclusive site of absorption of vitamin B_{12}, and is illustrative of the regional diversity of function in the gastro-intestinal tract. Debate raged over the function of bile salts. The chemists found them to be amphipathic substances having one end soluble in water and the other in fat, just like detergents. Was the detergent action of the bile salts the prime one, enabling enzymes to get at the insoluble fat molecules and break them down to soluble constituents, or did bile salts in some way solubilize the fat molecules and thus enable them to be absorbed? The American Alan Hofman resolved the debate in 1963, by showing that a combination of intact fat molecules, products of fat digestion and bile salts formed a suspension of small particles, micelles, soluble in water. The fat incorporated in these micelles is taken through the jejunal mucosa, whilst the bile salt component is left behind and finally reabsorbed in the terminal ileum.

Knowledge of the structure and function of bile salts has provided the clinician with the explanation for several puzzling phenomena. Crohn's disease, a condition usually affecting the terminal ileum, may cause substantial fatty diarrhea. Once it was realized that bile salts, vital to fat absorption, are reabsorbed by the terminal ileum, the reason for this diarrhea became clear. Instead of being reabsorbed, bile salts were lost in the feces and became scarce in the body, and fat malabsorption ensued. In obstructive jaundice bile salts also accumulate in the body causing intense generalized itching. Relief is only to be had by reducing the blood bile salt level. Chemists showed that certain resins could bind bile salts in the gut and so interrupt their entero-hepatic circulation, lower the blood levels and ameliorate the itching. Finally a physico-chemical approach to the constituents of bile by Small in the 1960s showed that the solubility of cholesterol in bile was dependent on the bile salt concentration. When the bile salt concentration is low cholesterol precipitates out, forming gallstones. Conventional treatment for gallstones is surgical but the possibility of dissolving them by feeding the sufferers bile salts is being explored, and may decrease the necessity for these operations.

Coeliac disease. As with the bile salts, many disciplines have aided our understanding of coeliac disease which may cause severe malabsorption, with diarrhea, vitamin deficiencies, anemia and stunting of growth. Dicke, a physician working in German-occupied Holland, observed that his 'coeliacs' got better on their war-time vegetable diets, whereas Swedish coeliacs still eating cereals did not improve. He subsequently showed that it was the gluten, a protein present in cereals, which caused the destruction and flattening of intestinal villi, the hallmark of coeliac disease. As the villi are vital to absorption it is hardly surprising that malabsorption ensues. Villous flattening in coeliac disease had in fact been recognized from post-mortem studies since 1904, and tissue confirming the diagnosis was occasionally come by at laparotomy. Major advances in understanding coeliac disease were however made possible only

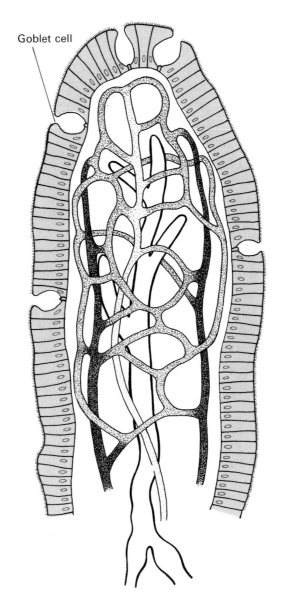

Goblet cell

when a simple biopsy technique was pioneered. In 1956 Dr Margot Shiner, working at the Hammersmith Hospital, London, designed a per-oral biopsy capsule which could be positioned in the intestines by viewing with X-rays. The original capsule was rather cumbersome, and we now use a modified form designed by the American W. H. Crosby in 1958. This easy biopsy technique has transformed the gastro-intestinal scene in a number of ways. First, other rarer conditions characterized by specific abnormalities of the intestinal lining have been identified. Second, by introducing gluten into the gut of coeliacs and taking biopsies at short intervals our basic understanding of the disease has advanced. Changes, probably due to a reaction between gluten and the body's immunological defence system, take place within a few hours. Cells at the top of the villi die and the ones below come up to take their place. This happens in normal conditions, but the rate of the cycle is accelerated in coeliacs and the villi become first blunted then flattened. The lining cells are also immature and of poor absorptive

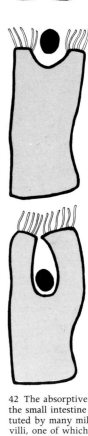

42

42 The absorptive surface of the small intestine is constituted by many millions of the villi, one of which is shown on the left of the diagram. The fine, finger-like projection is covered with cells overlying a rich network of fine capillary blood vessels, with a lymph vessel at the center. The soluble small molecules pass through the cell membrane and are transported, sometimes after local biochemical processing, to the base of the cell, whence the product is discharged into the bloodstream to be carried for further processing to the liver or directly to the organs and tissues of the body. The mucus-producing goblet cells interspersed among the other cells on the surface of the villus can be readily recognized. To the right, greatly magnified, another process of absorption is illustrated, where a larger molecule is engulfed and passes in a tiny vacuole into the interior of one of the cells lining the villus. The very fine hair-like projections, the so-called brush border, which have a selective and directive function of their own, are also illustrated.

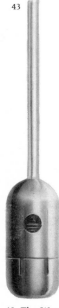

43 The Watson per-oral biopsy capsule, a later development from the Crosby capsule referred to in the text, used for taking small samples of the mucosa which lines the small intestine in the diagnosis of coeliac and other diseases. The capsule is swallowed by the patient and positioned under X-ray control. Suction is then applied through the tube so that mucosa is drawn into the circular window. A spring-loaded knife is then released and the capsule withdrawn with its sample inside.

44, 45 The samples taken by the biopsy capsule are examined under a dissecting microscope and later sectioned for examination under the ordinary microscope. 44 shows a picture taken through a dissecting microscope of a sample of normal small-intestinal mucosa, showing the slender, finger-shaped villi. In contrast, 45 shows mucosa from a patient with coeliac disease where the mucosa is flat with a mosaic pattern. The smaller pits which cover the surface of the specimen represent the crypts from which the villi normally grow, rendered visible in this disease by the absence of the villi which normally luxuriantly cover them. Here, as described in the text, villus formation is greatly restricted or absent, resulting in a seriously reduced surface area for absorption.

capacity and the combination of loss of absorptive surface and poor quality cells gives rise to all the symptoms. When gluten is removed from the diet the villi return to normal and the patient recovers. The rapid cell turnover in the villi may account for an increased incidence of cancer found in coeliacs who do not stick to their diet, and is obviously a fruitful field for investigation into the development of malignancy.

Basic research work, clinical acumen and the development of new techniques such as the Crosby capsule, liver biopsy, fiber-optic gastroscopy and arteriography have all helped our understanding of the upper end of the gut. What about the lower end?

Ulcerative colitis, a disease of Western civilization, in which ulceration of the colonic mucosa causes severe bouts of bleeding, still taxes clinicians greatly. It has to be differentiated from dysentery by careful stool culture. Specific diagnosis has only been made possible by the development of sigmoidoscopic, radiographic and bowel biopsy techniques. The first endoscope was developed by Dersomeaux in 1853, who used it to look into the uterus, bladder and rectum. The light source was an alcohol and turpentine lamp, with a suitably placed reflecting mirror. From this start the present sigmoidoscopes in use for over fifty years were developed. They allow a clear view of the bowel's lining, and changes characteristic of the whole range of bowel diseases have been observed by clinicians over the years. In ulcerative colitis, the typical picture is of reddened fragile mucosa which bleeds on contact, and which may be severely ulcerated. Biopsy through the sigmoidoscope, following the work of Sidney Truelove in Oxford, became a routine procedure after the Second World War and provided histological back-up of this clinical picture. Sigmoidoscopy and biopsy have enabled us to make a precise diagnosis, but to assess the extent of the disease radiography is used. Radio-opaque substances, given as enemas, have been used since the early 1900s. First bismuth, then barium was used, and in the 1920s, Fischer observed that a barium and air mixture showed up the bowel's lining more effectively, and that is essentially the mode employed now.

A recent adjunct to the barium enema is the colonoscope, a fiber-optic instrument about one meter long and highly flexible, making it possible for the entire colon to be viewed and biopsied. Its use is still being evaluated, but that it will enhance our diagnostic precision in large bowel disease cannot be doubted. Precise diagnosis of ulcerative colitis has placed treatment on secure foundations and carefully carried out clinical trials in the 1950s have shown that corticosteroid drugs can be life-saving in acute attacks.

Furthermore, clinicians have been able to define circumstances which require surgical removal of the colon. When this is necessary most surgeons prefer to remove the colon and rectum, leaving the end of the ileum as an artificial anus on the abdominal wall (an ileostomy).

Mechanical problems arising from this have been virtually eliminated since Bryan Brooke, Professor of Surgery at St George's Hospital, London, devised in 1954 a new method of fashioning ileostomies which prevented the scarring, narrowing and retraction which had hitherto occurred. He affixed the ileal mucosa directly to the skin, thus everting a small segment of bowel. His surgical ingenuity has had great benefit and ileostomy patients can now lead a normal life.

A major residual problem in colitis is the development of cancerous change in some sufferers. Basil Morson, a pathologist in London, showed in 1971 that regular biopsies may give a warning of malignant change and so prophylactic removal of the colon can now be undertaken on rational grounds in selected patients.

Gastro-intestinal tuberculosis. Epidemiologists have played an important role in gastro-intestinal disease, particularly in the virtual elimination of gastro-intestinal tuberculosis. Hippocrates recognized this to be a fatal malady, observing that death followed the onset of diarrhea in cases of tuberculosis. He also noted that the patient's hair all fell out. The first specific case reported was by Viordt, who diagnosed it as the cause of death of Louis XIII of France. Both these accounts were of secondary gastro-intestinal tuberculosis, due to the patient swallowing infected sputum. The incidence of this disease has declined with that of pulmonary tuberculosis (see chapter 6). Primary gastro-intestinal tuberculosis usually develops following the ingestion of infected milk. Koch, who discovered the tubercle bacillus in 1882, made a serious mistake when he said in 1900 that milk containing bovine tuberculosis was non-infective. Fortunately the Great Britain Royal Commission on Tuberculosis (1904-7) questioned Koch's view and showed that not only was contaminated milk infective, it was also the major reservoir of the disease. The Commission suggested that identification and slaughter of infected cows, coupled with pasteurization of milk, which kills the tubercle bacillus, would effectively eliminate bovine tuberculosis. Pasteurization of milk was implemented in the British cities anyway by the 1920s, but the farmers took a great deal longer to organize. In 1940, when the campaign finally got under way, it was estimated that 40 per cent of all cows were infected. By 1955 62 per cent of cows were in attested (or tubercle-free) herds, and by 1960 the whole cow population of Great

Britain was declared free. The table shows the remarkable efficacy of these preventive measures.

Incidence of gastro-intestinal tuberculosis in children under five years old in England.

Year	1921	1930	1944	1953
Total	1191	407	143	16
No. of Deaths	1007	363	112	12

Preventive diets. Having tackled most of the infectious diseases, epidemiologists are now concentrating on ways to prevent degenerative and carcinomatous disease. Comparative studies in Western and 'primitive' societies show that carcinoma of the colon, which accounted for 13 per cent of the 138,316 deaths from cancer in England in 1971, is very rare in primitive societies. Sir Denis Burkitt, an English doctor with many years' experience in East Africa, drew on the theories which Campbell, Painter and Cleave set out in their book *Diabeties, Coronary Thrombosis and the Saccharine Disease* and attributes this to a change in dietary habit. He argues that any carcinogenic substances in the feces would be both more dilute and pass through the bowel faster if the Western low roughage diet was replaced by a 'primitive' high roughage diet. Diverticular disease, in which pockets or bulges of the colonic mucosa are extruded through the colonic muscle wall because of unnaturally high intra-colonic pressures, has a similar geographical distribution to colonic cancer. Experiments recording colonic pressure in animals and humans have shown that low roughage diets cause high pressure. The symptoms of diverticular disease can also be relieved by a high roughage diet. In their book Campbell, Painter and Cleave extend the concept of the preventive potential of high roughage diets to appendicitis, diabetes, varicose veins, herniae, and even heart disease. This may be excessive, but it contains the possibilities of a real epidemiological advance, the benefits of which have yet to be realized. High roughage diets have, incidentally, revolutionized the treatment of constipation, which is nearly always relieved by this appropriate dietary adjustment.

Cholera. Although by applying long-established epidemiological criteria, cholera can be prevented, there are countries whose inhabitants have failed, through ignorance, poverty and oppression, to eliminate the disease. For them, basic research has opened up the possibility of a simple and cheap cure. In healthy people there is a large daily flux of fluid between the body and the gut lumen. The overall balance is in favour of the body, and so there is a net overall absorption each day. Cyclic AMP, a compound found widely in biological systems, controls this flux. Increased levels cause net excretion of fluid, giving rise to profuse water diarrhea. The cholera bacteria

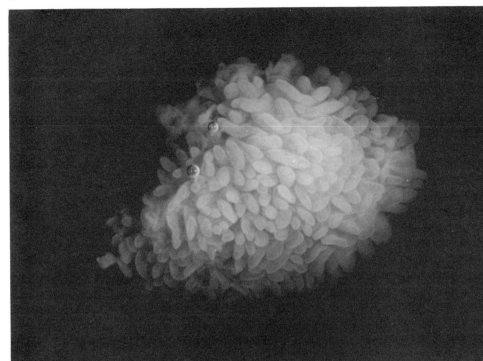

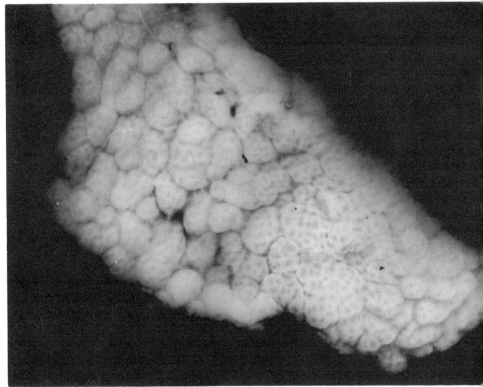

45

cause just such an increase in the cyclic AMP concentration and hence the classical watery diarrhea of cholera. Aspirin is an inhibitor of cyclic AMP, and may have a place in cholera therapy. In the meantime, the effect of cyclic AMP can be reversed by an oral solution of salt and sugar, and this simple treatment has been used very successfully in recent cholera epidemics. It is much more appropriate and practical than intravenous infusion of sterile fluid, which up till recently was the standard treatment for cholera.

3 The Body's Chemistry

Many routes have been traversed in the quest for more knowledge concerning nutritional diseases and its application to therapy. First, considerable emphasis has been placed upon devising an appropriate diet which will prolong life. Secondly, attention has been paid to modulating both the quality and quantity of nutrients in the diet to avoid excesses. Finally, with the acquisition of biochemical knowledge of the processes of the body, information has accrued about the precise role of nutrients in the body's metabolism.

We still lack precise knowledge concerning the action of some essential nutrients. While we know that trace metals are of considerable importance and that their absence leads to specific diseases, we do not understand their exact locus of action in the regulation of body chemistry. Similarly with the action of some of the vitamins, it is still uncertain whether their action is simply limited to the relief of their own deficiency or whether in addition they may have positive therapeutic actions. Thus we have the recent controversy on whether vitamin C will prevent the common cold and the increasing use of excess amounts of vitamins D and C in an attempt to prolong life.

It is beyond the scope of this chapter to consider all the advances which have been made in the understanding and treatment of nutritional diseases. In such a vast area of knowledge the author has had to be selective and dwell on those events in nutritional science which he deems most important in advancing our overall knowledge.

Nutrition was initially thought of as a means of survival only. Only later was it appreciated that certain diseases were related to the absence of special critical nutrients in the diet.

Scurvy is one of the diseases longest known to man and the discovery of its treatment presents one of the first examples of a controlled experiment in nutritional science. It is also, unfortunately, an example of the failure to employ expeditiously the information gathered.

Early descriptions of the disease exist as far back as 1500 B.C. but it did not become important until after the discovery of America when it presented a formidable problem during the long sea voyages. One finds many references in the nautical literature to the use of lemon juice to prevent scurvy, even as early as 1600. In 1753, James Lind, a surgeon in the English fleet, published his book *A Treatise of the Scurvy*, which outlined the famous experiment in which he showed that patients given citrus fruits recovered while others treated at the same time, but without citrus fruits, failed to do so. It was not, however, until 1795, some 42 years later, that limes or some form of citrus fruits were provided by regulation on ships of the British Navy, attracting to the British sailors the nickname 'limeys'.

Beriberi. The next 'deficiency' disease to be recognized was beriberi and that not until almost the end of the 19th century. About the year 1896, Christian Eijkman, a military doctor in the Dutch East Indies, was conducting certain investigations on chickens. To economize on their food he fed them on scraps from the wards at the military hospital to which he was attached. These scraps consisted chiefly of cooked, polished rice. On this diet the fowls developed paralysis which was at first obscure, but nevertheless bore some resemblance to the disease beriberi seen in humans. Serendipity revealed the true nature of this nerve disease in birds when a newly appointed director of the hospital refused to allow Eijkman to feed his birds on scraps from the ward. Henceforth, the chickens were fed on gava (rice still in the husk) and with this diet they recovered, almost miraculously. Eijkman's identification of this 'polyneuritis gallinarum' with human beriberi was, at first, rejected by physicians. However, after much research and co-operation with other investigators, Eijkman came to the conclusion that a diet of polished rice was the chief cause of polyneuritis in fowls as well as of beriberi in human beings. In 1901, Gerrit Grijns, Eijkman's successor, suggested that the disease was caused by the absence from the diet of some unknown substance normally present in the outer coat of the grains, and lost in the milling process.

Thus, the concept was rapidly growing that certain foods contained critical nutrients which, if lacking, resulted in specific diseases. In 1906 Gowland Hopkins, Professor of Biochemistry at Cambridge, expressed the belief that scurvy and rickets were disorders caused by diets deficient in unidentified nutrients, and in 1912 Casimir Funk brought this whole concept to the forefront by propounding the theory that beriberi, scurvy, pellagra and possibly rickets were caused by a deficiency of 'special substances . . . which we will call vitamins'.

As each new vitamin was discovered it was given a letter. It proved not a very good notation, however, because several were later found to be composed of a number of different compounds. Now that all the known vitamins have been analyzed, they are often given their chemical names. Thus vitamin C, the antiscorbutic (antiscurvy) material, is ascorbic acid and vitamin B_1, lacking in beriberi, is thiamin.

Other substances. David Marine demonstrated the relationship of iodine deficiency to thyroid enlargement and followed up his studies on animals and fish by instituting iodine treatment of patients in Cleveland, Ohio. In 1917, he initiated one of the first large-scale controlled human experiments that demonstrated the efficacy of the addition of iodide to drinking water as a preventive of simple or non-toxic goiter over a three-year period. In school children in Akron, Ohio, he was able to show that those children who were deficient and not taking additional iodide developed thyroid enlargement. After this clear demonstration of the value of iodide, the program for use of iodized salt was adopted.

Proteins. As far back as 1839 the Dutch chemist Mulder suggested the name 'protein' but, although he stated that proteins were probably the most important of all known substances in the organic kingdom, the growth of knowledge about their role in nutrition has been painfully slow. In the late 19th and early 20th centuries there was considerable debate as to the optimal quantity of dietary protein which should be recommended. The controversy was not without substance. Proteins and carbohydrates both supply similar caloric needs, so the substitution of lower-priced carbohydrates for the more expensive protein would seem to have considerable merit. The controversy still exists although all agree that extremes of protein deprivation or high-protein diets should generally be avoided. Human beings can tolerate widely different quantities of protein in their diets without sustaining any untoward consequences—how much they really *need* still

46 Two children show the disfiguring and permanent effects of rickets resulting from lack of vitamin D in the diet, in a photograph taken in Budapest in 1920. The bow-leggedness of the girl is due to the bending of the softened ricketty bone as it carries her weight. The boy shows the bossing of the bones of the skull, often called the 'hot cross bun' skull, caused by an abnormal accumulation of soft, inadequately calcified bone precursor in the flat bones of the skull. Teeth as well as bones may be irreparably damaged by this early deprivation, in this case probably resulting from the effects of civil strife and general malnutrition. Recognition of the therapeutic effects of sunlight, which forms vitamin D in the light-exposed skin, and the systematic addition of vitamin D and calcium to foodstuffs, have virtually abolished this disease of childhood, though dark-skinned people emigrating to less sunny latitudes remain at special risk.

47 This X-ray picture clearly shows the bending of the ricketty bone and also the characteristic expansion of the growing end of the bone due to the frustrated accumulation of excessive quantities of the soft bone precursor which fails to be converted by the normal laying down of calcium phosphate crystals into strong supporting structure. Subsequent treatment with vitamin D has led to healing and adequate ossification, though the architectural deformity of the early deficiency state will always remain.

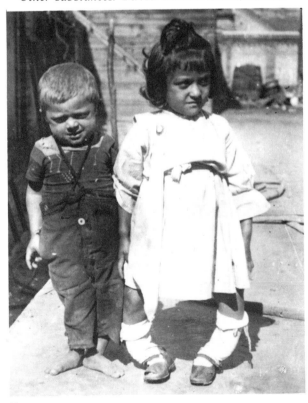

46

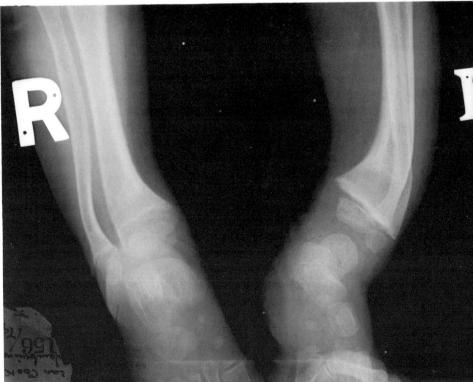

47

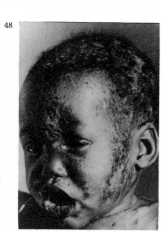

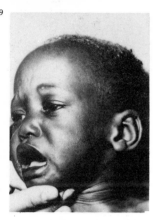

48, 49 Malnutrition and sub-nutrition are responsible for widespread and sometimes permanent changes of mind and body. However, the deficiency disease kwashiorkor can be effectively treated by the provision of a diet adequate in protein and calories. The comparison between the two pictures shows the extraordinary improvement in the condition of the skin and mucous membranes in a child with this disorder following just ten days of improved nutrition at a British Medical Research Council infantile malnutrition research unit in Kampala. Unfortunately some of the less readily visible but socially more devastating effects of malnutrition on brain development are probably irreversible.

remains a largely unanswered question.

Proteins are composed of long chains of amino acids, comparatively small chemical compounds which are identified by their content of nitrogen. Experiments started by the American W. C. Rose in 1942 indicated that ten of these amino acids cannot be synthesized in the body and must therefore be provided in sufficient quantity by proteins of the diet. They are known as the essential amino acids. Although we do not understand the exact role that each amino acid plays in the body chemistry, we recognize their enormous importance. For instance, a diet composed principally of maize is short of one amino acid, tryptophan, and also the vitamin nicotinamide. This combined deficiency causes the development of pellagra.

When the roles of the essential amino acids have been established it may then be possible to define more precisely the protein requirement of man and its relationship to health and disease.

Obesity. The accumulation of excess adipose tissue results from the consumption of more calories than are expended. Over and above the considerations of esthetics and personal vanity, obesity has clearly been shown to diminish life expectancy and predisposes particularly to coronary heart disease and diabetes. Recent evidence suggests that obesity alone may not be so threatening to life expectancy, but the combination of high blood pressure and being overweight is particularly devastating. Because eating represents a life-long experience associated with psychological and social factors as yet somewhat poorly understood, it is difficult if not almost impossible to convince people to follow a weight-reducing diet even when their apparent life expectancy is being threatened by their being obese.

Today, studies are being undertaken in many laboratories to determine the relationship between obesity during childhood and adult obesity. Investigations are in progress to determine whether or not there has occurred some change in fat cell size or number, which makes it difficult for the obese patient to lose weight in those years following childhood. The fat child so often becomes the fat adult and, as obesity is so difficult to lose once present, the image of the 'bonny baby' is perhaps one that we should change.

Atherosclerosis. In atherosclerosis the inner walls of the arteries are affected by deposits of fatty material and these may lead to fibrous changes. Through narrowing of the artery and by predisposing to local thrombosis atherosclerosis can cause various kinds of disease due to impairment of blood supply. The presence of fatty deposits in the lining of the arteries suggests a malfunction in the fat metabolism and/or an imbalance in the proportion of fat in the diet. The two principal factors in the individual which predispose to atherosclerosis are the level of the blood pressure and the level of cholesterol in the blood. However, in comparing populations it is the blood cholesterol level which seems to be the major determinant. The chief, but not the only, factor determining the blood cholesterol level is the nature of the diet.

The major effort in prevention has been to modify diet by reducing the proportion of fat and increasing the content of unsaturated fats (mainly vegetable) as opposed to saturated (animal). The presence of foods which contain highly unsaturated fats, such as corn oil, seems to be beneficial insofar as one can achieve progressive lowering of blood cholesterol levels. The optimal proportion of unsaturated to saturated fats in the diet is thought to be 2:1. Caloric restriction alone will produce some lowering of blood cholesterol levels, particularly in obese patients, though the effect is small and unpredictable.

The other important fat carried in the blood is triglyceride or neutral fat. It, too, has some relation to atherosclerosis, but it is not known whether it has a causative role. Following a meal containing a moderate amount of fat, triglyceride-rich large particles known as chylomicrons appear in the blood. A special enzyme is needed to 'clear' (dispose of) these chylomicrons. In certain patients this enzyme is either lacking or not fully effective. For a prolonged period following a meal, these patients' sera remains creamy and rich in ingested fat and their treatment is simply to avoid meals which are high in fat content and which would therefore produce a large amount of circulating triglycerides.

On the other hand, there are other patients for whom a meal rich in carbohydrate content will produce an increase in circulating serum triglycerides. The treatment of these patients is not to avoid fat, but rather to adjust the diet so that it is lower in caloric content and, specifically, contains a lower proportion of carbohydrates.

The composition of the blood may affect not only the arterial wall but also the clotting property. High fat levels increase the clumping and stickiness of the blood platelets—tiny white bodies much smaller than red cells—and these sticky platelet clumps may set off a clotting process within a narrowed artery. Controversy still continues as to how much we accomplish in the prevention of atherosclerosis by altering the diet. Perhaps changes in diet should be introduced at a much earlier age to achieve major beneficial effects. Until we gain more definitive information, the consensus is to treat obvious abnormalities in fat metabolism, rather than to promulgate recommendations for the general population.

Nutritional standards. Perhaps one of the

greatest advances which has occurred in the area of nutritional science during the past 30 years is the increasing recognition of the socio-economic and political importance of food.

In 1932, the British Medical Research Council and the Lister Institute published a report, *Vitamins—A Survey of Present Knowledge*, in which they laid down standards of vitamin requirements for mothers and infants. In 1936, John Boyd Orr described in explicit terms the relationship between income, food and health in Great Britain. He set out the nutritional composition of the average diet for each income group and showed that between a third and a half of the population had inadequate intakes of calcium, iron and vitamins A and C; the lowest income group had insufficient protein, and the two lowest groups insufficient calories, to maintain a healthy life. The League of Nations in 1935 addressed itself to the same theme and appointed a committee to deal with the problems of nutrition encountered in various countries.

In May 1941, as part of an effort to recognize the need for recommended dietary allowances, a committee devised an extensive table (on the basis of data and evidence present at that time) giving daily caloric values, protein, mineral and vitamin content for various populations performing at different levels of activity. This table of recommended dietary allowances was presented at the American Institute of Nutrition and the American National Nutritional Conference, and the recommendations were formally accepted as *goals* at which to aim until further research would justify making changes. Although one may question the wisdom of attempting to dictate nutritional requirements on the basis of consensus, nevertheless this initial effort was to have tremendous impact insofar as it set guide lines (and also made a commitment) for good nutrition for vast population groups. This work is still being continued by the Food and Agriculture Organization of the United Nations.

In summary, the concept of nutrition has changed from a concern with diets and nutritional necessities to a realization of its value for the maintenance of health among all peoples of the world. As a large proportion of the world's population is suffering from lack of food (i.e. total calories, not just specific nutrients), nutrition has become more and more associated with the *provision* of food and the kinds of food which can be grown in abundance while preserving good nutritional qualities. Discussion of this topic is, however, outside the scope of this book.

Inherited disorders of metabolism. In the years to come, people will look back upon the 20th century as a period in which the doors to the understanding and treatment of familial or

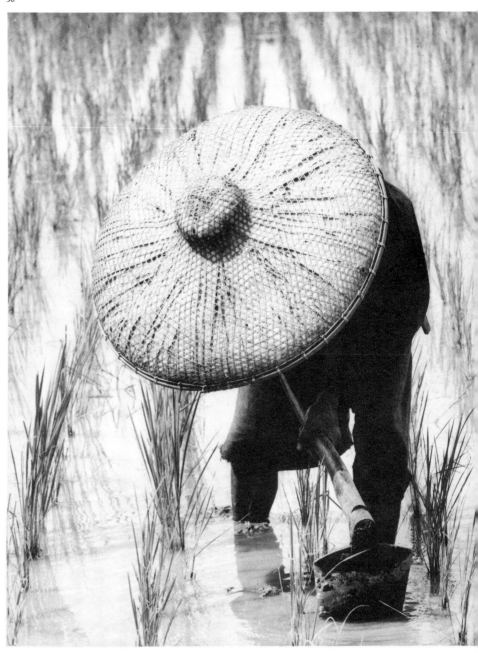

inherited disorders of metabolism were opened. During the 20th century not only has the precise defect been defined in a number of diseases of metabolism, but we have also gained considerably in understanding the mechanism of inheritance, the role of genes and chromosomes in transmitting genetic information. The story of genetic coding, information transfer and protein synthesis constitutes one of the major advances in basic science (as contrasted with applied science) and will ultimately have vast implications for clinical medicine.

Let us, however, return to the beginning of the present century when Sir Archibald Garrod began his studies on a rare disorder known as alkaptonuria. In 1908 in his classic Croonian lectures, Garrod related the disease to an inborn error of metabolism. He later extended his observations and studies to other unusual diseases such as albinism, cystinuria and

50 Some of the problems of malnutrition are being met by the development of new strains of cereal by agricultural scientists. Vegetable protein often lacks certain essential amino-acids and breeding experiments have produced new strains, in which certain of these amino-acids, such as lysine, are present in greatly increased abundance. The picture shows an Indonesian peasant tending his rice crop in a paddy-field, in an area which not long previously had been laid low by poverty, hunger and disease.

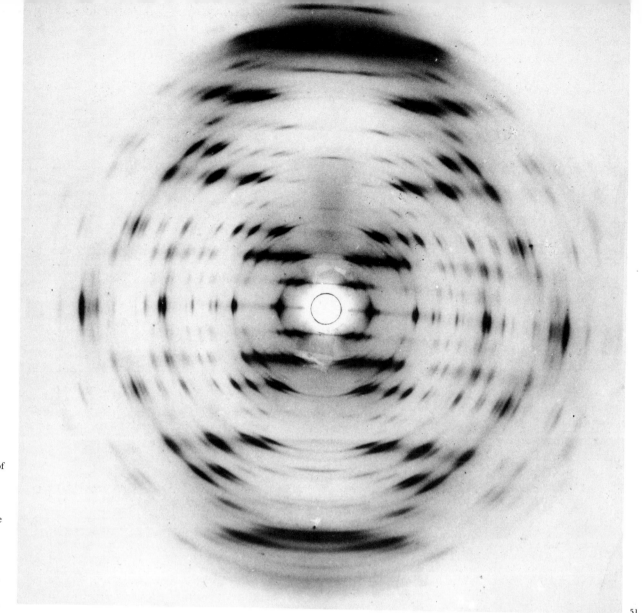

51, 52 This historic picture
shows a pattern which was
responsible for unlocking one of
the great mysteries of genetics.
When a beam of X-rays is
passed through a crystal of
DNA (deoxyribonucleic acid) a
characteristic diffraction picture
is formed as a result of the
bending of the rays as they
travel through the crystalline
structure. It was this picture
which suggested the structure
of the twisted double strand of
DNA illustrated in the
molecular model below–the so-
called 'double helix'. Each
strand of DNA encodes the
characteristics of the cell in
terms of both structure and
function, and the separation of
the strands enables this
information to be carried
intact into the next generation
of cells, where a further com-
plementary strand is rapidly
assembled. This genetic material
can withstand nutritional deprivation of the host in a remarkable way, carrying on to the
successors the potential for
normal development when
conditions improve. However,
small changes in the structure
of this 'genetic code' may cause
major disturbances in the capacity of the cell to metabolize
nutrients. Starved of an essential product, the cells may
become subject to a state of
inherited malnutrition. The
dramatic advances of recent
years in the understanding of
the structure and function of
DNA have explained many
metabolic disorders in man and
have opened the possibility of
repairing or avoiding a number
of them. The region of the DNA
molecule which carries the code
for the formation of an essential
enzyme is defective in children
suffering from phenylketonuria,
described in the text.

pentosuria (passage of an abnormal sugar, pentose,
in the urine) and developed the concept that
certain complex disease states arise from a single
defect in metabolism, which itself was the result
of unknown abnormalities of inheritance.

One cannot give sufficient emphasis to the
importance of the original observations and
thoughts of Garrod. While these disorders by and
large do not occur very frequently, nevertheless
the recognition of this class of diseases is of
tremendous significance to physicians.
First, we are now aware that if certain of these
diseases are recognized early in life, particularly
during infancy, one can prevent or modify their
subsequent clinical manifestations. Secondly,
one can, knowing the pattern of inheritance,
advise families of the risk of having a child
bearing one of these particular abnormalities.
Not all inherited errors of metabolism are of
serious consequence; the clinical manifestations
may range from the totally trivial to the gravest
forms of physical and mental disability. Within
the past few years, it has become possible to
diagnose certain of these inherited disorders in
the fetus in the very early stages of development.

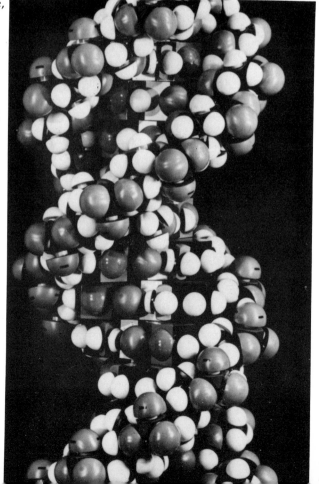

If the results indicate that the infant would be born with a crippling or lethal disease, the pregnancy can be safely cut short. The decision to end a pregnancy is not made lightly and involves considerations which are discussed elsewhere in this book.

Phenylketonuria. In 1934, a doctor named Følling described ten patients who excreted phenylpyruvic acid in their urine and were mentally deficient. Subsequently, a characteristic disease was recognized and given the name phenylketonuria, detectable soon after birth by a simple chemical test of the urine.

This disease develops during infancy, although there is universal agreement that the infant with phenylketonuria is not clinically abnormal at birth. The biochemical basis of this disease was found to be the absence of an enzyme for dealing with the amino acid phenylalanine, a component of many proteins. An excess of phenylalanine accumulates and in some unknown way affects the nervous system. However, if the affected child is fed on protein food from which phenylalanine has been removed, the brain develops normally.

With the recognition of phenylketonuria and the use of a simple test to establish the diagnosis, a new concept evolved in our diagnostic approach to inborn errors of metabolism. Thus, during the 1960s considerable efforts were made to devise a number of tests to diagnose various inherited defects. The screening of both blood and urine of children at birth or soon thereafter has achieved a striking degree of refinement and can now detect a number of diseases.

Wilson's disease. In its classical presentation Wilson's disease is a rare hereditary disease, characterized by cirrhosis of the liver and degenerative changes in the brain producing spasticity, rigidity, tremor, and difficulties in swallowing and in speaking. This disorder usually manifests itself under the age of ten years, and only recently have its frequency and significance been appreciated. The pathophysiology of Wilson's disease remains unclear and somewhat controversial. The signs and symptoms are best explained by the abnormal accumulation of copper in various critical organs of the body, though there is considerable disagreement about how the copper comes to be deposited.

The treatment of choice in Wilson's disease involves the removal of copper from tissues, either by excluding copper from the diet or by enhancing its excretion with various drugs. In 1956, Dr J. M. Walshe, a Cambridge physician, reported that penicillamine was very effective in enhancing copper excretion in the urine. The mode of action of penicillamine is to combine with copper by a process known as chelation, in which the copper becomes gripped within the penicillamine molecule and is then excreted.

The natural course of untreated Wilson's disease is progressively downhill. Dramatic improvement, particularly in the neurological manifestations, frequently follows the use of penicillamine. Those patients with predominantly the hepatic form of the disease may also show considerable improvement in liver function when given penicillamine therapy.

As already implied, in many patients a presumptive diagnosis of Wilson's disease can be made before the onset of symptoms. Although the evidence is still being accumulated, it is believed that if this disorder can be detected in the asymptomatic stage, its disabling symptoms can be prevented.

We thus have a disease which can be recognized early, before symptoms of clinical disability occur. In the use of penicillamine to withdraw excess copper deposits from various tissues we have a very effective therapy, which can reverse or prevent the tragic complications of the disease. Despite these conditions it still remains for the astute clinician to recognize Wilson's disease in its early stages and to initiate appropriate therapy.

Gout. Unlike most inherited disorders, gout (see chapter 8) is relatively common. A 'crystalopathy', it is caused by the accumulation of crystals of insoluble salts of uric acid in joints, kidneys and tendons. Notwithstanding our present limited knowledge concerning the mode of its inheritance or its pathophysiology we have made reasonable progress in its treatment. Most patients are able to lead relatively normal lives without having much in the way of disability.

A look into the future. It is difficult even to guess at the advances which will be made in the diagnosis and treatment of inborn errors of metabolism. This is an area of tremendous interest amongst researchers today and many new techniques are being developed. We have already mentioned the value of genetic counselling in the hopes of decreasing the prevalence of various inherited disorders. We shall certainly hear, year by year, of more of these mysteries being explained.

Studies are in progress to determine whether one can alter the individual's complement of genes in given metabolic disorders but a more direct approach has been to utilize enzyme replacement in the treatment of various inborn errors. In general, three approaches are being explored. First, the direct administration of a purified enzyme; second, the utilization of an enzyme which has been protected by a microencapsulation or entrapment; and third, the transplantation of an organ which can itself supply the critical enzyme that may be missing.

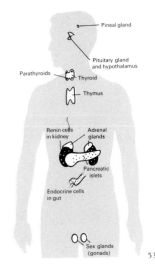

53 All of the chemical activities of the body are under the control of the endocrine (or ductless) glands indicated here. These glands, which manufacture chemical messengers or hormones, discharge their product directly into the circulating blood, in contrast with the exocrine glands, which secrete through a system of ducts into a body cavity such as the stomach and intestine. The importance of the diffuse endocrine function of the mucosa of the stomach and gut is increasingly recognized (see illustration 35). It is also likely that certain cells in the lungs (not indicated here) may have an endocrine function. The tiny pituitary gland in the head has an overriding controlling influence on most of the other glands depicted. It regulates the action of the thyroid gland and the cortex, the outer layer, of the adrenal glands. It also regulates the activity of the sex glands or gonads. Though small, it is composed itself of two distinct lobes, the anterior and the posterior, which function independently of each other. The parathyroid glands and the medulla, or inner core, of the adrenal glands are not directly under pituitary control. The islets of Langerhans, representing only about one-hundredth of the volume of the pancreas, which is shown in toto, are largely controlled by the level of glucose and other nutrients in the blood.

The data is as yet preliminary, but organ transplantation does seem to be feasible for the treatment of a number of inherited disorders, provided the problems inherent in organ transplantation can be resolved.

The endocrine system. The endocrine system consists of a number of small ductless glands, such as the pancreas, scattered throughout the body. These glands release minute quantities of chemical messenger molecules directly into the blood and also regulate and co-ordinate the activities of the main parts of the body. When one or more of the glands becomes overactive or underactive, more or less grave abnormalities of metabolism, growth, sexual development or body functioning occur.

The term 'diabetes' was first recorded by Aretaeus in the 2nd century A.D. and although classical physicians were able to render elegant descriptions of the symptoms, their understanding of the disease was limited. One thousand years had to pass before the advent of a major advance in the understanding of this disorder. Paracelsus in the 16th century performed the classical experiment of evaporating the urine from diabetic patients and obtaining a white material, which he termed a 'dry salt'. It remained for Thomas Willis in 1679 to show that this material indeed was not salt but sugar (he tasted it!). Soon it was recognized that the basic fault in diabetes was a high level of sugar in the blood which showed by the presence of sugar in the urine. Sometimes we can learn the cause of disease by producing a similar malady in animals. In the experiment performed by Joseph von

Mering and Oscar Minkowski in Strasbourg in 1889, the pancreas was removed from a dog and the animal became severely diabetic. The distinguished German pathologist Paul Langerhans had already discovered within the pancreas clusters or islands of cells which were distinct from the remaining pancreatic tissue. Finally the British physiologist Edward Sharpey Schafer, impressed by the American Eugene Lindsay Opie's observations of the abnormal appearances of the islets of Langerhans in diabetics, postulated that those islets must secrete a substance which controls carbohydrate metabolism. In 1916, he proposed the name of 'insulin' for this hypothetical internal secretion of the pancreas.

Unfortunately, in the medical literature there exists an everlasting controversy as to who discovered insulin and first utilized this material in the treatment of diabetic patients. In 1921, however, the famous Canadians Sir Frederick Banting and C. H. Best, following the observations of Dr Moses Barron that ligation of pancreatic duct would produce atrophy of all pancreatic tissues except the islets, utilized this approach to isolate relatively pure insulin. In August 1921 they showed that, whereas extracts of spleen, liver and other tissues were without effect in lowering the blood glucose in a diabetic dog, their preparation of insulin produced significant lowering of the blood and urine sugar.

Imagine the sense of excitement throughout the world when the first patient received insulin therapy in January 1922. The physician who earlier had felt so helpless as he waited for the

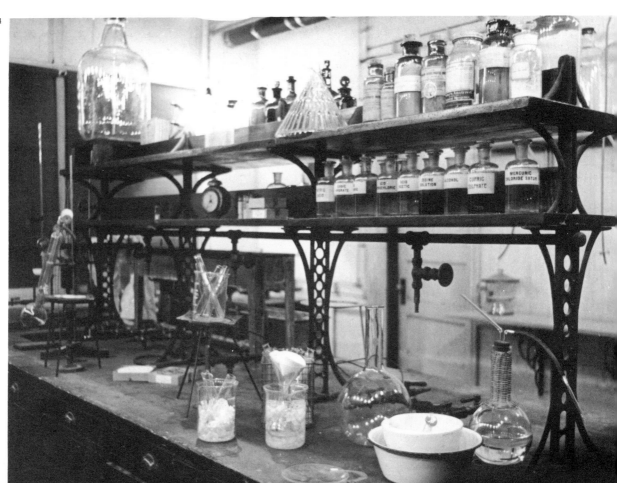

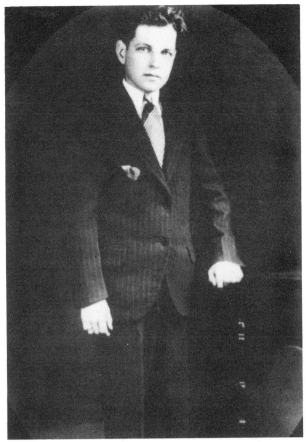

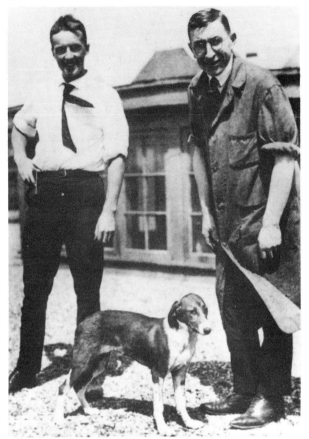

inevitable death of his diabetic patients, now saw in the advent and availability of insulin the placing of a miracle drug in his hands.

The thyroid gland—hypothyroidism. Although Pliny the Elder (23-79 A.D.) referred to the frequent occurrence of goiter, particularly prevalent in certain districts of Switzerland, it remained again for Paracelsus to proclaim that only some patients with goiters behaved abnormally. Although Paracelsus did not appreciate that the primary problem in these goitrous patients was insufficient function of the thyroid gland, he did recognize the fact that not every patient with a goiter was necessarily afflicted with behavioral abnormalities.

Another distinguished physician, from Basle in Switzerland, Platerus, was responsible for a very concise description of cretinism. He emphasized the mental retardation of some goitrous children.

The clinical breakthrough, however, came with Sir William Gull who, in a paper read on 24 October 1873, described the disease hypothyroidism in adults and suggested that this was essentially the same disease as cretinism in children.

The experimental work of Sir Victor Horsley in the latter part of the 19th century led to the conclusion that the condition of hypothyroidism and its variants are due to loss or absence of function of the thyroid gland. In 1920, George Redmayne Murray, a physician at Victoria University in Manchester, was the first to treat hypothyroidism by the administration of an

extract of animal thyroid glands, a treatment much refined but still highly successfully used today. Many a person has since been rescued from a life of dull apathy.

The dramatic restoration to normality by treatment is one of the most satisfying acts of therapy. It is particularly important for the physician to recognize hypothyroidism if present at birth or early infancy. The newborn cretin is usually a normal baby presumably because he has received the hormone from the mother's thyroid. Untreated, mental and physical development is severely retarded but if such a child is given adequate amounts of thyroid hormone from an early age he develops entirely normally.

Endocrine overactivity. During the early epoch of descriptive medicine (the late 18th and the 19th centuries), physicians described various endocrinopathies in which the defect was not due to absence of any particular hormone, but to the fact that certain critical glands were hyperfunctioning and secreting excessive amounts of hormone. Hyperfunction of the thyroid gland, hyperthyroidism, is a good example.

A number of physicians in various countries, including Caleb Hillier Parry (British), Robert James Graves (Irish), and Carl A. von Basedow (German), at approximately the same time described a group of patients, predominantly female, who demonstrated the characteristic symptoms of hyperthyroidism—nervousness, weight loss, rapid pulse and prominent eyes. It

54-6 A great triumph was scored in 1921 when Frederick Banting and Charles Best, the former a young postgraduate and the latter an undergraduate medical student in Toronto, succeeded in isolating insulin from the pancreas gland and so brought the chance of survival to many millions of diabetics. The primitive conditions under which they worked are shown in the photograph of their laboratory, preserved as an exhibit in the National Museum of Science and Technology. The two scientists themselves appear with the dog which received the first extracts of insulin, and illustration 55 shows Leonard, a 14-year-old boy who was the first human to be kept alive thanks to the discovery of insulin.

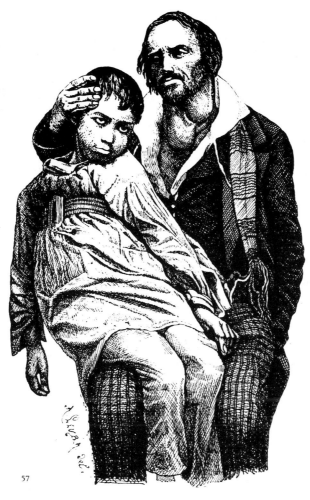

57

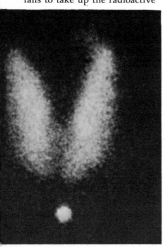

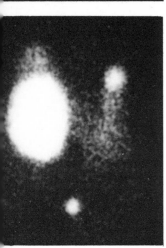

was early recognized that the administration of iodine was helpful in the treatment of some patients with hyperthyroidism. Unfortunately, while some patients do respond rapidly to iodine treatment, a number of patients do not and may even become more hyperthyroid than before. Then, too, there were some toxic reactions observed with iodine therapy including severe rashes, fever and enlargement of the parotid or salivary glands.

With improvement in surgical techniques it became possible to treat hyperthyroid patients by partial removal of the thyroid gland and, indeed, this procedure is still being performed in certain selected cases.

In 1943, however, a group of drugs was developed, thiourea and 2-thiouracil, which specifically interfered with the synthesis of the thyroid hormone. These agents, administered at relatively frequent intervals, result in remarkable control of the patient's hyperthyroidism. After a year or two's treatment with drugs, about 50 per cent of the patients go into a permanent state of remission and will require no further therapy. It is not clear whether or not the drugs have themselves produced the remission, or if it simply occurs spontaneously during the treatment period.

A radioactive isotope of iodine is specifically picked up by the thyroid and so can be used to

suppress the overactive gland by 'auto-irradiation'. This major advance in the treatment of hyperthyroidism means that now the patient can simply take a single drink which returns the thyroid function to normal. No surgery is required, nor a year or two of medication. The procedure is without morbidity or mortality. Patients so treated must, however, be followed closely for years as they may eventually develop abnormally low function of the thyroid gland and require treatment for this.

The adrenal glands. In 1855, Thomas Addison, a physician at Guy's Hospital in London, described the characteristic symptoms of the disease that now bears his name, and related it to a failure of the adrenal glands. We now know that affected patients cannot secrete normal amounts of cortisone and other corticosteroids, which are made in the cortex of the gland. Later, in 1932, the American neurosurgeon Harvey Cushing drew attention to the existence of adrenal cortical overactivity, in contrast to Addison's disease. This disorder is characterized by hypertension, purplish lines across the abdominal wall, the existence of diabetes mellitus, obesity involving predominantly the trunk, and a defect in bony architecture known as osteoporosis.

The treatment of chronic adrenal insufficiency is to give replacement hormones. Initially, it was necessary to give a somewhat crude extract of the adrenal cortex, in order to maintain these patients in a reasonably healthy state. Over the past 40 years, the various steroid hormones of the adrenal cortex have been isolated and identified and their specific properties delineated. This enables us to utilize more specific compounds in the treatment of chronic adrenal insufficiency and has led to the production not only of cortisone, but also of other similar steroid drugs for the treatment of a wide variety of diseases.

The treatment of excess adrenal cortex activity involves determining the exact cause of the disorder, and then instituting appropriate therapy. It may arise from over-action of the adrenal gland itself or be due to an increased drive on the adrenal gland from the pituitary gland, within the skull, which regulates glandular function. It secretes a factor which in turn stimulates the adrenal cortex to hyperfunction.

The most significant event which has occurred in the past 20 years in the field of endocrinology does not specifically relate to the treatment of various endocrine disorders, but to their diagnosis and an understanding of their pathophysiology. A problem for endocrinologists had been the very tiny quantities of hormones in the body. The amount of insulin in the blood of a man, for example, would weigh about as much as a grain of salt. In 1955, Solomon Berson and Rosalyn Yalow developed a *radio*

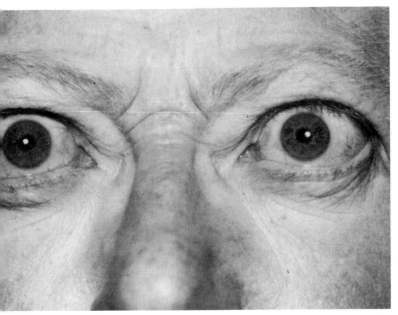 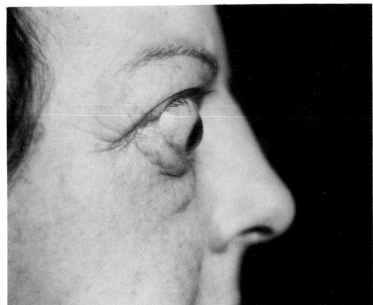

immuno-assay for the measurement of insulin levels in tissue and in tissue fluids. Subsequent to this, there became available a large number of assays for the measurement of various hormones. These techniques have provided a tremendous impetus in endocrinology and have given rise to a wealth of investigations of both a pure and a clinical nature. The diagnosis of specific endocrine diseases can now be made with far greater precision and patients have benefited not only in terms of therapy but also because diagnostic procedures have been simplified.

Corticosteroids—use in clinical medicine. Throughout the 1940s there was intense interest in defining the physiological roles of the various hormones present in the adrenal gland, particularly the adrenal cortex. It was appreciated in 1942 that there were perhaps a total of 26 distinct steroids in the adrenal cortex. These various compounds were soon identified and their specific metabolic effects defined.

Against this background, the Americans Philip Hench and Edward Calvin Kendall in 1949 announced the dramatic effect of cortisone and ACTH in the treatment of rheumatoid arthritis. As early as 1929, Philip Hench had noted the fact that when arthritic patients became pregnant or jaundiced, they experienced a temporary remission in their arthritis. He believed that there might be some substance in the blood possessing anti-rheumatic activities. The impact of this work on clinical medicine can be assessed from the fact that in the year following the first published report of the effect of cortisone in the treatment of rheumatoid arthritis, the Nobel Prize in Medicine was jointly awarded to Kendall and Tadeus Reichstein (who were responsible for so much of the basic chemical research that led to the synthesis of this steroid), and also to Hench who realized the applicability of steroid hormones in the treatment of rheumatoid arthritis.

For a short time the corticosteroids were widely acclaimed as the greatest of wonder-drugs and were used in a number of conditions where they were not always warranted and in doses that were not altogether appropriate.

Consequently serious disabling side-effects were observed, which caused the medical profession to become over-cautious in the use of these agents in the treatment of diseases. As may be expected, the pendulum has swung back, and these drugs have finally come to assume an appropriate and rational place in our clinical armamentarium.

The success of this marriage of basic investigation with clinical skill and knowledge reminds us once again that both elements are important if we are to continue to make substantive advances in the diagnosis and treatment of disease.

The chemistry of life is at times complex, almost mystifying to the uninitiated. New discoveries continue to be made. The acquisition of knowledge at times exceeds our capacity to apply these new ideas in the treatment of disease. To quote Sir Isaac Newton

'I do not know what I may appear to the world but to myself I seem to have been only a boy playing on the sea-shore, and diverting myself in now and then finding a smoother pebble or a prettier shell than ordinary, whilst the great ocean of truth lay all undiscovered before me.'

iodide as a result (59). The emergence of an unregulated secreting nodule of thyroid tissue will feed back on the pituitary control of normal thyroid tissue, leading to a progressive shut-down of pituitary drive to the remainder of the gland, which however remains responsive. The point will come when the nodule just usurps the function of the whole gland, which then becomes totally inactive. Further increase in the activity of the nodule will lead to the condition of hyperthyroidism, when acceleration of the body's metabolic processes leads to dramatic increase in food consumption and heat production, and a rapid weight loss. Localization of a hot nodule may assist in its surgical excision. More ominous is the single cold nodule, which may be the first indication of thyroid cancer.

60, 61 Overactivity of the thyroid gland is often accompanied by a characteristic change in the eye, illustrated here. The upper lid is drawn back, exposing the white of the eye above the pupil, and the globe of the eye itself is pushed forward by an accumulation of tissue in the orbit, both tending to give rise to the appearance of exaggerated shock or surprise in the facial expression of the person affected.

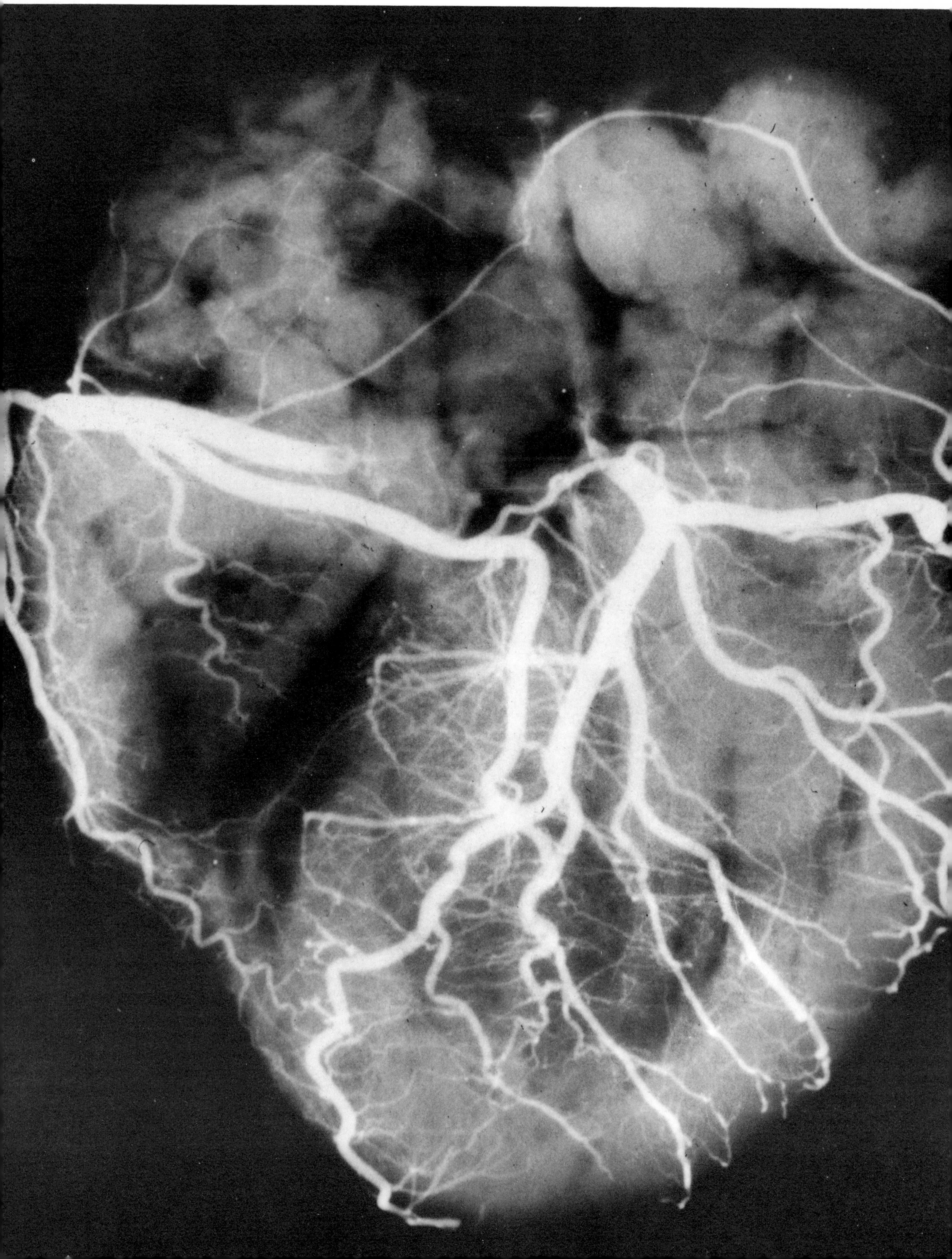

4 Circulation and the Heart

Approximately half of the present population of the 'first' and 'second' worlds is destined to die of disease of the heart and blood vessels. The fate of the peoples of the 'third' world is at present less well defined although, if the premature deaths from starvation, infestation with parasites, and infectious diseases are reduced, the effects of degeneration and failure of heart and blood vessels will be unmasked.

There is no branch of medicine in which triumphs and achievements are more urgently needed. There is certainly no field where the potential rewards are greater. Until recently the history of medicine has consisted of advances based on small increments of knowledge from within the discipline. True, there have been previous periods of accelerated advance due to outside influences. In the 16th century, for example, many of the ablest men of the time—Vesalius, Copernicus, Galileo and William Harvey—were attracted to Padua because of the freedom of thought there which resulted from over a century of anti-clerical rule. Later, in the mid-19th century, the railways and telegraphy made scientific meetings, and the transference of knowledge between doctors, much more easy. Over the past two decades medicine has been undergoing massive changes due to the effects of the growth of science and technology, plastics, electronics, computers, the wide use of antibiotics, and the products of fundamental thinking in the pharmaceutical industry ending in drugs like cortisone, the Pill and beta-blockers. All these factors and many others have introduced changes so rapidly that the results are revolutionary and we are still in the midst of them. The medical establishment has scarcely experienced the discomfort in adapting to one new concept before another arrives to sweep away the new as well as the traditional. Nowhere

has the process been more rapid than in the cardiovascular field.

The hitherto significant hazard of cardiac surgery has become an acceptable risk with improved diagnosis, new techniques, the heart/lung machine and intensive care. In turn the advances in cardiovascular surgery have had repercussions throughout medicine. Almost all branches have been affected; immunologists have been asked to maintain viable transplants, hematologists to cope with blood changes after surgery, psychiatrists to study the effects of stress in recovery rooms, physicians to treat new abnormalities of cardiac rhythm: the examples are limitless.

To many, death from cardiovascular disease conjures up a picture of a person who, in the prime of life, suddenly drops dead, in the middle of some activity such as driving or making a speech. Every day in a city the size of London, New York or Tokyo approximately 100 people have a coronary attack. Of these only about a dozen will die dramatically during the working day. Another dozen or so will die in an ambulance or hospital. Sudden death results from failure of a coordinated heart beat or cardiac arrest following blockage of a diseased coronary artery. Acute failure of the circulation causes loss of consciousness in seconds and clinical death in minutes. The remaining 75 will survive with varying disability, usually to succumb later to another heart attack or to another manifestation of the disease.

It would perhaps be fortunate if all sufferers from heart disease could have a swift end to their lives. Anyone who has witnessed the lingering death of a relative or friend with heart disease will remember the emaciated patient, breathless on the least exertion, the sallow jaundiced skin contrasting with the congested

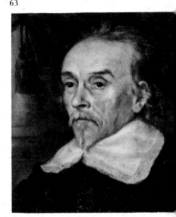

63

62 The heart is a strong muscular pump and it is nourished by the coronary blood vessels demonstrated in this X-ray photograph in which the vessels are outlined with radio-opaque material. The two coronary arteries can be seen emerging from the aorta, the large artery carrying the blood from the left ventricle (compare illustration 75). In a similar technique the coronary circulation is studied by a process known as cine angiography, in which pictures are taken at rapid intervals, so that a dynamic picture of the coronary circulation is obtained.

63 William Harvey (1578-1657). Harvey discovered the circulation of the blood and the function of the heart as a pump. The ancient teaching of Galen was still in Harvey's day the established belief about the workings of the body, accorded a status comparable with that of the Christian religion. In Galen's system purple venous blood was enriched with 'natural spirit' in the liver, and the scarlet arterial blood with 'vital spirit' by the lungs. The heart simply warmed the blood. The challenge faced by Harvey in overturning the established orthodoxy of centuries was tremendous, but he had irrefutable logic on his side.

and blue face, the legs grossly enlarged with excess fluid. Apparently the patient's distress emanates not from the heart but from almost every other system in the body. Digestion, dependent upon the liver, has failed. The fluid balance depending on the kidneys is awry. Ultimately the heart cannot maintain its own blood supply and the death spiral commences.

Medical treatment. Before the advent of practical and routine cardiac surgery the only method of interrupting the inevitable progress down the death spiral was to administer medicines. Some of these act on the heart muscle to improve its function, others act on the kidneys to reduce fluid retention and there are also drugs which prevent the formation of substances essential for blood clotting. Finally and importantly, there are the traditional medicines used to make the terminal patient's life less unpleasant.

Digitalis was the first to be used and remains the most important of the drugs in the cardiologist's armamentarium. In the 1770s an English physician, William Withering, experimented with a folk remedy for dropsy. It soon became clear that the active ingredient was an infusion of the leaves of the foxglove, *Digitalis purpurea*. He found that this extract increased the urine output and sometimes for a time the patient's cardiac condition improved. In structure digitalis is a cardiac glycoside. We now know that the improvements produced by digitalis were in part due to a still not fully understood direct stimulant effect on the cardiac muscle, and more importantly to the reduction in heart rate in patients with atrial fibrillation. This observation is not new either. John Ferriar in 1799 described the effect of the foxglove in 'Diminishing the frequency of the pulse'. By 1810 he realized that this was not a constant effect and that its power lay in slowing and strengthening the action of the heart. The innate rhythmicity of the heart muscle is different for various parts of the heart. The ventricles, the main muscular pumping chambers, have a slow innate rhythm. If disconnected from the remainder of the heart they beat at a natural rate of between 12 and about 30 beats per minute. In life their beating is constantly kept at a higher rate thanks to the faster impulse generation transmitted from the atria, the smaller, upper chambers which, despite their size, play a dominant role in the regulation of heart rate. These impulses are conducted to the ventricles by a pathway composed of specially modified muscle fibers. The atria, which also have a slower innate rhythm than that of the beating heart, are in turn triggered by impulses arising from a specialized node of tissue, known as the sinoatrial node.

In health, every impulse arising from the atria

stimulates the ventricles. This is not the case with disease of the bundle of special tissue causing a partial block, when the ratio may drop to 2:1 or 3:1. When the ventricular rate is too slow to maintain a good cardiac output an artifical pacemaker has to be used.

In atrial fibrillation the atrial muscles only pass on irregular and rapid impulses to the ventricles. As a result of this the ventricles contract too quickly and ineffectually before they have had time to fill properly. They can only eject what is in them. A rapid pulse rate due to atrial fibrillation responds well to digitalis and other cardiac glycosides which reduce conductivity through the bundle and slow the rate.

Diuretics. One of the most helpful series of drugs introduced into the treatment of cardiovascular disorders has been the diuretics. They enhance the flow of urine and, in so doing, lighten the burden of the circulating blood volume on the heart and blood vessels. Most diuretics act on the kidney. Most of the fluid component of the circulating blood filtered out in the glomeruli (see illustration 180) is reabsorbed in the network of fine tubules which eventually join and drain via the ureters into the bladder. Diuretics interfere with this process of tubular water reabsorption. The increased water loss in the urine may be accompanied by a depletion of certain of the circulating salts (and undue potassium loss may be particularly troublesome). This problem may be overcome by using diuretics which 'spare' body potassium by affecting only a specific region of the renal tubule. Unfortunately such diuretics tend to be weaker in their capacity to enhance the desirable water loss. Stronger diuretics are therefore often given with a potassium supplement to compensate for the unwanted loss and so avoid body depletion.

Heart failure can be greatly relieved by the reduction of the circulating fluid volume. Another important therapeutic use of diuretics is to 'unload' the circulation in high blood pressure. Recent research has shown that diuretics also have a direct relaxing effect on the walls of the constricted small blood vessels which cause the blood pressure to rise.

Antidysrhythmic drugs. Sudden changes in heart rate and rhythm, some of them described above, can be a major cause of disability and probably account for the sudden deaths from 'heart attacks' so common in our society. The control of these dysrhythmias has been a major area of therapeutic advance in the treatment of heart disease.

The antidysrhythmic drugs act on the heart muscle itself, its nervous connections and its response to circulating control hormones. Digitalis and quinidine were founding members of this class of drug. Both of them were potent, valuable but sometimes dangerous remedies. Quinidine was used to convert the chaotic irregularity of the heart in atrial fibrillation back to a regular, orderly rhythm, but in its earlier use sometimes had the catastrophic effect of stopping the heart entirely. Digitalis imposed a partial blockade on the transmission of the barrage of impulses from the fibrillating atria to the overstimulated ventricles and so slowed the ventricular rate. This slower rate, allowing the ventricles to fill more effectively between contractions, did much to restore the heart as a pump. An additional effect of digitalis is to render muscle more irritable and sometimes the drug itself caused irregularities. We are now better able to exploit the advantageous effects of these drugs while avoiding the disadvantages. This has been helped by our ability to measure the levels of digitalis in the blood and so to monitor the dosage needed more accurately.

The rate and rhythm of the heart are much affected by direct nervous stimulation and by epinephrine and nor-epinephrine (adrenaline and nor-adrenaline), hormones released into the circulation from the medulla of the adrenal glands. These substances increase the heart rate as well as affecting the skin, producing pallor and a cold sweat—a reaction familiar to most people when they are anxious or frightened. Certain of the cardiac effects of the adrenal hormones and the cardiac accelerator nerves can be blocked by drugs known as beta-blockers. The blocking action of these drugs arises from the fact that they closely mimic the naturally-occurring substances in their molecular shapes but do not have the same effects; they thus prevent the action of the natural hormones by occupying their receptor-niche on the muscle cell

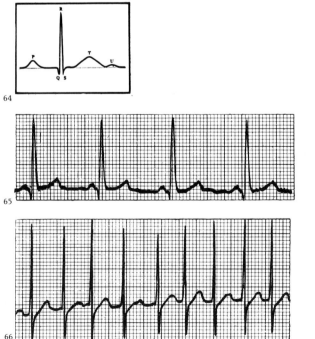

64

65

66

wall, a sort of competitive usurper function. (The accelerator effect of nervous stimulation is brought about by the release of nor-adrenaline at the nerve ending, affecting the same receptors in the muscle wall.)

Similarly, when the need is to speed the heart, the deceleration of the heart brought about by the vagus nerve can be blocked by the use of atropine, the active principle of deadly nightshade. Its other name, belladonna, derives from its use by women in ancient times to dilate the pupils (by paralyzing the pupil muscles) so as to produce a fashionable wide-eyed appearance. Many similar substances have been produced which block vagal action in the heart or, selectively, elsewhere as well. Vagal block is an important part of the pre-medication before a surgical operation involving anesthesia.

High blood pressure (hypertension) can lead to damage of the arteries and their finer ramifications, the arterioles, in various parts of the body—the major clinical manifestations being strokes, heart attacks and kidney failure. One rare variety, called malignant hypertension, is so called because in the past it was so lethal that no patient survived more than about 18 months from diagnosis. The outlook was transformed by the advent of drugs which could dramatically lower the blood pressure and maintain it at safer levels for long periods. The early examples of these were relatively crude and unselective, so that patients, while saved from death, were subject to unpleasant side-effects. Now we have a very varied range of drugs which, singly or combined, can control blood pressure with no, or in most cases relatively mild, side-effects. The most common variety of hypertension, called 'essential' because the cause is not precisely understood, is often symptomless, remaining undiscovered until a stroke or heart attack occurs. It is now known that treatment of what was once regarded as mild hypertension can greatly reduce the risk of a stroke occurring, though it is not yet certain that heart attacks can be similarly prevented. Thus screening of middle-aged people for hypertension is a justifiable exercise and should lead to a considerable reduction in disability and death due to strokes.

Research into the causes of hypertension has been furthered by a number of innovations and improvements in diagnostic procedures. These include the injection of radio-opaque substances to outline the interior of arteries, the use of radioactive substances to test kidney function, and the injection of other radio-opaque materials which are excreted via the kidneys, so outlining the kidney and the renal tract. Development of biochemical measurements has led to the identification of several endocrine and metabolic causes of hypertension, including hyper-secretion

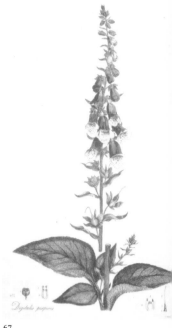

67

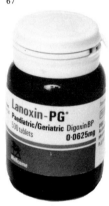

68

67, 68 The common foxglove, *Digitalis purpurea*, and a modern preparation of the active ingredient digitalis. It was discovered as a means of steadying and strengthening the action of the heart by the 18th century English physician William Withering (1741-99), and is still in use today in the treatment of heart failure. Withering's observation of the effectiveness of an extract of the foxglove was important in the history of scientific drug development for the way in which Withering used observation and deduction to isolate the one effective constituent of a folk remedy. Withering also systematically studied the effects of the drug at different dosages so as to enable him to establish the correct dosage and to sort out its real mode of action from the effects of overdosage, such as vomiting, which had been thought to be part of its curative action. It is in fact a highly potent drug, and the greatest care has to be exercised in its use. The exact nature of its direct effect on the heart muscle is still imperfectly understood, but it remains an important cardiac drug.

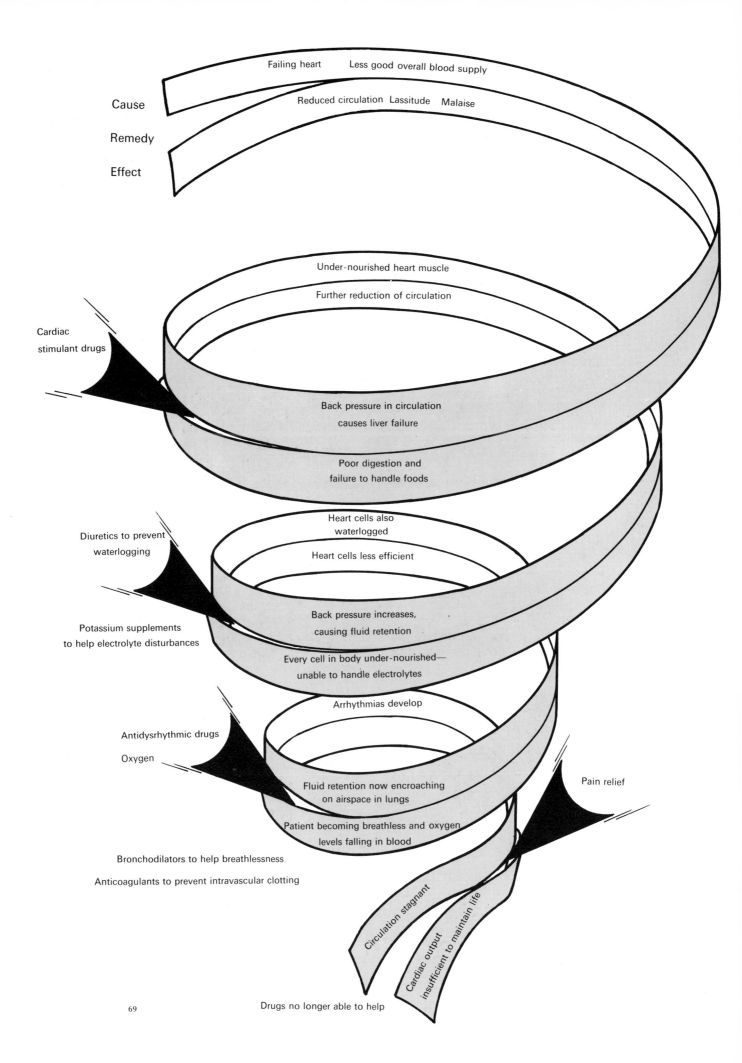

Cause

Remedy

Effect

Failing heart   Less good overall blood supply

Reduced circulation Lassitude   Malaise

Under-nourished heart muscle

Further reduction of circulation

Cardiac
stimulant drugs

Back pressure in circulation
causes liver failure

Poor digestion and
failure to handle foods

Heart cells also
waterlogged

Diuretics to prevent
waterlogging

Heart cells less efficient

Back pressure increases,
causing fluid retention

Potassium supplements
to help electrolyte disturbances

Every cell in body under-nourished—
unable to handle electrolytes

Arrhythmias develop

Antidysrhythmic drugs

Oxygen

Fluid retention now encroaching
on airspace in lungs

Pain relief

Patient becoming breathless and oxygen
levels falling in blood

Bronchodilators to help breathlessness

Anticoagulants to prevent intravascular clotting

Circulation stagnant

Cardiac output
insufficient to maintain life

69   Drugs no longer able to help

of hormones from the adrenal gland. Although these specific kinds of hypertension are uncommon, their importance lies in the fact that they may be curable by surgery, without the need for prolonged or life-long treatment with drugs that reduce blood pressure.

Anticoagulants. These are another group of substances frequently used in cardiac and vascular disease but with debatable efficacy. The therapeutic goal in their use is to produce a patient sufficiently anticoagulated for no unwanted clot to form, but at the same time retaining sufficient of the clotting mechanism for him not to bleed to death every time he shaves or brushes his teeth. Since the balance is a fine one there is a tendency to err on the side of undertreatment rather than overtreatment. Many physicians believe anticoagulants to be a great boon whilst many surgeons, because they find clots in a supposedly anticoagulated patient, think that they are of little value.

The discovery of anticoagulants came by pure chance. A farmer in Wisconsin in 1934 noticed that some of his cows were bleeding to death from the slightest cut. The distraught farmer took a dead cow and a bucket of unclotted blood to the local university where Dr Karl Paul Lent became interested. He and his team eventually traced the trouble to bishydroxycoumarin, a substance in spoiled clover closely related to coumarin which gives new mown grass its attractive smell. Dicoumarol, as the resulting drug was named, diminishes the formation in the liver of substances necessary for the clotting mechanism. It is interesting that this discovery arose from a lucky meeting. One cannot imagine how a farmer would be received now at one of our older universities after hours with a dead cow and a bucket of liquid blood. The Wisconsin

70

farmer's success lay in the fact that, in arriving after normal working hours, he was naturally selecting a dedicated worker.

Antibiotics. Antibiotics are not generally thought of as substances valuable in heart disease. They may well be life-saving when a patient has a major infection within the heart or great vessels. This condition, known as bacterial endocarditis, used to be a uniformly and rapidly lethal disease. Organisms, often quite harmless bacteria, may grow as large colonies, on defects in the heart or on abnormal vessels. A decade ago if someone with a valve congenitally abnormal or diseased as a result of rheumatic fever were to get an infection into his bloodstream from some small wound such as vigorously brushing his teeth, the bacteria could grow rapidly on the diseased part of the heart. If this colony was established in a turbulent area where the vortices protected the growing bacteria from the antibodies within the blood stream, death would follow, both from destruction within the heart, and from masses of septic tissue and organisms flying off into the circulation and lodging in the brain, kidney or some other essential organ. Now, if the diagnosis is made correctly it is possible to identify the organism in the blood and to administer the antibiotic to which the organism is sensitive. As a result of this it is frequently possible to eliminate the disease completely before severe local or peripheral damage has occurred. The underlying lesion, the diseased valve or the abnormal connection between two chambers of the heart, can then be operated upon at leisure.

Sometimes, unfortunately, the doctor will miss the diagnosis initially and treat the patient with one or more antibiotics which will suppress, but not kill, the invading organisms. The disease may then go on, relatively benignly, for some considerable time and when it is correctly diagnosed two things will have happened. First, most circulating organisms will have been killed off, making it extremely difficult to isolate the offending organism; secondly the delay in treatment and the necessity for treatment of the bacterial endocarditis by very large doses of wide spectrum antibiotics, which hopefully will kill any organism which may be present, means that destruction within the heart may be severe.

Another very important aspect of the advance in the use of antibiotics is that until recently any major overwhelming infection could get into the bloodstream in the form of circulating live organisms, septicemia. Now, because it is possible to treat almost any septicemia with antibiotics, bacterial endocarditis can be prevented.

These two examples of bacterial endocarditis and the treatment of septicemia with antibiotics are examples of the direct effects of antibiotics on the circulatory system. In many ways the indirect

69 Like most organs in the body, the heart has enormous reserves. Only when these are all overwhelmed by disease which either damages its muscle or valves, or increases the pressure against which it pumps, or increases the volume which it has to pump, will its output fall. The dramatized diagram shows the steepening descent to total failure of the circulation and death. The upper ribbon represents diagnosis, and the lower, symptoms. At each stage of the spiral is shown the treatment which attempts to minimize the effects of each condition and to slow progress down the spiral. Although the kind of progression is similar in different varieties of heart disease, the rate of progression varies enormously, as does the response to particular treatments.

70 Regular contraction of the muscular ventricles of the heart is essential for adequate circulation of the blood through the lungs and through the body as a whole. The electrical impulse to contraction is normally transmitted by a specialized bundle of muscle tissue running from the atria to the ventricles below, known as the Bundle of His. Disease may interfere with the orderly generation and transmission of this impulse to contract, and abnormal rhythms may supervene. In such cases, an artificial pacemaker may be implanted in the heart wall to take over the regulation of the heart beat. This requires the placing beneath the skin of a small battery, connected by fine wires which pass through the veins and make contact with the muscle wall of the ventricles. By complex electronic circuitry, an electrical impulse can be delivered to the heart wall at a prearranged rate, and even programmed so that, if the normal heart beat should pick up again, the artificial pacemaker impulse will be suppressed. Batteries with very long life, some of them nuclear-powered, have been devised, but even these require replacement every two or three years.

repercussions of the use of antibiotics are more important.

One very important manifestation of disease which has almost completely been eliminated since the advent of penicillin is the cardiovascular effects of syphilis. Syphilis has assumed varying importance throughout the history of man. In some civilizations it has been a major scourge, whereas in others the disease itself has waned and its effects, though pandemic, have been less severe.

Now, with a population where syphilis, though still fairly frequently contracted, is nearly always effectively treated in its early stages, we find that by the time the patient reaches old age the organisms have been dead for many years, whereas in the pre-antibiotic era the syphilitic organisms would have survived in and ultimately destroyed the vascular system of the arteries themselves, causing large aneurisms and leaking valves. Thus, one indirect effect of antibiotics on cardiovascular disease is to reduce the ravages of syphilis.

Another much more important example of the preventive effects of antibiotics is on the late manifestations of rheumatic fever. Repeated severe streptococcal sore throats were very common in children, and have almost completely been eliminated in Europe by the use of suitable antibiotics to destroy the streptococcus early on in the course of the disease. This results in a reduction of the allergic effects on the heart and nervous systems. The disease is still common in India and in some Eastern countries and its eradication is probably not entirely related to the use of antibiotics. It is certainly partially related to better public health measures, better housing, less exposure to damp climates and better nutrition. Nevertheless rheumatic fever and rheumatic hearts, which formed the major part of the cardiologist's practice and still provide many subjects for the surgeon's knife, are gradually becoming less common.

Even so, when reviewing medical triumphs we should not give credit for this reduction in the incidence of rheumatic heart disease and advanced syphilis entirely to antibiotics. There is no doubt that since reliable records have existed the virulence of these diseases and many others has waxed and waned. At the moment these two diseases, with the aid of antibiotics, are in a quiescent phrase, but we must be on guard for their re-emergence.

Cardiac surgery

Historically the physician has been the first, and until recently the only, person to treat people with cardiovascular disease. Cardiac surgery only dates back to the late 1950s when the heart/lung machine became safe enough to be acceptable for general use. It is true that

Sir Henry Souttar attempted to open the mitral valve in 1923. Other pioneers soon followed this operation and closed heart operations became commonplace in the early 1950s. Surgery on the major peripheral blood vessels and operations on the great vessels around the heart became frequent in the 1940s. There has been a continuous refinement of technique and improvement in results, and the whole emphasis of traditional medical treatment for cardiac disease is now changing. Accurate diagnosis with initial conservative drug therapy followed by surgery in the situations where operative intervention is possible is now accepted practice. Patients, until recently, were referred for operation late in the progress of their disease with consequent poor results—a story repeated throughout the history of surgery even to the recent examples of transplantation of kidney and heart. Gradually surgical intervention is becoming more routine. If only cardiac surgery could offer a comprehensive set of alternatives to the often ineffectual medical treatment, the situation might radically improve for the patient with heart disease. It is apparent however that contemporary heart surgery, except in limited areas, does not by any means offer a practical alternative to medical care. Surgery at the moment can only deal with a very limited range of congenital and acquired heart disease. Some congenital disease is so complex as to be beyond reach. Most acquired and degenerative disease is so diffuse that surgery can only offer palliation and even then at great expense with arguable benefit. Nevertheless there are areas where the duration and, more important, the quality of life can readily be improved.

Heart valve replacement has become common. Mechanical valves have been refined as a result of 10 years' combined efforts of manufacturers and dedicated surgeons and research workers. It is now possible to buy several reliable makes and models of mechanical valves; true, they all share fundamental shortcomings in that they cannot incorporate perfectly in the body, nor can they operate in an entirely physiological way without obstruction to flow and without requiring back-flow to close them. None has a potential life approaching the three score and ten of a normal human being, none is able to repair itself, or resist infection and all carry the risk of thrombus formation: yet many thousands are inserted each year with immediate success, transforming the life of the cardiac cripple into an extended life of reasonable quality before some require replacement. In view of mechanical breakdown the alternative biological transplant valves offer architectural and mechanical advantages and can resist infection but are not self repairing unless inserted as living grafts and require more surgical expertise to insert.

71 Many secrets of the heart and circulation were uncovered by the use of the cardiac catheter, a flexible tube which can be fed along vascular channels into and even beyond the heart itself. Through it, X-ray contrast medium can be injected to outline selected regions of the circulation. This X-ray photograph shows a catheter which has been passed up through the vein of the right arm, down through the major collecting vein of the heart (the superior vena cava), through the right atrium, into the cavity of the right ventricle. Radio-opaque contrast medium injected into the ventricle has in this radiograph outlined the pulmonary arteries supplying both lungs. Obstruction of a pulmonary artery or its main branches (for example, after a pulmonary embolism) can be displayed in this way. A catheter passed through an artery into the left side of the heart can similarly be positioned so as to fill and outline the coronary arteries, obstruction of which is responsible for heart attacks. An obstruction so located may then be bypassed at surgery with a vein graft (see illustration 75). The fine catheter used does not interfere with the function of the heart or of the valves through which it passes.

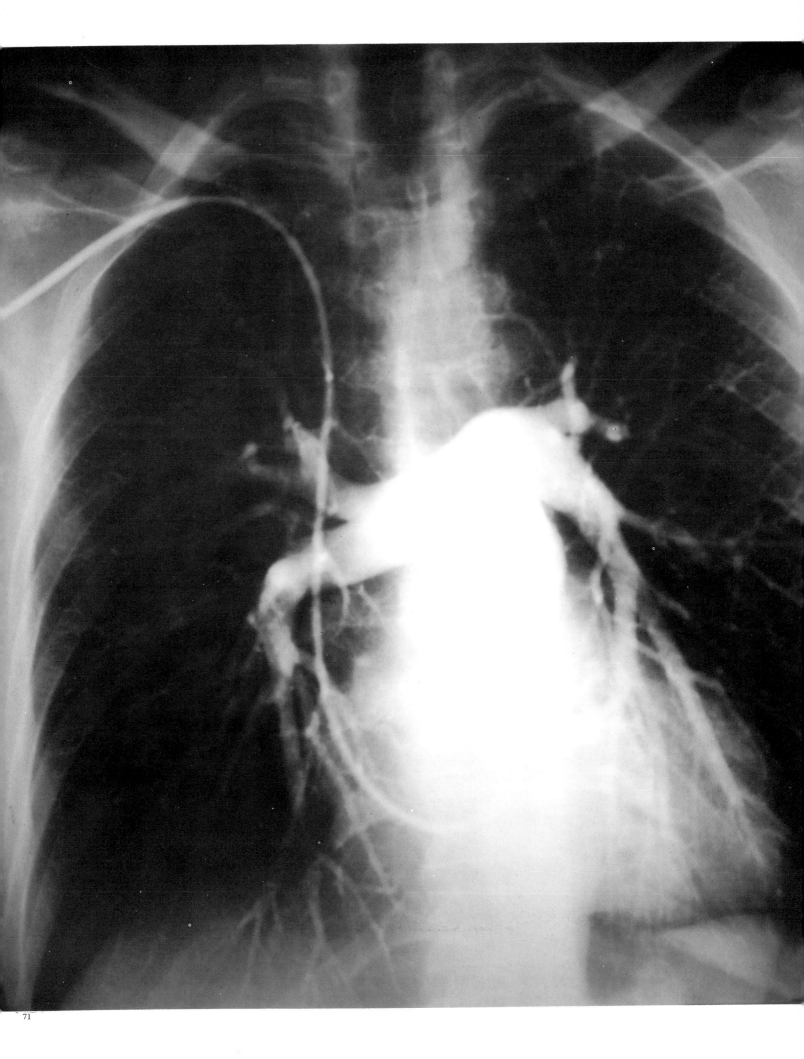

72 A heart-lung machine. In some operations it is necessary to arrest the heart's action so that surgery can be performed. The circulation must then be maintained by a machine and because blood cannot in these circumstances pass through the patient's lung, the machine also has to perform the functions of the lung as well. The machine therefore incorporates a pump and an oxygenator. The large circular shapes on the sloping top of the machine are the main arterial pump and other pumps for recovering the blood spilt in the operating field.

73, 74 The onward passage of blood through the pumping chambers of the heart and out into the body depends crucially on the efficient operation of the valves between the chambers, which prevent backward flow. The heart valves were frequently susceptible to serious damage in the past by rheumatic carditis (part of rheumatic fever), which led to distortion which both obstructed the onward flow of the blood and permitted backward leakage. This mechanical inefficiency led inevitably to pump failure and medicine had little to offer apart from rest and support with digitalis for the failing heart muscle. The situation was revolutionized by the first successful attempts at cardiac surgery, splitting of a contracted valve with the surgeon's finger or with a small knife attached to that finger. Now total replacement of the diseased valve is often carried out. The aortic valve may be replaced by a preserved, freeze-dried human valve taken, for example, from an accident victim. Artificial valves have been constructed from stainless steel and synthetic fabrics capable of uniting completely with body tissues. Two types of valve are shown here. Illustration 73 shows a ball and cage valve, used to replace the diseased aortic valve. When the ventricle contracts, it expels its blood from below upwards into the aorta by raising the ball. As the ventricle relaxes, the ball settles firmly back into its seating, preventing backward flow. Illustration 74 shows the three billowing curtains of an artificial tricuspid valve, seen from above. The pressure generated by the atrium pushes the curtain-like cusps aside to discharge its contents into the ventricle. A moment later, as the ventricle contracts, the cusps are forced into close apposition with each other, preventing backward flow into the atrium.

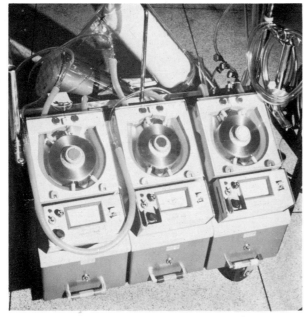

It is difficult to see how real advancement in cardiovascular surgery can take place on the basis of tiny improvements. A new philosophy is needed before real inroads can be made into the massive mortality rate resulting from cardiac and vascular disease. Examination of the evolution of cardiac surgery reveals some of the constraints which have determined the apparently pusillanimous approach to cardiac disease.

Souttar's pioneer operations to relieve mitral stenosis (blockage of the valve) were not successful. Two vital areas of expertise were lacking at that time; accurate diagnosis, and an understanding of post-operative management in patients who had had their chests opened.

Before surgical intervention became routine simple classical clinical methods of diagnosis of heart disorder known to every practising doctor were allowed to serve. It did not matter to the dying patient whether his valve was tight, or leaking, or both, and there was no point in questioning the diagnostician, for nothing in treatment would be altered. Early cardiac surgery provided a need for greater diagnostic accuracy. Surgeons wanted to know as much as possible about the heart before using the limited safe operating time available to them. Some surgeons even connected the mother's vessels to her child's circulation while they operated on the now bypassed heart. In this situation particularly, a mistaken diagnosis had the potential of the death not only of the infant but of the mother as well.

In the early days of cardiac surgery cooling the patient, cross circulation with a human volunteer or attachment to a heart/lung machine of limited performance all allowed only a few minutes' circulatory arrest to repair a simple defect. If the cardiologist presented a patient with a mistaken diagnosis, at best the surgeon would be able to close the heart and the patient

would not be materially harmed: but death frequently followed an operation for an uncorrectable lesion.

Before routine cardiac surgery, cardiodiagnosis depended partly on careful examination of the X-ray shadows of the heart and empirical analysis of the electrical activity of the heart, but mainly on the clinical judgment, skill and experience of the cardiologist. That diagnosis—using such simple methods—was ever accurate is remarkable, yet really competent diagnosticians generally achieved remarkable accuracy. The large numbers of patients awaiting cardiac surgery soon overwhelmed even the doyens of the art and many new physicians entered the field. For them a new science had to replace the old art. Mechanical measurement of pressure changes inside the heart and visualization of what was happening in the heart became important. Threading a catheter into the right side of the heart was soon shown to be a relatively safe and simple procedure. Coincidentally, the aerospace industry provided miniature electronic transducers which enabled pressure information to be obtained from within the heart. At this stage diagnostic hunches could also be reinforced by taking samples of blood from areas where it was thought that arterial blood might be leaking to the venous side; and tight valves and leaking valves could be explored by measuring the pressure gradients across them.

Angiography. The same catheter made it possible to visualize the heart by injecting radio-opaque dyes into the various chambers and taking serial or ciné X-rays to follow the flow of radio-opaque medium follow the flow of radio-opaque medium through them. It was also possible to inject the medium into peripheral vessels and to take quite simple X-rays to visualize blockages. At the same time as the invasive diagnostic procedures were developing, pioneers like Starr in the United States were trying to extract more information about the heart than could be obtained from the mechanical measurement and visualization of what was going on within it. He was interested not only in finding out how much blood the heart was ejecting with each beat but also in measuring how quickly the heart was ejecting it, by assessing the recoil of the patient applying Newton's third law of motion, 'Every action has an equal and opposite reaction'. The first ballisto-cardiograph as it was called became a diagnostic tool which had a brief fashion. Its potential was never realized. This was partly because of the pressing demands of conventional cardiology for anatomical information in order that the patients could be reliably referred to surgeons. The new information which became available was not in a form which could be readily interpreted and its significance was not appreciated at that time. It is unfortunate that we have to admit that even today this is still the situation and that nearly all the cardio-diagnostic techniques are invasive, involving surgery and a small but substantial risk to the patient, and they do not give any real information about the price the heart has to pay in order to pump its blood. They tell us little about the state of the heart muscle, nor do they give any inkling as to whether it is drawing upon irreplaceable reserves to do its work. Artificial means of circulatory support are now within sight of practical use and there is a growing appreciation that the information from non-invasive techniques is better not only because of the safety and lack of pain, but also because it indicates the performance of the heart muscle. Catheterization and angiography yield information about a patient at a single point in time, whereas non-invasive techniques can be monitored continuously. Continuous information adds a new dimension to time-related trends.

Since the beginning of medical practice patients and relatives have asked doctors for predictions about the future. Many doctors exceed their knowledge and make confident statements about the future of their patients. The term prognosis is used for medical forecasts, but the acquisition of a term does not immediately make the management of the desperately sick patient any less crucial. The new non-invasive techniques for the first time tell us at least whether the patient is getting better, staying the same, or getting worse.

When dealing with the larger peripheral vessels of the heart many workers now use ultrasonic techniques to examine the flow through diseased vessels. We are on the threshold of a new era. The two major problems facing Souttar and other pioneers are overcome and cardiovascular diagnosis is improving rapidly. Don Harrison and his team at Stanford University, Leon Resnekov and his group in Chicago, and many others, have applied computers to the information coming from cardiac catheterization and intensive care units. New non-invasive techniques will soon supplement, then replace, catheterization. Post-operative management is becoming better understood and more efficient. These two areas have both become 'super-specialties' in their own right.

These triumphs in the diagnostic and intensive care areas have abolished surgical constraints in the treatment of cardiovascular disease throughout the circulation. Vessels to the heart, brain, kidney and limbs can now be assessed and unblocked or bypassed.

Coronary vein grafting is creating a bridgehead into the enormous problems of hitherto untreatable degenerative disease of the arteries

supplying the heart itself. This operation is the most recent in a series intended to revascularize the heart. In itself it is not particularly difficult but it does illustrate the principles of vascular surgery, all of which are based on simple logic.

It consists of taking a living vein from the patient's leg and using it as a conduit to bypass a blocked artery to the heart. In a patient with symptoms such as heart pain the site of the blockage can be located using angiography. A ciné X-ray film using an image intensifier clearly delineates the site of occlusion after an opaque substance has been injected via a thin tube threaded along an artery into the suspect artery. It is also important to establish whether there are disease-free vessels past the blockage to allow sufficient 'run off' to prevent the graft from clotting.

The operation itself is done with the patient

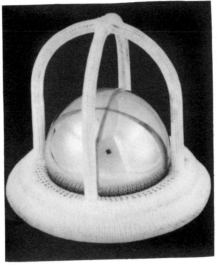

73

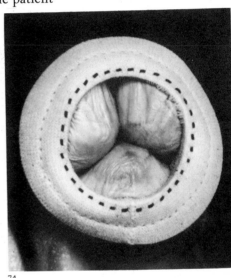

74

75 This diagram shows vein grafts of the three coronary arteries. The vein graft passes from a newly-made opening in the aorta to the healthy artery beyond the blocked part.

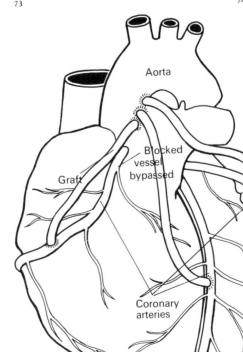

Aorta

Blocked vessel bypassed

Graft

Coronary arteries

75

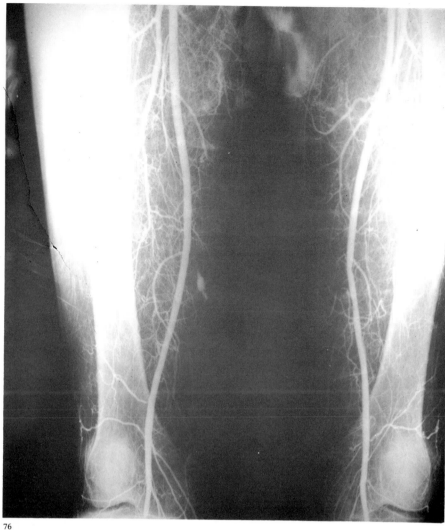

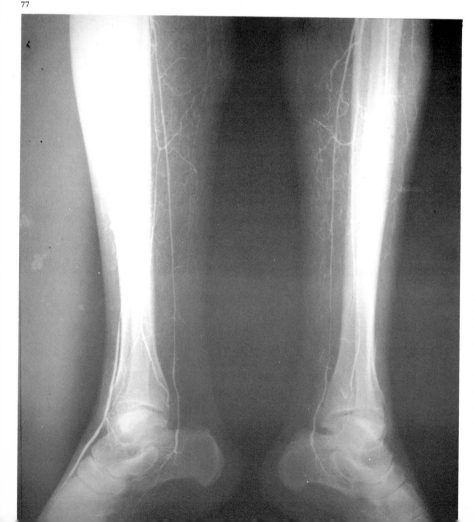

connected to a life-supporting heart/lung machine. Lengths of vein are sewn to the three matchstick-sized main arteries of the heart as required: one is at the front, one on the left, and one at the back to which access can only be gained by lifting the heart. When these difficult junctions are complete and bloodtight the heart is allowed once again to take over the circulation. The upper ends of the grafts are then sewn to the aorta just above the heart. These joins are made while blood is flowing through the aorta using special curved clamps to isolate the one side of the aorta temporarily making it into a double-barrelled vessel. This allows normal circulation whilst giving the surgeon a dry field to make this difficult junction.

As with all its predecessors an assessment of the results of this operation is difficult. The act of opening the layer of tissue surrounding the heart is itself sufficient to eliminate heart pain, so that pain relief is no index of increased blood flow. Electromagnetic flowmeters can demonstrate a flow through the graft, but where that blood goes and whether it does any good before it enters the venous system frequently remains in doubt. Post-operative angiocardiography can be used to demonstrate the patency of the graft, Real success can only be measured in terms of increased survival time, reduced breathlessness and improved quality of life; data about these is accumulating slowly. The global benefit of this operation does not lie in the modest number of clinical successes but in its indication of the hopelessness of the contemporary treatment of many patients who just do not have enough heart muscle to maintain life, yet who are otherwise fit. No one disputes that heart replacement could be the answer to this problem; opinions differ about how best this should be done. There are two alternative philosophies. Many believe that mechanical devices should be used though the story of implanted mechanical prostheses has been an unhappy one. When artificial heart valves became a surgical proposition the problems and shortcomings of mechanical implants were highlighted. We do not have materials which are non-thrombogenic; we do not have materials which can cope with the 40 million annual flexions which are necessary in some valve components. We are not within sight of an ideal design which will not cause turbulence or cavitation and which will not cause significant resistance to flow. We cannot match the perfection of natural valves which after thousands of million years of evolution can float together without any regurgitation. For a mechanical heart the problems are several orders of magnitude greater. We cannot truthfully even envisage power sources capable of producing sufficient clean energy for implantation to drive a mechanical heart. No one has seriously considered the problem, let alone the solution of linking a mechanical heart to the nervous and chemical mechanisms which normally control the heart's output and its response to circulatory needs. Engineers now suggest that if the mechanical heart is not feasible it might still be possible to support the circulation in other ways. Theoretically an inadequate circulation might be assisted in three ways: by mechanically boosting it, by reducing the demands made upon it, or by a combination of both.

Various methods of cutting down the metabolic processes dependent upon millions of enzyme-chemical reactions have been suggested or tried. A reduction in body temperature of 5° centigrade should, if normal chemical laws are obeyed, reduce the metabolic rate by 25 per cent. It would do so if all the enzymes involved had a linear response to temperature changes. However some enzymes work more efficiently at 25° than at 37° centigrade, other are inhibited almost completely at this temperature; consequently abnormal metabolic pathways and bizarre intermediate products result. Cooling is always accompanied by a certain amount of cumulative biochemical disturbance, increasing with the duration and depth of hypothermia. A logical extension of hypothermia is to attempt to mimic hibernation. Hibernating animals which are normally homeothermic can progressively lower their body temperature in conditions of reduced external temperature to a low temperature requiring minimal circulation to support life. The mechanism by which this progressive metabolic slowing down is achieved is not understood, nor is the absence of clotting in the stagnant blood vessels. Although there have been attempts since 1952 to produce hibernation-like states, we are no nearer to achieving genuine hibernation.

If oxygenation were the only function of the circulation, high pressure oxygen should succeed in providing a suitably enriched environment. High pressure oxygen chambers have been in use for over a decade without any conclusive demonstration of their value to patients, other than those with bends or gas gangrene. They also place a physical barrier between patient and attendant with increased risk.

Relieving the patient from the burden of breathing by using a mechanical ventilator reduces cardiac work slightly. None of the currently available methods of resting the circulation has much advantage over the time-honoured medical tradition of giving morphia, raising the foot of the bed, and keeping the patient peaceful and quiet.

Many methods of boosting the heart have been tried. Some, such as the DeBakey pump bypassing the left side of the heart, are simply engineered devices requiring major surgical

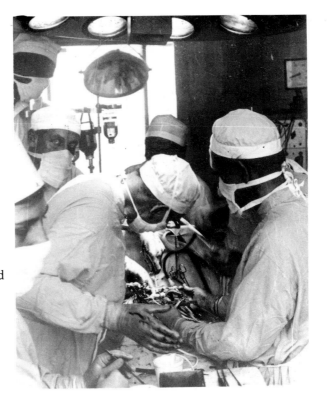

78

interference to connect them to the patients. Others such as inflatable balloons in the aorta, which ensure an adequate coronary flow and are synchronized so that they collapse just before the heart pump contracts, are more complex but require less surgery. All interfere with the physiological state of the patient, already rendered abnormal by circulatory inadequacies. That no single circulatory support technique has any clear advantage over the others suggests that they may all have failed to turn promise into performance. If we are seeking an explanation of this we have to remember that the possible circulatory benefit of an operation in any particular case has to be weighed against the cost to the patient of the surgical intervention and the physiological disturbance it induces.

Every day thousands of sound organs are cremated or interred, and tons of human fetal tissues are incinerated annually. The potential value of animal donors has not yet been realized. The arguments in favor of living tissue to replace or repair the heart are much more powerful than the mere failure of the mechanical heart as a viable alternative. Biological tissues repair themselves, resist infection, are powered by highly efficient metabolic energy sources, are perfectly designed, are non-thrombogenic, have perfectly smooth blood surfaces, incorporate well and have a reliable longevity unapproached by mechanical hearts. Just as within the concept of mechanical methods of supporting the circulation there were several options, so with biological replacement there are three main alternatives worthy of consideration.

76, 77 The combination of X-ray photography and the injection of radio-opaque material is also of great value in the diagnosis of obstruction of arteries throughout the body. These X-rays show the arterial supply to the legs. The main arterial pathway is open, though, on the right, indentations of the column of radio-opaque material betray the presence of arteriosclerotic plaques in the arterial wall. In the picture of the lower part of the limbs, attenuation of the column of contrast medium suggests areas of partial obstruction due to arterial wall disease.

78 The scene in the operating theater with an open heart operation in mid-course.

Homotransplantation. If the mechanical heart was pie in the sky, surely heart transplantation should have shown itself to be the elixir of life to the thousands of patients currently denied treatment. Rejection by society of this procedure is related to unfair publicity, for which those involved in the American artificial heart program are partly to blame. In the 1960s surgeons wishing to replace the heart by mechanical means deliberately sought attention: television, radio, newspapers and magazines were wooed for favored time and space, hopefully to aid funding of the artificial heart program. For the first time the media were able to witness the problems associated with a growing point of medicine. What was previously a private affair between the dying patient, the research worker, the clinician and the patient's close relatives was presented to the millions who seek entertainment from the media. They had their appetites whetted by real life-and-death dramas. It became obvious to any producer or editor that if he wanted to gain prestige he could look at the medical scene and find willing enthusiasts prepared to talk about their work, many of them failing to point out that they were talking about things which they wished for, rather than about established fact. It was not surprising that the television companies and the newsmen, their techniques already established for finding out what was happening in the hospital environs, should have been well prepared for the early clinical application of a quarter century's research work in heart transplantation. As a result of this an unprecedented amount of publicity surrounded the first human heart transplantation. Every minority opinion— frequently uninformed—was voiced. Political response, important in countries with centrally organized medicine, bows to public opinion rather than guiding it. The clinical results of heart transplantation were never compared with established medicine. The media did not tell the statistics of heart transplantation. They did not point out the initial disasters which complicated other operations now perfectly acceptable such as kidney transplantation. Apparently there is total unawareness of the high failure rate of many established operations for potentially lethal conditions even after nearly a century of experience. It is only in the private universities in the U.S.A. that this work continues.

The use of heterotransplantation. In the United States a chimpanzee's heart has been transplanted into a human with some initial success. A primate kidney transplant has secreted urine in a human. In this country two attempts have been made to use a pig's heart/lung preparation to boost the circulation in parallel with the patient's own heart which was connected to a heart/lung machine. These attempts failed because the blood chemistry of the animal donor differed widely from that of the recipient. The animal kingdom has never really been surveyed properly as a potential source and bank for organs for human beings. The electrolytes, biochemistry and tissue groups are not known to us. They could be, in return for a modest research investment, thus answering the vital question: could we use living heterograft organs?

Fetal homotransplantation. Another line of research in heart replacement which shows promise is the use of fetal material. This may be one of the most valuable of all the methods available to us for repairing the heart. The biological facts on which this form of treatment might depend are all well known. The fetus in its development goes through stages comparable to our ancestral stages. In its early development the fetus is simple and primitive. Primitive animals are capable of complete regeneration even after halving. More complex animals can completely regenerate a complex structure such as a limb after amputation. Recent Russian work on amputated amphibian limbs shows that in an animal which would normally heal an amputation by scar, regeneration can be complete if the skin sheath is left almost intact. Some adult human tissues such as the liver, blood, bone, blood vessels, gut, lymphoid tissue, etc. have considerable powers of repair and regeneration, whereas adult heart and brain do not. After a heart attack there are sometimes transient attempts at regenerative repair around the lesion which soon disappear. The nucleus of every adult cell probably contains sufficient information, not just to replicate itself, but to build a complete individual. This has been beautifully demonstrated by Dr Gourdon at Oxford who, by removing the nucleus from a fertilized frog egg and replacing it with the nucleus from an adult frog gut cell, produced an animal indistinguishable from those produced by normal sexual reproduction. Embryo extracts are rich in growth factors, there being an interplay between fast dividing cells, in embryonic tissues, which results in differentiation and organization of their neighbors. It may well be that the use of fetal material is not a remote concept. The use of adult cadaver material, animal or human, implies that part of the life-span dictated by the biological time clock is used up, whereas human fetal cells have a greater potential life span before them. In addition, fetal tissue could be available in quantity, and can be banked for up to a month. Thus, should tissue matching be important, it will still be practicable.

These interesting properties of fetal heart tissue, along with its availability, do not alone make its future application obvious. If parts of fetal hearts are placed in apposition in organ culture, fusion takes place and a complete heart results. More significant is the beating performance of these hearts, which will coordinate to assume the beating rate of the fastest component. The line of fusion between separate parts is often difficult to find even with the microscope. Fusion of cells to give functional continuity is interesting biologically and of great relevance to the purposes discussed here as it can take place across the species barrier. A composite heart of cat/mouse, rat/mouse, rabbit/mouse, or dog/rabbit will behave in the same way as hearts made from fetuses of the same species. The performance and survival after fusion are not influenced by the composite nature of the specimen. These facts, coupled with the apparently weak antigenic properties of early fetal tissues, suggest that immediate application might be in the treatment of heart block—a biological pacemaker, in fact. If the experimentally demonstrable fusion of fetal tissue could be made to work in a clinical situation the changing of worn-out battery units will become unnecessary. Instead an injection of fetal cells will fuse with the ventricular wall and pace the heart, responding to all the physiological stimuli. Advances such as those involving fetal cellular or extract implantation will require a careful public education and preparation to avoid hostile responses. The cost of carrying out such treatments for the large number of patients who could benefit from them is a problem which society constantly faces. This merely highlights society's general dilemma in attempting to decide on the allocation of less than infinite resources between health, education, housing, defense etc., and, within medicine, between, for example, dramatically pain-relieving operations for the otherwise unimportant problem of piles on the one hand, and keeping alive totally dependent, brain-damaged vegetating accident victims on the other. It goes without saying that respect for life must be paramount, but what does this mean in the face of an unavoidable choice between improving the quality of life for those for whom this is possible, and preserving a life which has no quality?

Practical difficulties have already arisen when new, initially expensive and numerically potentially important forms of treatment are translated from the laboratory to the clinical area. Some patients may be treated if, by geographical accident, they meet an enterprising doctor. In countries with centrally organized and funded medical services the patient is more likely to be referred for treatment, but little more likely to receive it. The availability of new and expensive treatments is determined by a complex interplay between the enthusiasm and advocacy of the professional and the cost/benefit approach

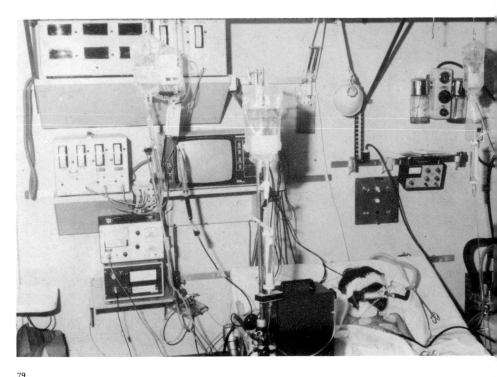

79

of administrators and politicians. The final court of appeal in most countries is the view of society as a whole, informed by the media and articulated via the ballot.

Conclusion. The reader might assume from this review of the treatment of cardiovascular disease that there are some grounds for complacency in the medical profession. *Diagnosis, treatment* and *after-care* are all advancing rapidly. But where are the triumphs in *understanding the causation* of disease of the heart and blood vessels and what is to be done in the field of *prevention*? Certainly there have been imaginative and thorough studies of whole communities. The most famous is the Framingham study in which a whole community in Massachusetts has been studied for almost 20 years. This concept of acquiring a data base about a representative population not undergoing any special treatment has been extended to the study of large population groups treated with new substances aimed at lowering blood lipids and blood pressure, in the hope of preventing degenerative arterial disease. The magnitude of this task can be appreciated only by those involved in unravelling the masses of information, and the financial cost is enormous. And not all the effort expended in treating the existing population is lost to future generations. The studies of the future leading to preventive regimes will rely heavily on non-invasive cardiodiagnostic studies. Posterity may thank this seemingly illogical generation, which bans cyclamates and yet allows cigarettes, for appreciating that cardiovascular disease is likely to remain the biggest killer.

79 The place occupied by technology in much modern medicine is most strikingly evidenced in this view of a patient receiving intensive care in the recovery room after a heart operation. The boxes on the wall at the top left of the picture contain equipment which gives constant monitoring and trend recording (through a computer) of the vital indicators of the state of the heart and circulation. Below left and above right are the amplifiers which magnify the impulses supplied by pressure, temperature and electrical current transducers. These are displayed in the continuous moving electrocardiogram, pressure wave forms, etc., on the screen of the memory scope (right below), and in the digital counters (left above) which show systolic and diastolic pressures (the pressure within the arteries during and before contraction respectively), venous blood pressure from two locations, and heart rate and body temperature. The patient is connected to a ventilator (out of picture), and suspended on columns are bottles for blood and saline, connected to a drip pump which monitors the rate of infusions. Finally, to the bottom left of the picture is shown the most up to date equipment which gives continuous visual monitoring of the state of oxygenation of the blood.

5 The Blood

Just as the nerves of the body are like telegraph wires rapidly transmitting messages, so blood is the highway and transport system of the body, and its function is even more vital to health and survival than any transport system in modern society.

Diseases of many other systems of the body affect the blood, and the bloodstream is a means of access for doctors to other organs and tissues— for instance by a simple injection into a vein.

The blood itself can be diseased, however, and then it must be treated. In the path to the understanding and conquest of blood disorders, scientists have eaten raw meat and regurgitated it for their patients, tested human blood against that of monkeys, treated children with some of the most powerful known cell-killing drugs, and resorted to the centuries-old technique of blood-letting.

These are among the hematologist's techniques, past and present, examined here, but first an introduction is necessary to the normal functions and composition of blood to see why it is so vital and what are its elements that must be maintained in health.

Blood carries the digestion products of food— carbohydrate, protein, minerals and vital trace materials—from the gut to the liver, which is the body's principal chemical plant. Here harmful elements are modified and forms of foodstuffs changed to meet the body's needs, before being released again into the blood for distribution. Where the bloodstream passes through the lungs, it takes up oxygen for distribution to the tissues. From all parts of the body, blood also picks up undesirable end products of biochemical changes and carries them for disposal to the kidneys, liver and lungs.

Another function of blood is to maintain within precise limits the composition of body fluids, both inside and outside cells. Any deviation in fluid, protein, carbohydrate or mineral content is immediately adjusted by exchange to or from the blood. This produces minor changes in the composition of the blood, which are monitored by special receptor cells strategically situated throughout the body, so that the blood's composition can quickly be returned to normal, for example by the release of a hormone.

Finally, the blood is the site of the body's defenses. Substances called antibodies in the blood specifically disable harmful bacteria, and white blood cells then engulf and carry off these invaders. Other travelling cells, the lymphocytes, detect foreign bacteria or foreign substances and make antibodies to attack them.

The amount of blood in the body of a person weighing 70 kg (154 lbs) is about five litres (nine pints). More than half of this is fluid, the complicated protein-rich plasma of the blood, and the remainder consists of cells. The most abundant cell in the blood is the red blood cell (erythrocyte): each cubic millimeter of blood— a very small drop—contains over five million of these cells. After its manufacture in the bone marrow, each red blood cell remains active for about four months. The spleen which filters out and destroys old and imperfect red cells sometimes gets over-enthusiastic and destroys many more than it should. This produces a form of anemia which can be cured or controlled by an operation for removal of the spleen.

A red blood cell is shaped like an automobile tire—a round disk with a much thickened edge which can be distorted into a long sausage shape as it is pumped at high speed through tiny capillaries. For a fraction of a second the wall of the red cell lies right up against the fine capillary lining and this is enough to allow exchange of oxygen, carbon dioxide and other materials.

The red color of blood is due to a complex protein substance called hemoglobin which packs the red cell. Since hemoglobin contains iron, it is easy to understand why lack of iron in the diet or loss of blood may give rise to anemia.

White blood cells (leukocytes) are fewer in number than red cells; only two for every thousand red cells. But there are several different types of white cell mainly concerned with defense. The lymphocytes, for example, which are made in the lymph glands, manufacture antibodies against foreign bacteria. Another type of white cell, the polymorph, moves like a pond amoeba. It is attracted to areas of tissue damage or of bacterial invasion and swallows up bacteria, particularly those that have been inactivated by antibodies.

In addition to red and white cells, blood contains 'platelets'. Each platelet consists of small particles shed from the edge of a large cell in the bone marrow called a megakaryocyte. Platelets are concerned with blood clotting.

Pernicious anemia. Red blood cells have to be manufactured continually by the trillion to replace the one per cent that are destroyed each day. Many materials apart from iron are required for the manufacture of normal red cells, and some of them are available in only tiny amounts in food. Among these are two of the B vitamins— vitamin B_{12} and folic acid. Inadequate supply of these vitamins means inadequate blood production—and hence anemia.

It was the German Paul Ehrlich, discoverer of white blood cells, who last century recognized the fatal type of anemia that results from lack of these vitamins. The disease had been described before by Thomas Addison, a physician at Guy's Hospital, London, but he could not pin down its cause. In 1855 Addison wrote: 'For a long period

80 A stereoscan picture showing the blood cells at 3,800 times magnification. The red cells look like automobile tires with a central hollowing. Towards the lower half of the picture are two cells more rounded in shape, with a slightly irregular surface. These are lymphocytes which are concerned with immunity (see illustration 81). The tendency for red cells when out of the body to adhere to each other like piles of coins ('rouleaux') is shown by the four cells in the top right hand portion of the picture.

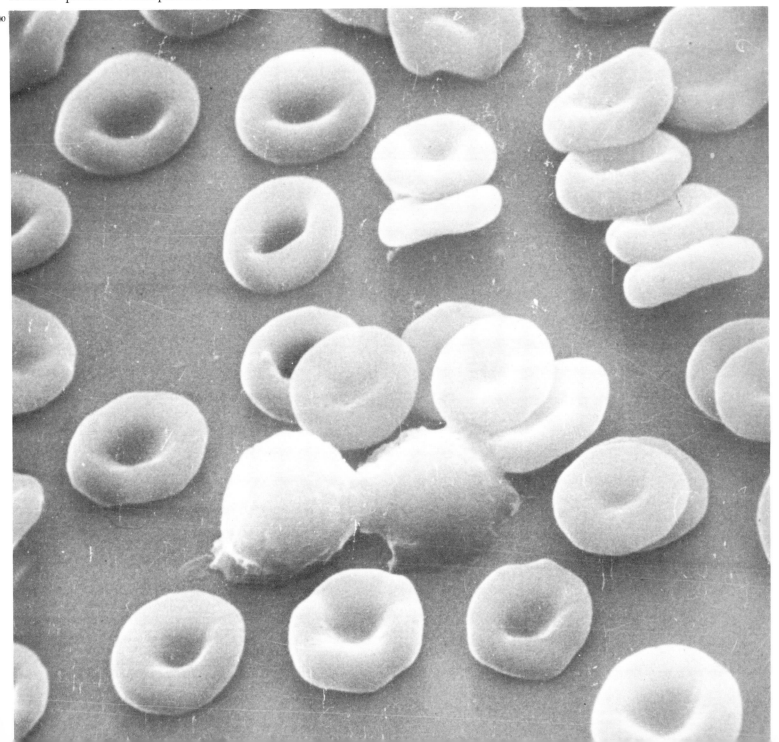

81 The system of defense against infection and against cancer cells is based on the role of a blood cell called the lymphocyte. This is produced in the marrow (1) from the same stem cell that produces all the other blood cells.

When the lymphocyte leaves the marrow it is processed for one of two major functions.

B cells. It can be altered to become capable of making antibodies. It is thought that a tissue in the gut, known as Peyer's Patches, is responsible; in chickens it is an organ called the Bursa of Fabricus— hence the name B or Bursa cells.

When such a lymphocyte comes into contact with a bacterium (or a fungus) it divides to produce a large number of lymphocytes, all of which now recognize this bacterium and produce antibodies against it. The lymphocyte changes in appearance at this point and is called a plasma cell (2). The antibodies are formed on the surface of the lymphocytes, and are shed into body fluids.

The antibodies latch on to the bacterium (3). In some cases, the bacterium propels itself with leg-like flagellae, and the antibodies immobilize these (4). The antibodies may be helped by other substances in plasma and body fluids called complement (3, 5).

Once the bacterium has been attacked by antibody and complement it is either killed or rendered very susceptible to ingestion by cells called macrophages (6). Complement itself can attach to bacteria or fungi and help combat infection (7). Some bacteria excrete toxins. These toxins are also recognized by B lymphocytes, which produce an antibody called an antitoxin (8).

T cells. Other lymphocytes pass through a gland situated in the chest above the heart, called the thymus gland (9), and become T lymphocytes (some of which are known as K cells). T cells can also recognize 'foreign' cells, such as fungi (10), virus-infected cells (11) and cancer cells (12). Some bacteria are also attacked by T cells (not shown).

K or killer cells are T cells which kill foreign cells directly, rather than through the agency of secretions. For example, cells which might become cancer cells are killed off in this way. It is these K cells which reject transplants or non-compatible tissues such as a kidney transplant, a skin graft or incompatible bone marrow.

Normally B and T cells collaborate in eliminating infection and in removing the clones or complexes of foreign cells.

When these processes are mistakenly directed against the body's own structures, a state of 'autoimmunity' develops. This may lead to the derangement or destruction of previously normal tissues, for example, the joint linings in rheumatoid arthritis.

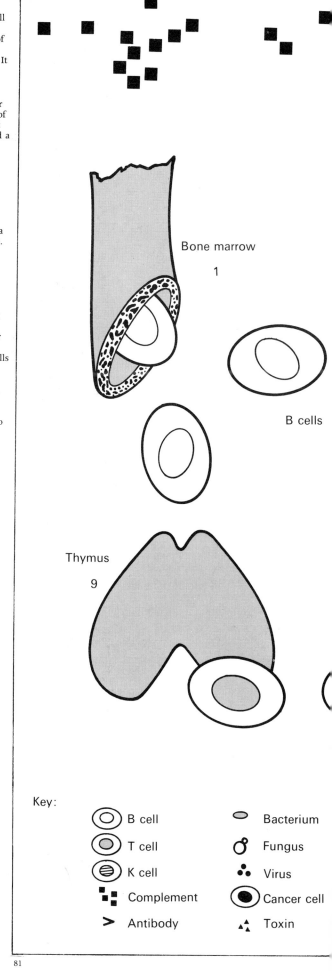

Bone marrow

1

B cells

Thymus

9

Key:

B cell   Bacterium

T cell   Fungus

K cell   Virus

Complement   Cancer cell

Antibody   Toxin

81

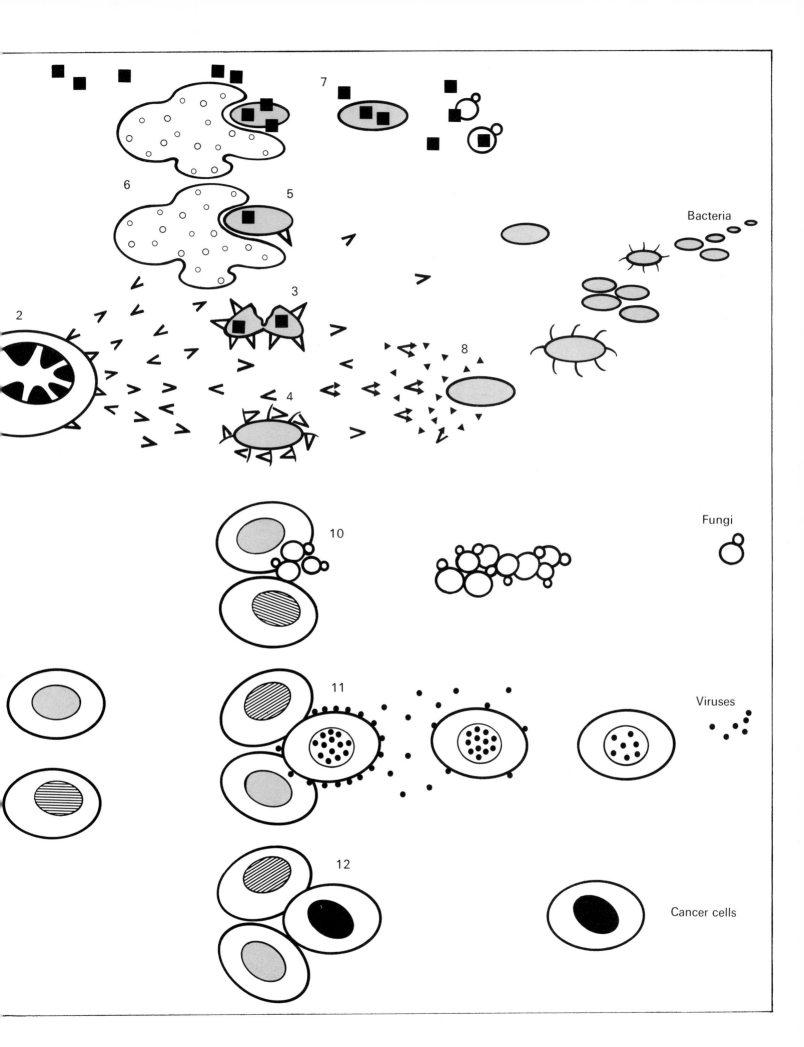

Bacteria

Fungi

Viruses

Cancer cells

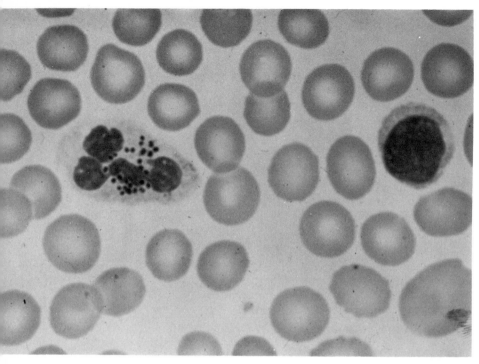

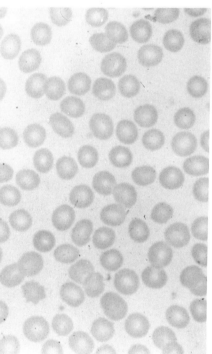

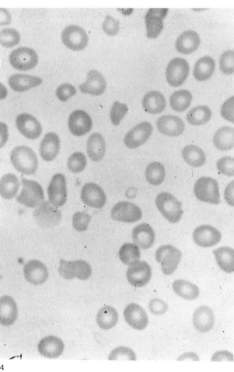

standby, arsenic was highly thought of, and the patient's diet might exclude beer and meat but include waste 'slops'.

The disease remained fatal until the 1920s. At that time Whipple in the United States was studying the effects of foodstuffs in overcoming anemia, and he found that liver restored dogs to normal after withdrawal of fairly large amounts of blood from a vein. This prompted George Minot and William Murphy at Boston in 1926 to see whether liver would be useful in pernicious anemia. Over a period of time they persuaded 45 patients to take half a pound (250 g) of almost raw liver each day. The fortitude of these patients was rewarded with a striking improvement in their symptoms and a substantial amelioration of the anemia.

In the next few years there were some remarkable efforts to improve the palatability of raw liver; a substantial section of one 1930 textbook on pernicious anemia would have been equally in place in a cookbook. But the demonstration of the efficacy of liver prompted a series of attempts to isolate the factor in this food that cured the anemia. Soon an injectable liver concentrate did away with the need to eat large amounts of liver.

Equally important was the research which reached its culmination 30 years later with the isolation of pure vitamin B_{12} from liver by Ernest Lester-Smith and his research group in England and Edward Rickes and his colleagues in the United States. The great obstacle in this work was that the only way to know whether a particular fraction of liver contained the antianemic factor was to try it on a patient with pernicious anemia. This required a continuous supply of patients. Fortunately, or unfortunately, pernicious anemia has a frequency of one to two people per 1000. Above the age of 60 the frequency is almost one in 100 in the U.K., and the researchers' problems were solved by H. G. Ungley in Newcastle-upon-Tyne. He used liver extracts prepared by Glaxo, and it soon became apparent that the potent preparations were always pink. At about this time American scientists developed a method which bypassed the need for testing

I had from time to time met with a very remarkable form of general anemia, occurring without any discoverable cause whatever. . . . It makes its approach in so slow and insidious a manner that the patient can hardly fix a date to his earliest feeling of that languor which is shortly to become so extreme. The countenance gets pale, the whites of the eyes become poorly, the general frame flabby rather than wasted. . . . The disease, in my own experience, resisted all remedial efforts and sooner or later terminated fatally.'

Small wonder that this anemia was called 'pernicious anemia'.

The remedial efforts referred to by Addison were bizarre by our standards; bleeding was a

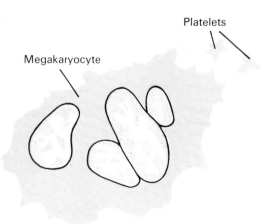

Platelets

Megakaryocyte

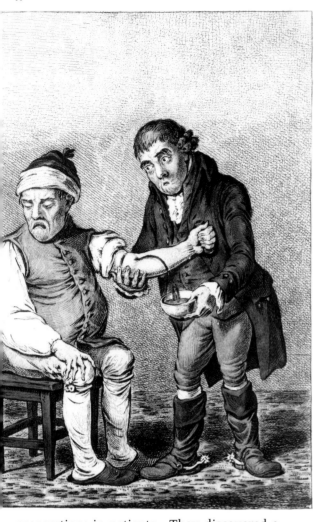

preparations in patients. They discovered a bacterium which needed the 'liver factor' as much as man. If no 'liver factor' was present the bacterium failed to grow; if it was present the bacterium flourished. Indeed, its growth was in proportion to the amount of 'liver factor' supplied. Eventually both groups isolated a red compound which they named vitamin B_{12} or cyanocobalamin. The red color was due to the metal cobalt, of which one atom was present in the center of each molecule. This pure substance, vitamin B_{12}, is used in the treatment of pernicious anemia today.

A spin-off from this research helped animal farmers. In many countries there was a wasting disease of sheep called 'pining'. This, too, was cured by vitamin B_{12}, because pining arises when sheep are grazed on cobalt-deficient pastures and their gut bacteria cannot make the vitamin. Spraying the fields from helicopters with cobalt salts prevents the disease.

While the research was continuing on the isolation of liver factor, other scientists were seeking an explanation of why some people developed a deficiency of vitamin B_{12}. Much of this work was carried out at the Thorndyke Laboratory in Boston by a group headed by Dr William B. Castle.

In 1860, a distinguished English physician,

Dr Austin Flint, had said 'I suspect, that in these cases, there exists degenerative disease . . . of the stomach. . . . I shall be ready to claim the merit of this idea when difficult and laborious researches of someone have shown it to be correct.' How right he was.

It was known that the stomach juices in pernicious anemia were subnormal. Normal gastric juice is acid, because of a considerable content of hydrochloric acid, but in pernicious anemia the gastric juice lacks acid and is neutral. Getting the pernicious anemia patient to drink dilute acid did not correct the anemia. Dr Castle and his colleagues swallowed raw minced beef, regurgitated it after a short period, and then introduced it via a tube into the stomach of pernicious anemia patients. They did this every day, and the results showed that while raw beef alone had no beneficial effect on pernicious anemia patients, raw beef regurgitated from a normal stomach produced a dramatic improvement in the patient's blood. Something in normal gastric juice was needed to prevent this anemia.

In this way, Castle showed that there was a protein substance present in normal gastric juice which is essential for the absorption of vitamin B_{12} from food, and that this factor was missing in pernicious anemia. This protein, christened 'intrinsic factor', was thus the key to the cause of pernicious anemia. The once fatal disease, now understood, is dealt with today by regular injections of vitamin B_{12} directly into the body. As with some other failures of absorption, our understanding of the cause of the disease is not matched by an ability to treat it at this level, but we are nevertheless able to bypass the defective absorption step.

Blood transfusions and the Rh (Rhesus) factor. Since 1900 it has been known that blood plasma often contains an antibody that makes the red blood cells from another person clump together or agglutinate. Someone whose red blood cells are of Group A has a plasma factor causing agglutination of Group B blood, and vice versa. In this way four blood group systems were recognized: A, B, AB and O.

Red Cells	Plasma
Group O	Anti A and Anti B
Group A	Anti B
Group B	Anti A
Group AB	Nil

But another breakthrough in blood groups came 40 years later. The Americans Karl Landsteiner and A. S. Wiener injected blood cells from rhesus monkeys into rabbits, which naturally made an antibody against the rhesus monkey blood cells. Now, when rabbit serum containing this antibody was tested on human

82 This picture has been prepared from normal human blood to which pathogenic bacteria have been added. Cells called neutrophil polymorphs have ingested these bacteria. The cell to the left of the picture is such a cell with a clump of dark-stained bacteria in the cytoplasm (the material composing the substance of the cell). There are no bacteria left free in the blood plasma. Enzymes within this white blood cell will kill the bacteria. To the right of the picture is a lymphocyte. The remaining cells are red blood cells. In addition a platelet is seen as a small speck near the bottom of the picture, about the middle. The magnification is about 3,000 times.

83, 84 The blood of a person with pernicious anemia compared with normal blood. 83 shows a normal blood film at a magnification of about 1,000. The red cells appear as uniform round rings. 84 shows the appearance of the blood taken from the patient with pernicious anemia. There is much more variation in the size and shape of the red blood cells, but many of them are oval in shape and larger than the cells from normal blood. In addition there are far fewer red cells in the anemic blood than in the normal blood.

85 A diagram showing a megakaryocyte, one of the giant cells in the marrow which are responsible for the production of platelets. Unlike most cells, this cell has up to sixteen nuclei (four are shown in this example). Platelets are formed by the shedding of fragments of the surface of the cell cytoplasm. Each megakaryocyte gives rise to about four thousand platelets before it reaches the end of its normal lifespan. Platelets are concerned with the normal process of blood clotting.

86 An 18th century print showing a doctor who has obviously just dismounted from his horse (and probably not washed his hands) carrying out a phlebotomy. Today this procedure is only rarely carried out with therapeutic intent, either to relieve stress on the heart, or to relieve symptoms in patients who have too much blood (polycythemia). Modern blood donors are bled under somewhat different conditions, as well as for a different purpose. Sets for removing the blood are designed so that the blood does not come into contact with air during its collection. The blood can be used as such, or it can be processed, still in an enclosed system, to take off red cells, platelets, plasma, or particular plasma proteins such as those required to treat hemophiliacs.

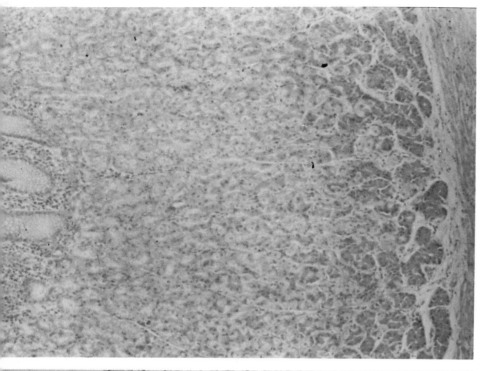

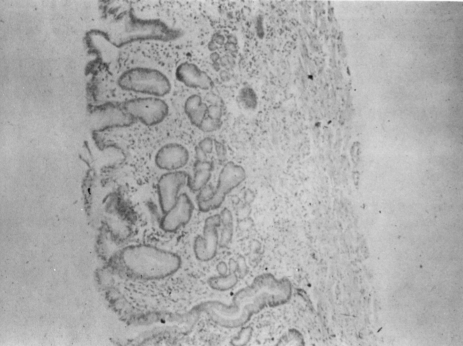

87, 88 87 shows a section through a piece of material from a normal stomach (magnification about 200), made up of a mass of cells which secrete the gastric juice. This consists of a solution of hydrochloric acid, enzymes that split proteins, and 'intrinsic factor', a protein essential to the absorption of vitamin B_{12}. B_{12} is present in liver and was shown by William B. Castle and his group to be the curative factor in pernicious anemia. 88 shows a similar piece of material obtained from the stomach of a patient with pernicious anemia. The stomach is much thinner than normal because of the almost total disappearance of the secreting cells.

had reacted with the transfused husband's red blood cells. They suggested that the link between husband and child was that the child had inherited a factor from the father (rhesus) which the mother lacked. For the antibody found in this woman's blood was the antirhesus factor.

It is now known that this state of affairs occurs when the mother lacks the rhesus blood factor (i.e. she is Rh-negative). The Rh-positive father passes on to the infant the rhesus factor. Small numbers of the developing baby's red cells escape into the mother's circulation. The mother responds to these 'foreign' blood cells by forming antibodies against them. Now the infant responsible for this initial stimulus to the mother's antibody mechanism is unaffected. But if the next baby is also Rh-positive, the already formed maternal antibodies will cross the placenta to the infant, attack his blood-forming cells and produce severe anemia. These events usually occur late in pregnancy and result in either a stillbirth or a very anemic, jaundiced infant. The situation can be anticipated by looking for rhesus antibody in the mother's blood during pregnancy. If this is present, the doctor is alerted to the possibility that the infant may be affected. A history of such an event in a previous pregnancy is of great importance.

Whether the infant is affected or not can also be gauged by looking at the amniotic fluid in which the developing baby lives while in the womb. Samples of this fluid can be simply and safely drawn off with a needle and syringe. If the infant's red cells are being destroyed by

blood, the red cells of most people were clumped by it, while about 20% were unaffected. The larger group we now call Rh-positive and the smaller group Rh-negative.

The vital application of these studies came from observations by Levine and his colleagues in the United States. In 1939 they found antibodies in the blood of a woman who had just given birth to a stillborn infant. They also knew that the woman had reacted violently to a transfusion of blood from her husband. In attempting to understand what was taking place, they suggested that the antibody in this woman's blood was directed against some tissue of her stillborn child, and perhaps the same antibody

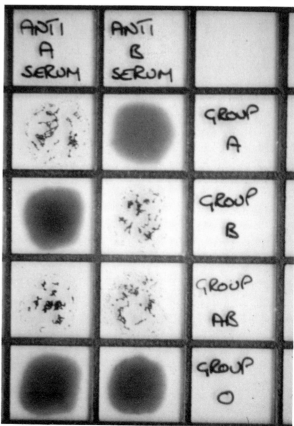

rhesus antibodies, an increase in the yellow substance (bilirubin) formed out of defunct hemoglobin is apparent in the amniotic fluid. This is a further indication that the infant is affected.

Since most of the damage is done in late pregnancy, the modern practice is to deliver these babies early, i.e. about a month before full term. The obstetrician needs very fine judgment since delivery too soon will produce a small infant with a poor chance of living and delivery too late may result in brain damage due to accumulation of the yellow bilirubin in the infant. Even after such an infant is born, a second major decision must be taken. All the infant's red cells are coated with the rhesus antibodies and are likely to be destroyed rapidly. This destruction would release harmful bilirubin which must at all costs be prevented from reaching high levels. So if this is likely to happen an exchange transfusion is carried out.

Progressively, over the course of a few hours, the infant's blood is removed and replaced by Rh-negative blood which cannot be attacked. Bearing in mind the small size of a baby's blood vessels, this is a very delicate procedure, often carried out under emergency conditions, but it has resulted in a dramatic decrease in the death rate of infants affected by rhesus antibodies.

A blood transfusion of cells that will not be damaged by the rhesus antibody can now be given when the infant, still in the womb, is severely affected. The blood is transfused directly into the unborn infant's abdominal cavity and finds its way into the circulation. If necessary, further transfusions can be given until the infant is large enough to be delivered.

At the same time as this momentous work was being done to save rhesus children, others were thinking how to prevent mothers at risk being sensitized in the first place. For all Rh-negative women with Rh-positive husbands are at risk. First, working on the old observation that the hemoglobin in fetal cells is more resistant to acids than adult hemoglobin, a technique was devised for demonstrating the presence of fetal blood cells in the mother's circulation: when blood containing a mixture of adult and fetal red cells was exposed to a weak acid, the adult hemoglobin was broken up but the fetal hemoglobin left intact. When the blood was then stained with a pink dye, the fetal cells took up the dye and were stained whereas the maternal red cells all appeared as poorly stained ghosts. With this simple method it was shown that some leak of blood from baby to mother was frequent not only during labor but during any procedure that disturbed the infant. The leak was very small—no more than 0·05 or 0·1 ml of blood.

Next, two groups of scientists, one in New York and the other in Liverpool, set out to see whether they could suppress sensitization in the Rh-negative woman by giving her a serum containing antirhesus. This would 'clump' the fetal cells and so hasten their removal from the circulation. Treatment of women at risk was preceded by experiments in Rh-negative male volunteers. (In America they were inmates of Sing Sing, while in the U.K. and Germany the volunteers were public-spirited men who had been rejected as blood donors for one reason or another.)

Some men were given small injections of Rh-positive red cells, and most of them produced antibodies. But when the Rh-positive red cells were injected along with an appropriate dose of antirhesus serum, no antibody formation took place. Thus the stage was set for a trial in women. Mothers known to have had a leak of infant's blood were alternately not given any special treatment—the customary treatment at the time— or given the new treatment, an injection of a concentrate containing antirhesus antibody. The mothers were followed to see if they became sensitized to the rhesus factor. Of 176 mothers not given any treatment, 38 became sensitized, but of 173 given the antiserum, only one became sensitized. These results have since been confirmed many times and it is now standard practice to give all Rh-negative women a dose of antirhesus serum after delivery. In this way doctors hope largely to eliminate the once-fatal hemolytic disease of the newborn. This is a good example of a clinical trial comparing an 'old' and a 'new' treatment. It would be wrong to try out a new treatment on all patients initially, since its benefits could not be assessed and it might even be harmful. Conversely, it would be wrong to deny everyone the potential benefit of the

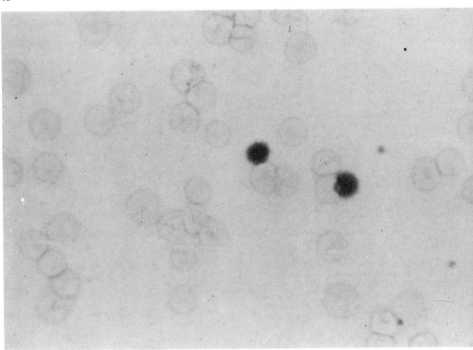

89 A typical experiment to show the effect of blood grouping sera on blood taken from people with the four common groups. A suspension of red cells has been placed on a glass tile and mixed with a drop of blood grouping serum (Anti A or Anti B). These blood grouping sera are obtained from normal blood donors, Anti A from a Group B person, and Anti B from a Group A person (see table in text). The photograph was taken 90 seconds after the addition of the antiserum. In the top line the Anti A serum has agglutinated the Group A cells. These cells were not affected by the Anti B serum. The Group B blood cells were unaffected by the Anti A serum but strongly agglutinated by the Anti B serum. The Group AB red blood cells were strongly agglutinated by both antisera. The common Group O red blood cells were not clumped by either.

90 Fetal hemoglobin withstands treatment with acids and alkalis more readily than does adult hemoglobin. This fact is used in demonstrating the presence of small numbers of fetal red cells that may have passed into the maternal circulation. The illustration shows a maternal blood film made after delivery. It has been exposed to weak acid and then stained. The weak acid has destroyed the hemoglobin in the maternal red cells, and the empty red cell envelope can still be seen. Two fetal red cells which have withstood this treatment and taken up the stain are shown in this illustration. This demonstration is important when the mother is Rh-negative. Should the fetal cells be Rh-positive the mother might form rhesus antibodies which could then harm the next fetus if it too inherited Rh-positive cells from the father.

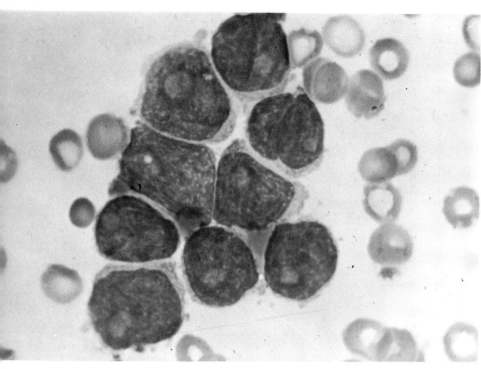

91 A clump of leukemic cells magnified one thousand fold from the blood of an affected child. The pale area in the nucleus of each cell, the nucleolus, is frequently seen in primitive blood cells, of which the leukemic cell is one example. These leukemic cells proliferate in the bone marrow in an uncontrolled manner and escape into the blood and other tissues. The other, smaller cells are red blood cells.

treatment. The treatment of alternate cases with the old and the new treatments is the only practical way to resolve the dilemma.

Acute leukemia. Leukemia is a 'cancer' of blood-forming cells. Unless treated it can be fatal within months of diagnosis. It involves an uncontrolled excessive growth of bone marrow cells which do not mature into proper blood cells capable of oxygen transport, body defense or control of bleeding. Because of a paucity of functional blood cells, patients are anemic and prone to infection (which can be fatal) and to disastrous hemorrhages.

The most common age group for acute leukemia is the first five years of life; and happily it is in this group that treatment has made the greatest progress. Some improvement has also been made in management of the disease in adults, but so far this is chiefly a prolongation of survival rather than a cure.

A large part—though not all—of the progress in the treatment of leukemia is due to the pharmaceutical industry's discovery of effective new drugs. Considerable effort has been spent in seeking the best way of using these new drugs to achieve maximum effect. Most of them are cell-killers that are slightly more lethal to leukemic cells than to normal cells. The use of such drugs requires both judgment and experience. Most of them interfere with the processes by which cells divide and reproduce themselves. Others, such as asparaginase, remove a building material that is needed by leukemic cells to make protein. (In this case the material is the amino acid asparagine, which normal cells generally do not need.)

The origins of antileukemic drugs are diverse: some are products of the skill of the organic chemist; others are extracted from plants—such as the blue periwinkle (vinca) which yields vincristine; and others are extracted from molds or bacteria.

In addition to the availability of drugs and better understanding of how they should be used, the success achieved recently in childhood leukemia is related to vast improvement in supportive measures. There has been much debate about whether leukemia has increased in recent years. Certainly many more cases are diagnosed, but probably some leukemic children in the past were killed by infections to which they were very susceptible without the underlying leukemia being suspected. Antibiotics like penicillin now overcome these infections and also enable doctors to deal with dangerous infections during the course of treatment. Another major source of support is the blood transfusion service: severe anemia can be rapidly reversed by transfused red cells and problems of bleeding by transfused platelets. Even transfusion of white blood cells is now a regular possibility.

A vital factor in the successful treatment of childhood leukemia is the availability of two drugs that are unusual in their lack of toxicity to the patient: synthetic cortico-steroids (see chapter 3) and vincristine. When given together, these cause a rapid disappearance of the leukemic process in most children and a return to apparent normality. However, if nothing more is done the disease will return within months.

Leading from this, the use of many combinations of drugs has been explored—with careful and methodical variations in the combinations and the timing. Are results better if drugs A and B are given daily, or once weekly, or for a whole week followed by a whole week off? What is the best dose of drugs A and B? Is the combination A and B better than A and C, and what about A, B and C together?

Unfortunately, these questions can only be answered in trials on patients with leukemia, although animals with the disease are used in preliminary studies. And since no single doctor sees enough patients to answer the questions by himself, international co-operative trials have been carried out, comparing various ways of using the drugs systematically. As soon as one combination proved superior the schedules were adjusted. Hence better understanding of the management of leukemia has brought longer and longer survival to such children, who were leading normal lives at school and at play during treatment.

Patients and doctors were encouraged to see children surviving a disease that was once fatal within weeks. Leukemia was being brought under control. Was eradication and cure possible?

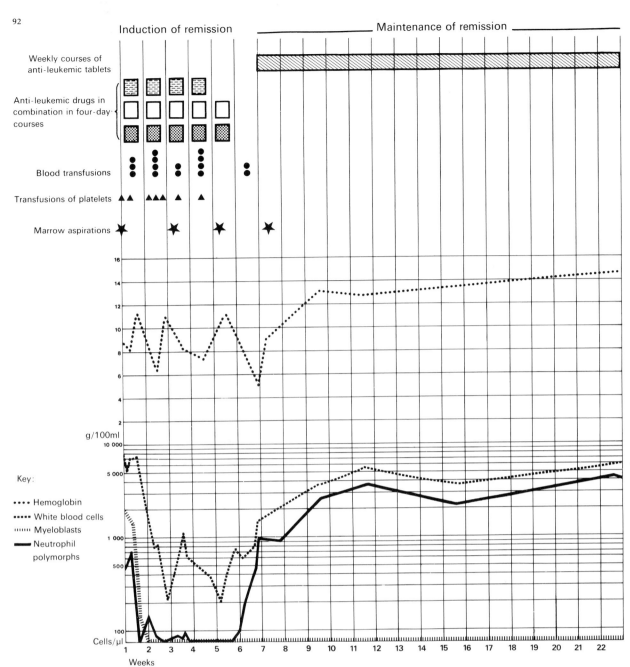

Induction of remission — Maintenance of remission

Weekly courses of anti-leukemic tablets

Anti-leukemic drugs in combination in four-day courses

Blood transfusions

Transfusions of platelets

Marrow aspirations

g/100ml

Key:

•••• Hemoglobin
▪▪▪▪ White blood cells
⁞⁞⁞⁞ Myeloblasts
—— Neutrophil polymorphs

Cells/µl

Weeks

1 2 3 4 5 6 7 8 9 10 11 12 13 14 15 16 17 18 19 20 21 22

Most centers looking after numbers of leukemic children in recent years had one or two children who did so well that after eight or ten years there was no evidence of the disease. This was rare, but it did indicate that at least in some children the disease had been cured. If there was a cure in some children, why did most relapse? Where were the surviving leukemic cells lurking? The answer to the last question lay in observation of the children. It was noted that some who did well as far as the blood was concerned showed evidence of relapse in the nervous system. The brain and spinal cord are wrapped in membranes within the skull and backbone and are surrounded by a clear fluid derived from blood. In effect the nervous system is insulated from the rest of the body, which means that drugs do not easily reach the nervous system from the blood. It was clear that leukemic cells were surviving behind this barrier when they had been eradicated elsewhere.

To deal with this problem, radiotherapy specialists were called in. They subjected the skull and backbone to carefully controlled amounts of radiation so that all leukemic tissue in the brain and spinal cord was eliminated.

When all these methods were brought into use—drugs, support and irradiation—leukemia was eradicated from half of all children with the disease. Furthermore, when after three years all treatment was stopped, the children continued to remain free of disease.

It is now possible to speak of a cure of leukemia in a substantial number of children.

Blood clotting. Complex mechanisms change fluid blood into a solid clot to prevent its loss from damaged tissue. Many biochemical reactions are involved, each one triggering off the next in a stepwise manner and eventually leading to the release of an enzyme which causes a soluble

92 This diagram records the treatment and progress to recovery of a 15-year-old girl with leukemia. The course of treatment extends over several months. The graph refers to the changes in her blood as treatment removes evidence of leukemia and restores the blood to normal.

At the time of diagnosis the patient was anemic (hemoglobin 9 grams per 100 millilitres of blood instead of a normal value of 13 g). Although the total number of white cells was normal (8,000 cells/µl: normal 4,000-11,000), the type of cell was abnormal, the predominant cell being the leukemic cell called a myeloblast or blast cell. The number of the white blood cells that normally combat infection (neutrophil polymorphs) is below normal (500 cells/µl: normal 2,000-8,000). The marrow, where the blood is normally made, aspirated with a needle, confirmed the presence of leukemia.

A series of 4-day courses during which antileukemic drugs were given was started. This phase is called the 'Induction of Remission' phase. A 4 to 5 day gap is allowed between courses. At the same time blood was given (15 pints over 6 weeks) and platelets (which prevent bleeding) collected from a total of 70 blood donors over this period.

With this treatment leukemic cells disappeared from the blood as shown by the rapid decline in the first week. At the same time the normal neutrophils disappeared because of the toxic action of the drugs on blood-forming cells. The marrow after 7 weeks showed no evidence of leukemia. Restoration of normal blood formation is shown by the return of a normal white cell count. The hemoglobin level is maintained after the seventh week without transfusion. The patient was discharged from hospital and returned to school. Maintenance of remission was achieved by a weekly course of antileukemic tablets.

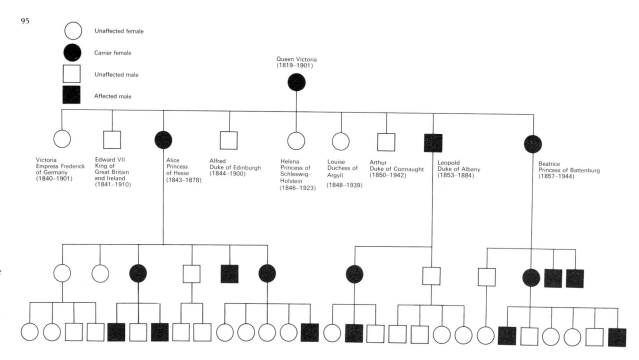

Unaffected female

Carrier female

Unaffected male

Affected male

Queen Victoria
(1819–1901)

Victoria
Empress Frederick
of Germany
(1840–1901)

Edward VII
King of
Great Britain
and Ireland
(1841–1910)

Alice
Princess
of Hesse
(1843–1878)

Alfred
Duke of Edinburgh
(1844–1900)

Helena
Princess of
Schleswig-
Holstein
(1846–1923)

Louise
Duchess of
Argyll
(1848–1939)

Arthur
Duke of Connaught
(1850–1942)

Leopold
Duke of Albany
(1853–1884)

Beatrice
Princess of Battenburg
(1857–1944)

93, 94 The drug Oncovin (vincristine) is an extract from the
familiar blue periwinkle.
Oncovin has been used in the
treatment of many forms of
cancer. One of its most valuable
applications is in the treatment
of acute leukemia in children.
The drug has a lethal effect on
some leukemic cells by interfering with certain phases of cell
division.

93

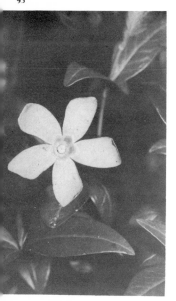

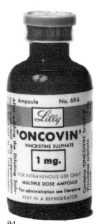

94

protein (fibrinogen) to form into a meshwork of
threads (fibrin) and thereby seal off the damaged
area. At the same time a different series of
substances exists to *prevent* clotting in undamaged
vessels—that is, to maintain the normal flow of
the blood; otherwise unwanted or even fatal clots
might form in normal blood vessels. When this
does happen, certain enzymes remove the clots
and restore the patency of blood vessels that
may have become blocked.

Part of our understanding of the complex
pattern of blood coagulation has come from
studying people who bleed excessively after the
most trivial injury, or even for no reason at all—
for example the condition called hemophilia.
Laboratory methods have been devised to find
out which of the essential blood coagulation
factors is lacking in a particular patient, so that
a precise diagnosis is usually possible. As a
result, more precise methods to treat bleeding
episodes have emerged. Even more important,
doctors can often take special precautions
during essential surgery, when for example a
boy with hemophilia has acute appendicitis.

These bleeding disorders usually are inherited
and run in families, of which the royal families of
Europe are the most famous example. Queen
Victoria was a carrier, and the disease ran
through her children and grandchildren to affect
her great-grandson Alexis, heir to the last Czar of
Russia, Emperor Nicholas II. In hemophilia there
is a lack (or a non-functioning form) of a
coagulation factor called the antihemophilic
globulin or factor VIII. The disease occurs in
males, while daughters of a hemophiliac are
carriers of the gene, without actually suffering
the disease. It cannot be cured but factor VIII
can be given when required, to restore
coagulation to normal for a number of hours.

The factor has a half-life of only about eight
hours in the body and so has to be injected
directly into the bloodstream, so permanent
restoration is impossible. But when a patient has
bled, perhaps into a knee producing acute pain,
an injection of concentrated factor VIII restores
blood clotting to normal for several hours, with
dramatic relief of pain. The injections can be
continued for several weeks if necessary to cover
major surgery.

Once again the blood transfusion services are
the main sources of factor VIII. If plasma—the
fluid part of blood—is kept at about 4°C, some
proteins precipitate out of solution. If this
precipitate is collected—by spinning the plasma
in a centrifuge and transferring all but the solid
part at the bottom of the tube—the precipitate
represents a concentrate of antihemophilic
globulin. Because of its precipitation in the cold,
the material is called cryoprecipitate. Thus the
concentrated factor VIII from five litres of fresh
blood can be given to a patient quickly in a small
volume of fluid via a syringe, to build up a
concentration in his blood that is sufficient for
normal blood clotting.

Polycythemia. It is also possible to have too
much blood. People with the condition called
polycythemia are rather plethoric or red faced.
A very common symptom is an intense itching of
the skin aggravated by bathing. Too much blood
is often accompanied by high blood pressure,
headaches, and a tendency to thrombosis
(forming blood clots). For all these reasons
treatment of the condition is desirable to restore
the blood volume to normal.

In the first place, however, the doctor must
make sure that the increased amount of blood is
not just a compensation for disease elsewhere,
such as in the lungs or heart. For if oxygenation

of the blood is poor because not enough is being pumped into the lungs—as in heart disease, or because of disease in the lungs themselves—the bone marrow will respond by increasing the output of red blood cells in an attempt to pick up more oxygen. When the marrow is overactive for no good reason and is making too much blood, the process can be controlled by periodically withdrawing amounts of blood from a vein—old-fashioned phlebotomy or 'blood-letting'. Red cell production can also be diminished by the effect of various drugs on the bone marrow, or by irradiation of the tissue. Irradiation treatment consists of giving a measured amount of radioactive phosphate which gets incorporated into blood-forming cells and for a week or two produces local irradiation to damp down the rate of blood formation. The effects are seen over the next three months as the numbers of red cells, white cells and platelets slowly fall nearer to normal levels. The benefit may last for several years before another dose becomes necessary. In general, radiophosphorus is used in older people and other treatments in young people. All methods relieve the symptoms: headaches disappear, skin irritation declines and other complications are ameliorated.

Much remains to be discovered and new knowledge is continuously being gained from many directions. At the molecular level the functions of many blood components are being elucidated. For example, the complete three-dimensional structure of hemoglobin has been determined so that the position of each atom is known. Even the curious change in shape of the molecule as it takes up oxygen atoms has been demonstrated. Tiny changes in hemoglobin composition give rise to a wide variety of massive changes in structure and function, of which some have been known for years but others are relatively new, and which have explained the causes and suggested treatments for a number of human blood diseases (such as sickle cell disease).

The abnormal formation of antibodies against

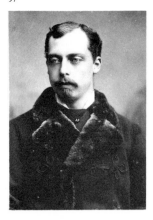

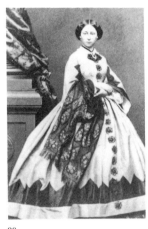

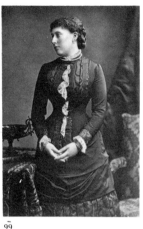

blood components represents another mechanism for the production of disease of the blood. These antibodies lead to clumping, abnormalities of function and even breakdown of the cells in the circulation. Methods of detecting antibodies formed against white cells, platelets and red cells are being developed. Further, the important question of why the body should start to make abnormal antibodies against its own tissues is the subject of active research by immunologists throughout the world.

Finally, the complex mechanism of blood clotting is being explored at molecular level and its understanding may help the control of arterial disease, which is one of the major killing diseases affecting modern man.

95-9 The bleeding disease hemophilia was present in the royal families of Europe in the 19th century and Queen Victoria (96) was a 'carrier' of the disease. Two of her daughters, Alice, Princess of Hesse, (98) and Beatrice, Princess of Battenberg, (99) were also 'carriers' but her son Leopold, Duke of Albany, (97) manifested the disease. The selective transmission of the disease to subsequent generations of Queen Victoria's descendants is shown in the diagram. The disease is not present in the British Royal Family since Edward VII did not inherit the abnormality and so was not affected. The gene for hemophilia is carried on the X chromosome, one of the sex-determining chromosomes (see illustration 211). There are two X chromosomes in the female and an X and a Y in the male. The gene for hemophilia is found on the X chromosome, but it is neutralized in the presence of a normal X chromosome. Since the abnormal gene is very rare it is therefore extremely unlikely that a woman will have two affected X chromosomes and so suffer from the disease. A woman with one affected X chromosome will, however, pass the gene to 50 per cent of her offspring. Daughters acquiring it will again be 'carriers', while sons to whom it is passed will have the disease. All the daughters of hemophiliac fathers must be carriers (the X he passes to them must be abnormal): all the sons must be spared.

6 Breathing and Health

There are five important diseases which occupy most of a chest physician's time: of these, two (pneumonia and tuberculosis) are caused by germs which are now easily controllable by antibiotic drugs; two (chronic bronchitis and lung cancer) are largely self-inflicted and virtually incurable; and the last (asthma) is an enigma more easily treatable than in the past but still posing many problems.

Besides the major advances in the antibiotic field which have substantially reduced the morbidity (discomfort, length of illness) of some chest diseases, improvements in X-ray and laboratory methods, with their greater availability, have brought earlier and more accurate diagnosis within the reach of most patients; while advances in anesthesia and blood transfusion have made major surgery of the chest much less risky.

In the U.K. respiratory disease accounts for nearly one quarter of all consultations in general practice, nearly one third of all absences from work, one quarter of deaths in males of all ages, and more than ten per cent of female deaths at all ages.

Pneumonia. This is an illness characterized by inflammation of the lung substance, due to infection by bacteria or viruses. The symptoms are usually those of fever, cough and phlegm, which may be bloodstained, some shortness of breath, and frequently pain over the affected area which is aggravated by deep breathing and coughing. The patient may be extremely ill, but in other cases the condition is comparatively mild with the patient walking into the consulting room. The diagnosis is made from the patient's account of his symptoms and from abnormal findings on examination such as crackles (crepitations) and sometimes a rubbing sound (pleural rub) over the affected area. Confirmation is by X-ray, the inflamed, solid area of lung throwing a shadow on the film. Bacteria may be grown on culture of the sputum (phlegm). This last investigation may be important because any germs grown can be tested for their sensitivity to different kinds of antibiotic. Those commonly found in this condition are pneumococci and staphylococci.

Before 1939, when sulfonamides became available, pneumonia claimed many victims, especially amongst the very young and the old. Since then penicillin, tetracycline, ampicillin (and the other new penicillins), the cephalosporins and the trimethoprim—sulfonamide combinations have all contributed to a decline in mortality from pneumonia. Gone are the days when one waited anxiously for the cyanosed, breathless, toxic patient to reach his 'crisis', the point when the body suddenly overcame the infection and with extraordinary rapidity it became clear that on this occasion at any rate the patient was going to recover. Now, with the appropriate antibiotic, improvement with settling of the fever is likely to occur within 48 hours, and it is unusual for anyone adequately treated to die of pneumonia. Failure to respond to treatment implies infection with an organism resistant to the antibiotic being used, in which case others may be tried and the sputum examined repeatedly to exclude tuberculosis. A partial failure of treatment is highly suspicious of underlying lung cancer. Virus pneumonias are not susceptible to treatment with antibiotics at present, but fortunately tend to be self-limiting and resolve spontaneously.

Tuberculosis. 'No patient should be regarded as cured of tuberculosis until he is safely dead of some other disease.' These words were written in 1930 by Dr R. C. Wingfield, the Medical Superintendent of the Brompton Hospital Sanatorium at Frimley, England, and remained

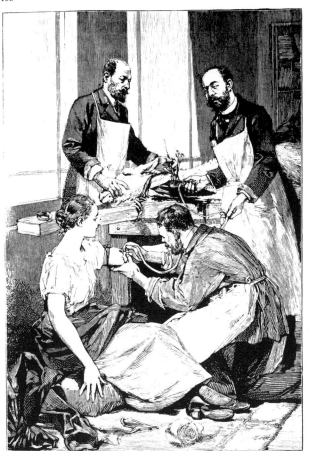

1895 was a further step in diagnosis, but there was no real treatment until the opening of sanatoria at the end of the 19th century, although Forlanini in Milan had initiated the first artificial pneumothorax in 1887. In London, the Royal Chest Hospital and the Brompton Hospital opened in 1814 and 1841 respectively but for many years housed their patients without really treating them. By 1900 advances in treatment had been made in these hospitals, and in this year the Trudeau Sanatorium in the Adirondacks was opened, followed by the Brompton Hospital Sanatorium at Frimley (1904), and the King Edward VII Sanatorium at Midhurst (1906). King Edward VII took a close personal interest in the building at Midhurst, and it is said that its beautiful site was chosen largely because it was near to the house of one of the King's mistresses. Swiss medicine had a corner in the treatment of tuberculosis in the first half of this century, for

basically true for the next 20 years. It is an index of the profound change which has occurred in the treatment and outlook of this disease since the early 1950s that such a sentence could not possibly be written today. Up to the introduction of satisfactory anti-tuberculous chemotherapy and B.C.G. vaccination, tuberculosis was a major scourge in all countries, and its control in the developed countries has been a considerable success story.

Caused by the mycobacterium tuberculosis (the tubercle bacillus), it is, in spite of the major improvements in treatment and prevention already mentioned, still the most important communicable disease now that malaria has been largely eliminated. It has been estimated that in the world there are ten to twelve million infectious cases of tuberculosis, and that approximately two million people die of it each year, the great majority of them in underdeveloped countries with inadequate medical services.

Tuberculosis is a disease of great antiquity, lesions having been found in Neolithic skeletons in Europe and in Egyptian mummies of 3700 B.C. In the 5th century B.C. Hippocrates described phthisis as a form of wasting due to ulceration of the lungs with cavity formation, and in 130 A.D. Galen considered it to be a contagious disease, but it was not until 1882 that Robert Koch identified the tubercle bacillus as the causative organism. The discovery of X-rays by Röntgen in

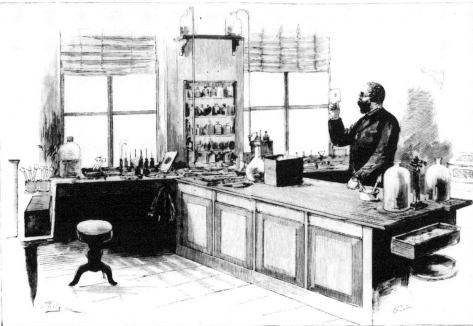

those who could afford the journey and the fees. The general regime appears to have been a mixture of rest and light activity in a beautiful climate with superb scenery.

At the Trudeau and at Midhurst the emphasis was on rest, followed by graded exercise, but at Frimley Marcus Paterson, a man of strong personality, introduced his regime of 'auto-inoculation' under which the patient was encouraged to take exercise to whip up his toxins, thereby stimulating his body's defenses against the disease. Fierce arguments were waged between the two schools of treatment, but in 1923 a carefully evaluated comparison of the results by Clive Rivière came down firmly on the side of rest as the regime of choice. From 1920 on, the artificial pneumothorax (temporary lung collapse) and thoracoplasty (permanent lung collapse by removal of parts of the upper 5-7 ribs

102 Many adults in the prime of their working lives were removed to a sanatorium for treatment of tuberculosis, like this one in the countryside near London. This fulfilled the dual function of ensuring optimal nutrition and hygiene and removing a source of contagion from the population. This sort of social isolation led to profound emotional responses in some patients, often wrongly attributed to the effects of the disease. These sanatoria, scattered throughout the western world, now lie empty or have been converted to other uses. Highly skilled centers of lung surgery often grew up around them and contributed greatly to advances in thoracic surgery whose benefits we continue to enjoy today.

103 The antibiotic streptomycin was isolated from a soil fungus, *Streptomyces griseus*, in 1944 by S. A. Waksman (1888-1973), a Russian who migrated to the United States as a young man. Since then many other anti-tuberculous drugs have been isolated or synthesized, a multiplicity of treatments which has been very valuable in meeting the problem of resistance to single antibiotics which emerges in the tubercle bacillus. Streptomycin and its successors offered the prospect of rapid eradication of infectious bacteria from the lungs of tuberculous patients and so greatly reduced the chance of infecting the innocent by-stander. These antituberculous remedies are also active against the non-pulmonary forms of the disease. Bone and joint tuberculosis accounted for many crippled youngsters. Much of this infection was transmitted in milk from tuberculous infection in cows. The eradication of bovine tuberculosis by herd control and by pasteurization of milk was the major contributor to control of the disease in humans.

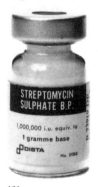

103

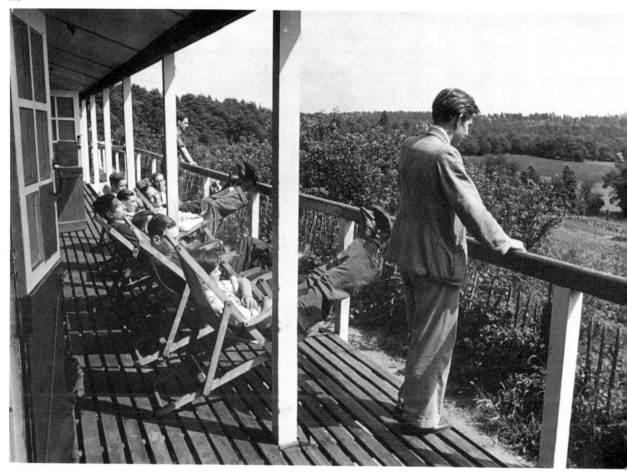

on the affected side) were developed and with bed-rest, fresh air and good food, were the main planks of treatment until the arrival of the anti-tuberculous drugs in the late 1940s.

There had been a steady fall in the tuberculosis death rate from the middle of the 19th century, due at first to better hygiene (housing, sanitation, and improvement in diet) and later to more rational treatment with rest and collapse therapy, coupled with earlier and more accurate diagnosis due to the development of diagnostic X-rays. But the real decline came with chemotherapy, especially with long-term treatment with at least two anti-tuberculous drugs which was developed in the 1950s. This revolution in treatment started with the discovery of streptomycin in the U.S. by Selman Waksman in 1944, and the proof of its effectiveness by clinical studies of Hinshaw and Feldman the following year. In 1946 Lehmann reported from Sweden the discovery of para-amino-salicylic acid, and in 1952 came the independent announcement by Fox in the U.S. and a group in Germany of the anti-tuberculous properties of iso-nicotinic acid hydrazide, isoniazid. For many years these have been the standard 'first-line' drugs, but gradually other effective drugs have been discovered and developed, such as pyrazinamide, prothionamide, rifampicin and ethambutol.

From the beginning anti-tuberculous drugs were subjected to clinical trials by the Medical

Research Council in Britain, and by the Veterans' Administration in the U.S.A., and early on it was discovered that using the drugs singly (at the time only streptomycin and P.A.S.) resulted in drug-resistant tubercle bacilli emerging after one to two months. Giving the drugs in combination prevents this drug resistance and it has for many years been standard practice to give three drugs initially (this takes care of the possibility that the patient's bacilli may be initially or primarily resistant to one of the drugs), for a period of at least three months until the results of sensitivity tests are known. Duration of treatment with drugs was originally in two to three month courses, usually in hospital, but during the 1950s it became clear that more prolonged courses, continuing after the patient's discharge from hospital, were much more effective in preventing relapses, and for the past 10 to 12 years two year courses using at least two drugs have become the norm. This is logical, as tuberculosis is a slow disease to heal and it would seem correct to continue treatment as long as the healing process continues. Certainly the results have been excellent, and it is unusual for relapses to occur if the patient has had a standard two year course with at least two drugs, provided that they have been taken regularly. Now that there is a range of drugs to choose from it is uncommon for treatment to be seriously disrupted by side-effects and with careful supervision of treatment the emergence of drug-resistant organisms can nearly always be prevented.

One important benefit of long-term drug treatment is the shorter time that the patient needs to spend in hospital and his much more rapid return to work. Surgical treatment is almost never necessary and the patient becomes quite quickly non-infectious so that the risk of spread to others is greatly reduced. Many patients fortunate enough to be picked up early with only small to moderate amounts of disease can be safely treated at home, and often do not even have to stop work. Similar treatment gives, on the whole, equally good results with tuberculosis affecting other parts of the body, e.g. the coverings of the brain (meningitis), the genito-urinary system, and the neck glands.

Coupled with chemotherapy as an important factor in the control of tuberculosis is B.C.G. vaccination. This stands for 'Bacille-Calmette-Guerain', which was originally a bovine strain of tuberculosis grown in the laboratory by these French workers for many years so that it gradually lost its virulence for both cattle and human beings. It was first used, by mouth, in infants in France in 1922 but its popularity received a setback in the Lübeck disaster of 1930 when contamination of a vaccine with virulent tubercle bacilli led to the death of a large number of infants in Germany. Since then the vaccine has always been prepared in special laboratories under very strict control.

The principle of B.C.G. vaccination is similar to that of smallpox vaccination, i.e. an artificially produced lesion due to a non-virulent organism raising the body's resistance to a subsequent infection with a virulent organism. B.C.G. is only given to those reacting negatively to the tuberculin test, i.e. non-infected individuals. Its efficacy has been shown by the work of Aronson and his wife on North American Indians which showed a high degree of protection, lasting over 20 years; similar results were achieved by Rosenthal and his colleagues in Chicago infants (1937-1948), and in the British Medical Research Council trial on 56,000 urban school leavers (1950-1952). A U.S. Public Health Service trial, in Puerto Rico and the southern states (1958 and 1966), showed less good results, the cause of which is not clear, but B.C.G. is generally accepted now as an important factor in the control and eventual eradication of tuberculosis. In the U.K., all school leavers and those at special risk (e.g. contacts of known cases, nurses, doctors, etc.) are vaccinated, but there is no comparable program in the U.S.A. In the underdeveloped countries B.C.G. has been found to be one of the cheapest and most effective methods of tuberculosis control.

Mass miniature radiography, i.e. the X-raying of large numbers of apparently healthy people,

has in the past been important in bringing to light cases of tuberculosis in an early and eminently treatable stage, but with the measure of control achieved by long-term chemotherapy and B.C.G. vaccination its value has now declined. But static camera units in hospitals and chest clinics have still an important part to play in making chest films easily available to the general public and their family doctors. Only by picking up cases early, before they become infectious, and treating them adequately, will the reservoir

104

104 The mobile X-ray unit, though now largely superseded in many advanced countries, is still a valuable method of case-finding in the village settlements of Africa, in one of which this photograph was taken. Tuberculosis in under-developed areas of the world has not yet been eradicated and remains not only a serious source of disease and death for them, but also a reservoir of infection which may be readily communicated to disease-free populations.

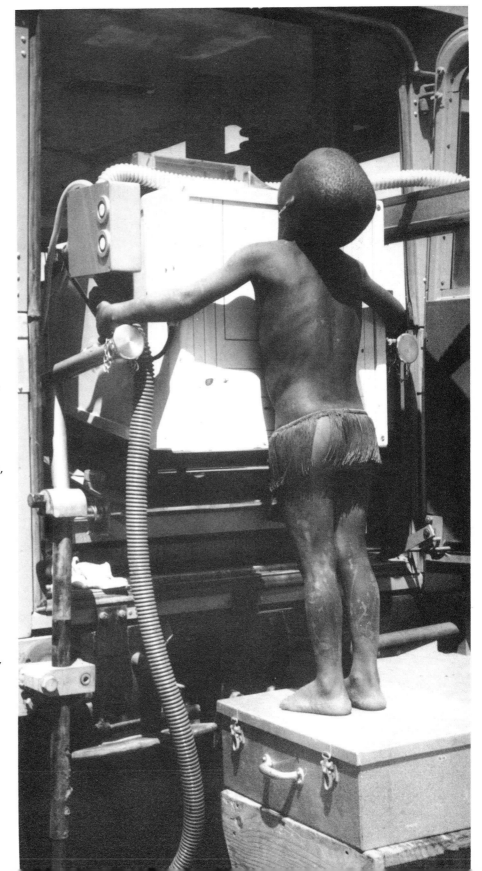

105 The poet John Keats (1795-1821) reflected the romantic image of the consumptive genius. His death from tuberculosis at an early age robbed the world of a remarkable talent; but he was not alone and the disease laid waste too many promising young lives. Ironically, it was his mother's death from tuberculosis which led Keats to seek to become a physician. One can only guess at the influence of the infection, with its fever and poisoning of the blood, on the flights of imagination so eloquently immortalized in his verse.

106 The lung is the organ of gas exchange. The blood coursing through it is brought into close contact with external atmospheric air, from which it extracts oxygen, and into which it discharges carbon dioxide. The diagrams show the gross anatomy of the lung (A), progressively magnified to show the fine terminal ramifications of the airway (B) and then the gas exchange surface (C) where an interlacing network of blood capillaries is separated from air by a very fine membrane. D represents diagrammatically the passage of blood cells through the capillaries. The de-oxygenated cells (white) take on their charge of oxygen (black) and pass back to the heart for re-distribution to the tissues of the body. The remarkable molecule, hemoglobin, responsible for this oxygen carriage has been subjected to very close study. The working out by F. Perutz and his colleagues in Cambridge of its three-dimensional structure has provided totally new insights into normal biological mechanisms and also explained the inherited disorder of sickle-cell disease.

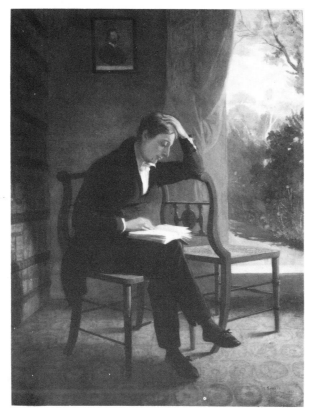

of infection be steadily reduced. These measures, combined with good nutrition and housing (prevention of overcrowding), the checking of contacts of known cases, and B.C.G. vaccination, are all necessary for the final eradication of tuberculosis. The bovine type is rare now, both in the U.S.A. and in the U.K., thanks to tuberculin-testing of cattle and the slaughter of positive reactors, coupled with pasteurization of milk. Between 1917 and 1940 in the U.S.A. 280 million cattle were tuberculin tested and 4 million positive reactors were slaughtered. The cost of this was 260 million dollars and the savings to agriculture were estimated to be 300 million dollars for each subsequent decade, quite apart from the benefit to the nation's health. Eradication of the human variety will be less easy but must energetically be pursued, for what a triumph that would be! 'There has never been much mystery about tuberculosis, except the mystery of why we have allowed it to remain with us for so long' (G. T. Stewart of Glasgow, 1969).

It is an interesting fact that many eminent literary figures have suffered from tuberculosis, for example Keats, the Brontes, D. H. Lawrence, and George Orwell; a tradition which was exploited by Bernard Shaw in *The Doctor's Dilemma* (1906), in which he also had a great deal of fun at the expense of the medical profession, guying at once the rigidity of approach and the multiplicity of 'cures' so characteristic of the period. In 1948 Betty (*The Egg and I*) McDonald published an account of life in a state sanatorium, *The Plague and I*, an interesting social document which amusingly

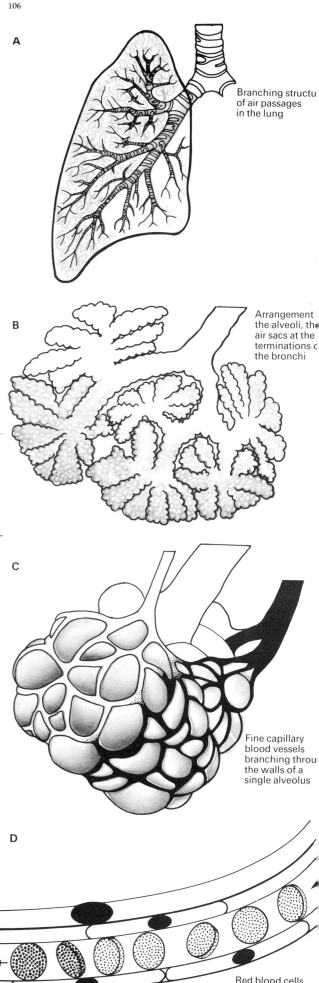

A   Branching structu of air passages in the lung

B   Arrangement the alveoli, th air sacs at the terminations c the bronchi

C   Fine capillary blood vessels branching throu the walls of a single alveolus

D   Red blood cells picking up oxygen as they pass throu the alveolar capilla describes the rigid regime considered necessary to restore patients to health in the pre-chemotherapy era.

Bronchitis. Acute bronchitis is inflammation of the larger bronchi or air tubes, caused by bacterial infection, commonly complicating influenza, the common cold, measles, whooping cough and, most importantly, chronic bronchitis. There is usually little difficulty in treatment with the range of antibiotics currently available, but if untreated it may progress to bronchopneumonia.

Chronic bronchitis. Chronic bronchitis is the term applied to the condition of patients who cough up phlegm on most days for at least three consecutive months in the year, excluding other causes such as tuberculosis. The condition usually starts with a slight morning cough associated with smoking, and gradually progresses with increasing cough and shortness of breath until there is serious interference with the enjoyment of life. Ultimately the patient becomes a respiratory invalid, balanced on a knife-edge between comparative well-being and severe illness, the latter being all too easily precipitated by infection, viral or bacterial, producing the dangerous state of respiratory failure. It is commoner in men, and mainly in those over forty.

Emphysema. Emphysema is a condition of the lung characterized by increase beyond the normal in the size of the air spaces (alveoli) beyond the final divisions of the bronchi, either from distension or from destruction of their walls. This results in a decrease in the surface area available for the interchange of oxygen and carbon dioxide between the air in the alveoli and the blood vessels (capillaries) in their walls, with a loss of elasticity in the lung tissue which gradually produces increasing shortness of breath. The cause of emphysema is not known but it may be due to an inborn error of metabolism. It may occur alone but much more commonly is associated with chronic bronchitis. Important joint studies by Burrows, Niden, Fletcher and Jones in Chicago and London in the mid-1960s did much to elucidate the respective roles of chronic bronchitis and emphysema in the development of airway obstruction in these patients.

The causes of chronic bronchitis are cigarette smoking, atmospheric pollution and infection. It seems that where individuals are exposed to both of the first two factors (including industrial fumes and dusts) the effects are likely to be particularly severe. The initial irritation of the bronchi stimulates a flow of mucus from glands in their walls, producing the cough and phlegm so characteristic of the disease. Infection of the mucus produces the attacks of acute bronchitis which are more an aggravating factor than an initial cause. They do, however, produce in the

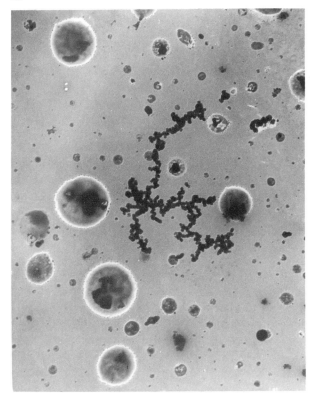

long run a good deal of damage to the lung tissue.

There have been several well-documented surveys showing that chronic bronchitis is almost confined to smokers, and that the death rate for chronic bronchitis is significantly higher in cigarette smokers than in non-smokers, and increases with the amount smoked. It has been found that cigarette smoking causes narrowing of the bronchi, thus increasing the effort needed to breathe. The respiratory tract is kept clear by the action of hair-like projections (cilia) attached to the cells lining the bronchial tree: these sweep mucus and particles upwards from the depths of the lungs and this action is inhibited by cigarette smoking. The failure of this mechanism leads to more frequent chest infections.

With regard to atmospheric pollution it has been shown that there is an increasing prevalence and mortality in chronic bronchitis with increasing urbanization; mortality is especially severe with seasonal peaks of fog, and exacerbations are closely correlated with increases in sulfur dioxide and smoke in the atmosphere. For example, two great smogs occurred in London in 1952 and 1962, both associated with increased death rates from chronic bronchitis, the mortality being much higher in 1952 before the passing of the Clean Air Act in 1954.

There is little evidence that infection is an initial cause of chronic bronchitis; 'chesty' children do not necessarily develop the disease in later life and probably do not have a greater predisposition to it than normal children. Exacerbations are usually associated with infections, upper respiratory infections (colds) nearly always descending to the bronchi and

107 If 'clean water' was the cry of the last century, then 'clean air' must be the call of this. A highly magnified sample (× 13,250) of material suspended in ordinary air and collected on to a thin copper film is shown in this photograph. The material consists of a mixture of spores, motor vehicle exhaust, fragments of vegetable fiber, and other unidentified flying objects. Fortunately the defense mechanisms of the lung are usually competent to protect against this aerial contamination, but even they may break down in time and this, with irritant gases, is responsible for the excess of chronic bronchitis in industrialized areas.

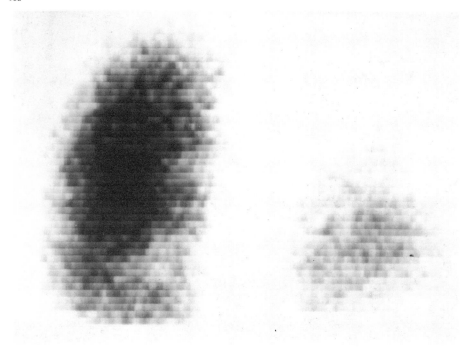

108 Circulation of blood through the lungs may be demonstrated by the injection of a radioactive emitter into the bloodstream. This is scanned as it circulates through the lungs by a rapidly moving detector rather like the scanner which produces the lines of which a television picture is built up. In the lung scan shown here, the dark emission pattern of the normal pulmonary circulation on the left contrasts markedly with the much less intense emission on the right, where the circulation has been obstructed by a clot in the main pulmonary artery supplying that side. Decreased blood flow also occurs in emphysema. Similar emission patterns may be recorded from the liver, the kidneys, the pancreas, and even the heart itself.

often the alveoli in these patients. Even with modern antibiotic drugs capable of clearing up bacterial infections rapidly, residual scarring tends to occur, and of course virus infections are unaffected by antibiotics and may take several weeks to clear completely in severe cases.

The interference with breathing in chronic bronchitis is due to generalized airways obstruction and the main factors causing this are mucus in the lumen of the bronchi, thickening of the mucous membrane lining the bronchi from chronic irritation and inflammation, and distortion of the airways by scarring and by emphysema. As the bronchi widen and lengthen on breathing in (inspiration), reversing the process on breathing out (expiration), it will be seen that increasing narrowing of the bronchi will eventually reach a stage where air flows in readily but may be trapped in the lungs on expiration. This produces impaired ventilation of the lungs, making breathing hard work and resulting in less perfect oxygenation of the blood than occurs normally. In many of these patients the interference with breathing is so severe that they cannot blow out a lighted match held a few inches from their mouths. In some cases bronchial narrowing is increased by wheezing (bronchospasm) which aggravates the situation. So, mucus produces cough and sputum, white or grey usually, yellow or green when infected; and airway obstruction plus emphysema produces shortness of breath. Increasing disability is commonly associated with rising levels of carbon dioxide in the blood producing cyanosis, until ultimately cardiac and/or respiratory failure supervene.

The term 'respiratory failure' implies that the lungs are not functioning adequately so that there is impaired gas exchange with a fall in oxygen

levels and a rise in carbon dioxide in the blood. Utlimately a stage of acute respiratory failure may be reached where the patient is cyanosed, drowsy and confused, with shallow breathing, ineffective cough, and high blood carbon dioxide levels. This is a dangerous state, necessitating hospitalization as deterioration may be very rapid. Expert nursing and physiotherapy to stimulate breathing and effective cough, oxygen, respiratory stimulants, antibiotics to combat infection, and treatment for the usually associated cardiac failure, are all essential for recovery. These measures usually produce improvement but it may occasionally be necessary to pass a tube into the trachea (windpipe), or do a tracheostomy, and connect the patient to a mechanical respirator. This treatment, involving as it does a good deal of discomfort, is only adopted if the ultimate outlook is fairly good with the prospect of a reasonably active life in the future.

How to prevent the disaster of increasing respiratory failure?

1. The patient must stop smoking.
2. Jobs should not if possible involve dust and fumes.
3. Weight must be reduced if necessary.
4. Wheezing must be treated with antispasmodic drugs such as salbutamol by tablet or inhaler.
5. Infections must be promptly controlled by antibiotics with the patient admitted to hospital if necessary.

Such measures, if strictly and conscientiously followed, will keep the majority of patients in a reasonable state of health for many years. They are the result of important surveys and investigations undertaken in the U.K. and the U.S.A. over the past 20 years, which have given not only a better understanding of the complexities of this condition but have also stimulated the public health authorities to demand better working conditions in factories, with adequate removal of noxious dusts and fumes, and improvements in housing especially concerned with dampness, warmth, and good ventilation.

The fact that atrocious living and working conditions have to a large extent been alleviated in the past 50 years underlines the importance of cigarette smoking as now the most important cause of this distressing condition. It is thus the first of the self-inflicted diseases to which reference was made at the beginning of this chapter.

Asthma. Asthma is an enigma: its causes are various and imperfectly understood, and cures are uncertain. It is characterized by paroxysms of shortness of breath and wheezing due to bronchial narrowing, which vary from mild to severe. It is slightly more prevalent in women than in men, tending to start at a younger age in the latter than in the former. There have been wide fluctuations in the mortality from asthma over the past 25 years, a marked fall in the 1950s due to the introduction of the steroid (cortisone) group of drugs being followed by a considerable rise in the late 1960s almost certainly due to over-use of inhalers containing isoprenaline. The death rate is now falling again.

The bronchial narrowing which can so severely interfere with respiration is caused by: contraction of bronchial muscle (bronchospasm); swelling (edema) of the mucous membrane lining the bronchi, due to allergy or infection; and plugging of the smaller bronchi with mucus, this last factor being encouraged if the patient is dehydrated.

What brings these mechanisms into action? Basically people wheeze for three reasons:

1. Allergy (hypersensitivity) to some external factor, e.g. grass pollen or house dust mite.
2. Infection by bacteria or viruses affecting the respiratory tract.
3. Psychological factors, e.g. tension, anxiety or depression. These are not often primary causes but frequently aggravate the condition.

There is also a small group who are sensitive to some dusts and fumes, e.g. toluene diisocyanate, used in the manufacture of plastics, volatile industrial glues, and enzyme material which is incorporated in some detergents. Such patients have no option but to cease contact with the offending material.

All of the three main factors mentioned above may operate in the same patient at different times, or occasionally at the same time. Thus asthma is what is called a 'multifactorial' illness, and this makes it essential that the physician should take a most careful history covering all possible causes of the patient's symptoms. It is now, since the control of tuberculosis, the greatest challenge in chest medicine in the developed countries. Great advances have been made in the past 25 years both in diagnosis and treatment, especially in the investigation and treatment of allergy, and drugs such as Intal and the steroids have revolutionized the outlook for many patients.

Allergy. Those patients in whom allergy is important will probably, though not invariably, be in the younger age range, say 10 to 30, may give a previous history of eczema or hay fever, and their symptoms will in many cases be seasonal, i.e. mainly in the pollen season, often accompanied by hay fever (running of the eyes and nose with sneezing). Grass is the main culprit here, causing symptoms especially in the months May to July in the U.K., but flower pollen and the spores of molds may also cause trouble. Sensitivity to grass is worse in hot, dry weather,

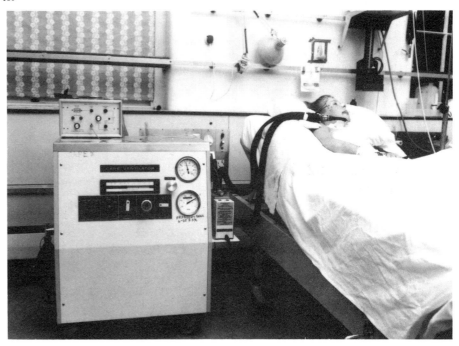

that to molds being worse when it is warm and humid. Pollen and spore counts are broadcast in America and Britain; these, referring as they do to a situation obtaining several hours before, are of little use to patients as a warning of a possible asthmatic attack, but they may help both patient and physician subsequently to track down the cause of such an attack.

Those whose symptoms are worse in the night and on waking are nearly all sensitive to house dust mite (*Dermatophagoides pteronyssinus*), the importance of which in asthma was discovered by Voorhorst and his colleagues in Holland in 1964. This microscopic mite is present in all samples of house dust and, as it lives largely off the scales of human skin, it is particularly common in the bedroom. We are shedding our outer layers of skin all the time, and whenever clothes are removed the room is showered with skin scales which also, during the hours of sleep, pass through the nightwear and bottom sheet into the underblanket and surface of the mattress. Here the mites thrive, and allergic subjects readily become sensitized to them.

Another allergic cause of wheezing is food, especially with small children who frequently have eczema as well, but occasionally this factor may operate later in life.

Skin testing may help to uncover suspected allergies, and the technique has been refined over the past 20 years largely through the work of Frankland and Pepys in the U.K. and Tuft in the U.S.A. Extracts are now available for testing patients against most substances which may cause allergic reactions but the ones used in any particular case depend on the history of the illness.

Once it has been established that allergy is a significant factor in the patient's asthma, the

109 A mechanical ventilator can take over the function of breathing when respiratory embarrassment is extreme and where asphyxia threatens the life of the patient. Often used during surgical anesthesia, this form of respiratory life support is now increasingly used in patients in whom the nervous control of breathing has failed or in those with such severe lung disease that the work of breathing is too much for them. Respiratory distress in the newborn, due to immaturity of the lung, previously often lethal, can now often be effectively treated with such a device and the baby tided over until the surface tension properties of the lung have developed adequately.

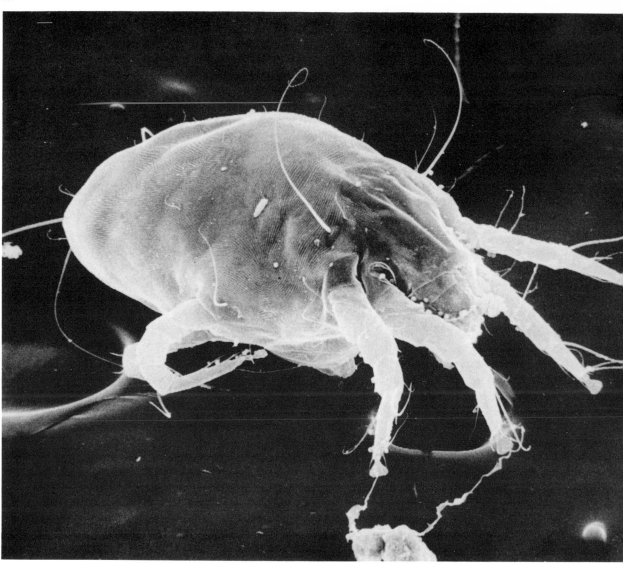

\110 The house dust mite, the tiny creature with the formidable name of *Dermatophagoides pteronyssinus* (shown here at 630 times magnification), is responsible for much allergic lung disease. The asthma that it may cause can often be cured by exercising strict dust control in the house, especially in the bedroom. Bedding may be thickly populated with these creatures and indeed it is surprising that so few people develop serious sensitization to them.

treatment consists of:

1. Removing contact with the offending material if possible, for example, dust control by vacuum-cleaning mattresses and pillows in house dust mite sensitization, or keeping off any article of food which is responsible for the symptoms.

2. Desensitization (hyposensitization) by giving weekly injections of gradually increasing concentrations of the allergen to which the patient is sensitive. Grass pollen sensitivity responds best to this treatment, with a success rate of about 75 per cent.

3. Intal (disodium cromoglycate). This interesting substance, discovered and first used by Roger Altounyan in the U.K. in 1967, is a powder which, when inhaled into the patient's bronchi, blocks the allergic reaction which occurs in the bronchial mucous membrane. It is particularly useful in cases where extrinsic allergens are inhaled from without, e.g. pollens, fungal spores, animal dander, or house dust mites. It is also useful in preventing wheezing due to exertion. It is *preventive* treatment and has to be taken regularly, the dose being adjusted to the smallest

quantity which will keep the patient well. It is a very great advance in treatment, but has also stimulated research into the mechanisms by which asthmatic wheezing is precipitated.

4. Bronchodilator drugs. These act by relaxing bronchial muscle and for many years the only drugs of this type available were adrenaline, given by inhalation (nasal spray) or by subcutaneous injection, and ephedrine which is given by mouth. They have over the past 20 years been replaced by more effective drugs, e.g. isoprenaline, orciprenaline, salbutamol and terbutaline. Isoprenaline is no longer in routine use because if over-used it can seriously affect the heart, causing abnormalities of rhythm, and it is almost certain that the increased mortality from asthma in the early 1960s was due to this drug. The other three drugs can be given by tablet or by inhalation and appear to be safe, especially if inhaler use is limited to four times in 24 hours. If not effective in this dosage medical advice is needed, as the patient will need other forms of treatment as a matter of some urgency.

5. Steroids (cortisone group of drugs). These are life-saving in the acute attack of asthma but have to

be given in adequate quantities both by mouth and by injection. They act to a large extent by decreasing the swelling of the bronchial mucous membrane caused by allergy (or infection), thus widening the air passages. They may also be essential in small doses as maintenance treatment to keep the patient free from symptoms. Because of side-effects the dosages are kept as low as possible. Prednisolone by mouth is the form generally used.

Infection. As a trigger for asthma, infection is more common in childhood and in middle age, but can affect any asthmatic. It is not usually, as far as is known, an allergic reaction to a specific infection, but the inflammation produced in the bronchial mucous membrane is sufficient to start off the asthmatic reaction in susceptible subjects. Certainly swelling will be present due to the infection, and this alone will produce some bronchial narrowing. This type of asthma is usually worse in the winter and is often associated with chest colds or bronchitis. The infection can be controlled by an appropriate antibiotic, but the patient may also need bronchodilators, and perhaps a short course of steroids as well.

Psychological factors. Many years ago Sir Arthur Hurst, the eminent Guy's Hospital physician, himself an asthmatic, used to teach that there is always an emotional factor in asthma. Few would quarrel with that dictum, for it is difficult to be dispassionate about one's own wheezing and the anxiety generated by an attack aggravates the situation in most cases. There is, however, the occasional patient whose symptoms are solely triggered by emotional causes, and sometimes by genuine depression. One survey has shown that a third of cases had stresses at the time of onset of their asthma which were significantly higher than those in a control group. These stresses included bereavement, threat to the security of a loved person, and family and marital problems. Marital disharmony covers a multitude of sins, but common complaints are of neglect of the spouse, especially by the husband ('He's always out at business/at the club/on the golf course.' 'He never talks to me.' 'He watches TV all the time.'), or of nagging of the spouse, especially by the wife of what she regards as an under-ambitious husband. Job and financial worries may cause stress and anxiety, as can concern about children, e.g. illness when they are small or at later ages trouble with the police. Over-protection is occasionally an important 'faulty parental attitude' conducive to the onset of asthma in a child, and antedates the first attack in some cases. Neglect is far less common, but rejection and/or lack of sensitivity to the child's plight can have devastating effects on an asthmatic child, and parental conflict is a potent source of tension throughout the family.

It is of course a great deal easier to identify difficulties and conflicts than to put them right. Simple explanation of the effects of conflict on asthma, whether of spouse or child, certainly helps but in most cases it is a question of working towards an adjustment by both parties to a difficult situation. With asthmatic children the basic need is for security, so that boosting the child's confidence is even more important than in adults. Parents must be helped to develop a sympathetically matter-of-fact attitude, encouraging the child to lead as normal a life as possible, and they must be taught exactly what to do in the event of an acute attack. This increases confidence all round and makes it less likely that the child will either exploit the parents' anxiety or be infected by it. Most asthmatic children lose their asthma as they grow older and this fact should be used to reassure parents.

Autohypnosis. Autohypnosis is an interesting form of treatment which was pioneered by Maher-Loughnan and Macdonald in London in 1959, and which is now used in other centers in the U.K. and in the U.S.A. It is essentially preventive and consists of teaching the patient to hypnotize himself for 15 minutes each day, to achieve a greater degree of mental and physical relaxation than is possible when fully conscious. The patient is taught this simple technique while hypnotized, and thereafter uses it on himself as a form of post-hypnotic suggestion. The importance of this treatment is that it is a form of self-help which works especially well where tension and anxiety are contributing significantly to the patient's symptoms.

The important thing in asthma is to *prevent* attacks of wheezing; it is not enough just to treat them as they arise. So causes must be energetically sought and all necessary forms of treatment employed to keep the patient well. All those mentioned above could be employed in any one patient at various times. We have moved on from the inhaler-dependent pigeon-chested patient of 30 years ago, even though some of our patients are steroid-dependent and perhaps moon-faced. Even though asthma cannot be cured, it can be controlled almost completely to enable the patient to lead a largely normal life. But what happens if the maintenance treatment breaks down and fails to control the patient's wheezing? The cardinal rule here is that large doses of steroids must be given both by mouth and by injection. If the attack is severe hospitalization becomes essential, as the patient needs expert nursing, an intravenous saline drip containing large amounts of hydrocortisone, oxygen, and possibly intratracheal intubation connected to a mechanical respirator to take the effort of breathing from the by now somewhat exhausted patient. This last measure can be

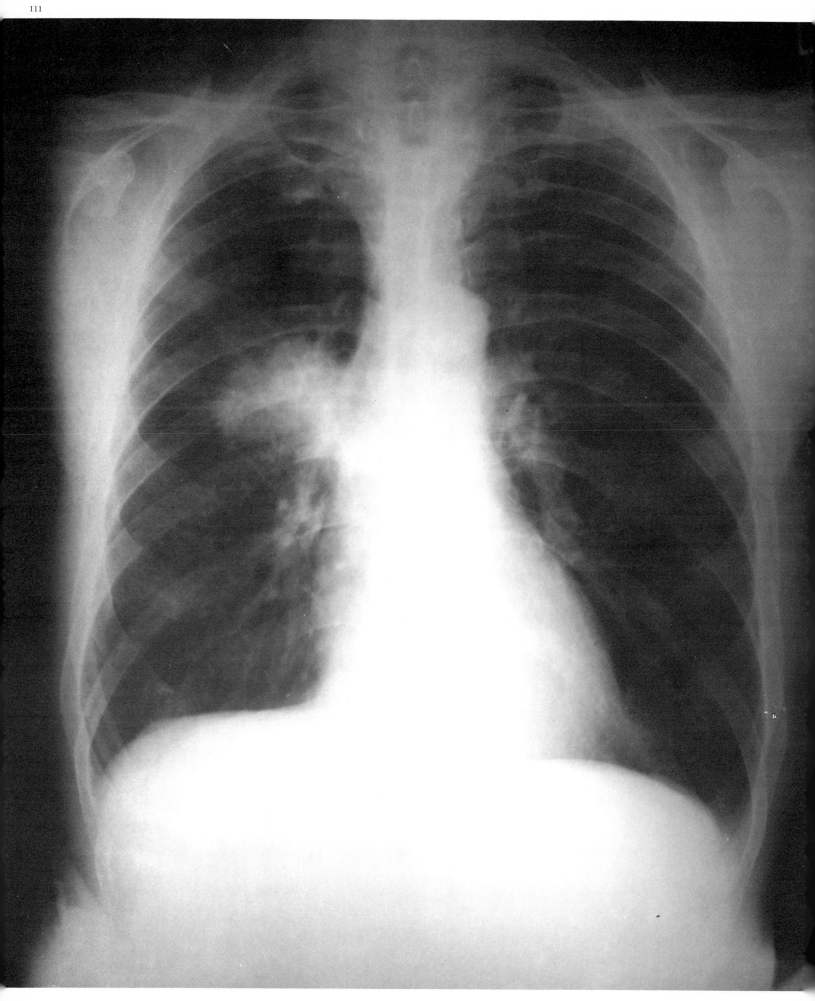

life-saving but is seldom needed if steroid treatment has been given early enough. No patient need die of asthma nowadays with all the facilities for treatment which are available but it is an illness where education of, and co-operation by, the patient are as essential as detailed and conscientious care by the physician.

Cancer of the lung. No up-to-date account of triumphs and less-than-triumphs in the treatment of chest-illness would be complete without some reference to the problems posed by cancer of the lung (carcinoma of bronchus). There has been a marked and steady rise in mortality from this disease over the past 30 years, greater in males than females, probably owing to the difference in smoking habits. Britain has the highest death rate from this disease, almost certainly due to very high cigarette consumption, and perhaps atmospheric pollution. The rate in the U.S.A. is less than half that in the U.K., and is thought to be due to the fact that Americans tend to smoke only about half of each cigarette. Many retrospective and prospective studies from several countries over the past 20 years have established a clear, quantitative relationship between the numbers of cigarettes smoked and the incidence of lung cancer. The risk is raised by habits, such as inhaling, which increase the exposure of the lungs to tobacco smoke; it is reduced by changing to filter-tip cigarettes, and declines rapidly during the 10 years after stopping smoking. Pipes and cigars play only a small part in the causation of lung cancer.

Carcinoma of the bronchus commonly arises in the wall of one of the larger bronchi, and besides growing into the surrounding lung tissue it tends to spread, often early in the illness, to glands in the center of the chest and in the neck, also to the liver and sometimes to the brain. The earliest symptom is usually cough and phlegm, frequently bloodstained, but the disease is insidious in onset and frequently in a moderately advanced stage before the patient seeks medical help. Because of this, treatment is unsatisfactory, surgical removal (the treatment of choice) being possible in only about 20 per cent of cases, and of these only about one-third are alive at the end of five years, making a five-year survival rate of less than ten per cent of all cases seen. Other treatments such as radiotherapy (deep X-ray treatment) and chemotherapy (e.g. cyclophosphamide) are almost invariably palliative and not curative.

Smoking. No wonder, after what has been said above, that doctors smoke much less than the general public, and that chest physicians in particular are so neurotic about people smoking. It is, after all, the one known controllable factor in both lung cancer and chronic bronchitis. Unfortunately it is a socially acceptable addiction, and although there is usually a fall in consumption after reports such as those issued by the Royal College of Physicians of England in 1962 and 1971, and by the U.S. Surgeon-General in 1964, after a few months the amount smoked creeps back to original levels. When it is realized that in the U.K. over 50,000 people die each year from carcinoma of the bronchus and chronic bronchitis, about twenty-eight thousand from each, often in the latter case after long and disabling illness, it seems incredible that the public are unwilling to give up this dirty, dangerous and expensive habit. No one is suggesting that smoking is the only cause of lung cancer, but that it is the most important known factor (as in chronic bronchitis) appears certain, and unless there is a considerable decrease in the number of cigarettes consumed no progress will be made in the prevention of cancer until the actual cause of cancer itself becomes known. Smoking is also known to double the liability to coronary thrombosis, and to delay the healing of gastric and duodenal ulcers. Mothers who smoke in pregnancy tend to have smaller babies, and are more likely to lose their babies from abortion, still births, and deaths in the first few days of life.

It is not difficult to stop smoking if the individual thinks it is important to do so. It is even more vital to persuade the young not to start. What a triumph it would be if that could be achieved on a large scale!

This review of the achievements and difficulties of chest medicine in the early seventies has shown that a great many chest illnesses are chronic, often causing many years of discomfort and disability before death supervenes. The fear of financial disaster due to such illnesses has largely been removed in the U.K. by the National Health Service, which has also ensured a more even distribution of medical resources throughout the country, so that nowhere is any patient far from skilled help. Coupled with this has been the work of the Government-sponsored British Medical Research Council and the U.S. Public Health Service who, with the Veterans' Administration, have ensured that chemotherapy, especially that of tuberculosis, has been used in an efficient and rational manner. Let us recognize these achievements for the triumphs that they are and hope that advances in the next 25 years will be equally spectacular.

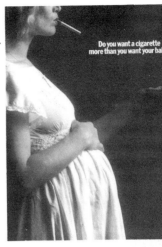

Do you want a cigarette more than you want your baby

112

111 The chest X-ray has almost become a part of the routine examination of the patient, particularly when there are any symptoms referable to the heart or lungs. The X-ray picture shown here exemplifies well the clear outlines of the bony structure of the chest wall and the central density of the heart with its apex lying to the left. The shadow of a moderately advanced cancer can be seen growing from the right upper part of the heart shadow and protruding out into the normally air-filled and radiolucent lung field (left of picture). Unfortunately, treatment at present available is of limited value. Most lung cancer is, in fact, potentially preventible and due to cigarette smoking.

112 Cigarette smoking has been identified as a contributing cause of much disease and death in modern society, and this has called forth a vigorous attempt on the part of health educationists to get people to abandon the habit and to prevent them from acquiring it in the first place. The photograph above has been used to deter the pregnant woman from smoking by drawing attention to the effects of inhaled carbon monoxide and nicotine on the growth of the developing fetus. There seems little doubt that the increasing incidence of lung cancer is largely attributable to cigarette smoking, and there is no doubt that chronic bronchitis and emphysema are aggravated, if not primarily caused by, the habit. However, the pleasures of smoking have such a grip on the population that anti-smoking campaigns have met with comparatively little success.

7 Orthopedic and Accident Surgery

Although the claim may appear outrageous, it is nevertheless true that for the past 50 years there is a record of greater achievement in medical science than for the millions of years of preceding human evolution. The astonishing rapidity of change within the particular field of orthopedic and accident surgery has resulted from the revolutionary developments in associated sciences such as physics, chemistry, metallurgy, etc., as well as from those within medical and biological science, which have increasingly explained the precise mechanism of different disease processes.

The refinement and precision of diagnostic techniques on the one hand, and the range and quality of the available therapeutic tools on the other, have combined to revolutionize the surgery of accident and repair within the past generation.

Orthopedic surgery has developed in this period from a narrow discipline which concerned itself with the correction of deformities in children (*orthos*, straight, and *pais*, child) to a major area of medical and surgical activity which is concerned with derangement of the locomotor apparatus in persons of all ages. The proper function of our body and limbs depends not only on the health of the person as a whole, but also on the detailed and coordinated efficiency of the muscles, ligaments, joints and nerves.

Operations which were designed to improve the function of limbs have been carried out for centuries: operations such as osteotomy (the division of a bone in order to correct deformity), arthroplasty (the reconstruction of a damaged joint) or major amputations of diseased limbs were all part of the repertoire of surgeons of the 19th century and earlier. However, the mortality was so enormous that each operation was transformed into something of a surgical lottery. The seeds of many important ideas were waiting to flower, but could not do so until the advent of anesthesia, antisepsis, asepsis, blood transfusion and non-corrosive metals. The ideas were always well ahead of the techniques that were essential for their success. As early as 1775 a broken bone was wired together, but the subsequent infection killed the patient. The great 19th century surgeon Langenbeck fixed a fractured hip with a metal nail, but the available metal corroded. The development of general anesthesia which was initiated by the Boston dentist William Morton in the middle of the last century, the subsequent discovery and use of antiseptic surgical techniques by Lord Lister a few years later, and the demonstration of the use of X-rays by Wilhelm Röntgen in 1895, each played an indispensable role which enabled orthopedic surgery to advance at a momentous speed once these techniques became generally available. To these early advances must be added the development of metallurgy which enabled surgeons like Venable and Stuck in the United States to study the problems of corrosion of metal when implanted into the body. In the early 1930s these surgeons developed the use of such a metal, biologically relatively inert, called Vitallium, to which they were introduced by a dental friend who had found that it did not corrode when used in the mouth.

The revolutionary advance occasioned by the discovery and development of antibiotic drugs has totally changed the face of medicine, including orthopedic and accident surgery. Not only are antibiotics able to control the everyday organisms which cause wound infection following accidents and in the operating theater, but they have also virtually conquered tuberculosis of bone and joint which in past generations led to so much disease, crippling and death amongst children and adults alike. Streptomycin, the earliest specifically antituberculous drug, virtually succeeded in eliminating the need for prolonged treatment in tuberculosis sanatoria (see chapters 6 and 15). Vaccines have changed the face of orthopedic and accident surgery. Tetanus vaccine came into being during the First World War and has now been superseded by active immunization with tetanus toxoid (see chapter 1). The dread complication of 'lock jaw' due to infection following accidental injury has been drastically reduced. In the early 1950s the U.S. virologists Salk and Sabin developed their vaccines against acute poliomyelitis, and the ravages of this disease are now rarely seen in economically developed countries. Hospital beds, as well as nursing, medical, surgical and ancillary skills, have been liberated to concentrate on entirely new problems.

It is self-evident that the greatest triumphs of medicine have been in the prevention of disease and in its early detection at a stage before permanent damage has been done. Bacteriology, virology, biochemistry and genetics have all played an important role against the general background of an improved economic environment in which the effects of malnutrition are now rarely seen in economically advanced countries. Although much remains to be done, the problems are now quite different. In accident surgery we have to deal with the

ravages of the automobile on the highway, and in orthopedic surgery the high proportion of imperative operations carried out in past generations have now been replaced by elective procedures to improve the quality of life.

The tradition of orthopedic and accident surgery has always extended its activity beyond the range of the immediate treatment of a patient to the stage of re-education and rehabilitation of the injured limb and the patient generally. These links with fields outside the immediate role of medicine, which were forged long ago, have now realized their full meaning and purpose, which is conditioned by the emphasis on the social aspects of disease and injury deriving its impetus from the social demands of the community. The surgeon not only has to straighten the crippled child, but has also to concern himself with the special problems of the child's education; not only to treat damage caused at work, but also to attend to the mechanical hazards of industry and transport; not only to undertake the surgical treatment of cripples, but also to be concerned with the social and legislative problems of vocational training and the resettlement of the physically handicapped. It was this varied and humanistic experience that was described by the doyen of British orthopedic surgery, Sir Harry Platt, as having determined the attitude of the orthopedic surgeon of today towards the art and science of medicine as a whole. This general attitude is beginning to permeate many disciplines of medicine and surgery and

113 An exaggerated, or not so exaggerated, picture of an 18th century operation for an amputation of a leg, in the possession of the Royal College of Surgeons of England, illustrating the terrors of limb surgery before the advent of anesthesia. Under these conditions speed was the hallmark of the successful surgeon. Limbs were frequently removed for severe injury, often with spreading infection which could threaten life even more than the amputation itself. The art of this classic amputation perhaps reached its zenith on the battlefield. The great French surgeon Ambroise Paré (1510-90) made his famous remark 'I dressed him. God healed him.' in relation to his ending of the horrifying practice of attempting to arrest bleeding by treating wounds with boiling oil. Nowadays amputation is most commonly performed because of obstruction of the arterial supply to the limb in older people. The frequency of this operation has been greatly diminished by the rise of arterial surgery. The obstruction can be cleared directly, or a tubular segment of vein or man-made material can be inserted in place of the blocked segment, or the obstruction can be bypassed with an artificial artery. Chronic or severe infection of soft tissue and bone, which so often threatened a limb, can now be dealt with by the antimicrobial antibiotics. In younger people accident and injury remains the commonest cause for amputation; the motorcycle is a chief offender.

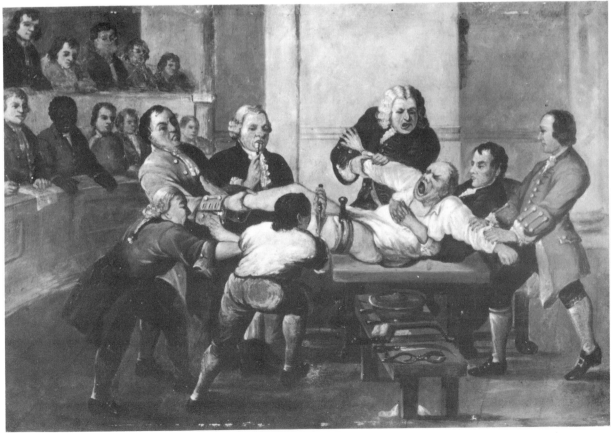

113

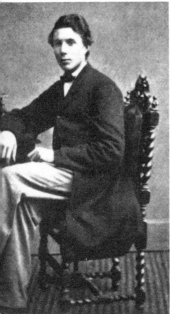

114 Wilhelm Röntgen (1845-1923), the discoverer of X-rays, as a schoolboy in Holland. Röntgen's discovery came, like the discovery of penicillin (see illustrations 234 and 235) quite by chance. He was studying cathode rays at the University of Würzburg in Bavaria in November 1895 when he noticed that the rays were causing luminescence in a sheet of paper coated with barium platinocyanide, passing through a sheet of cardboard which lay between the source and the coated paper. The effect continued when he took the piece of paper into the next room. He immediately settled down to intensive experimentation and made a fully-substantiated announcement of the properties of the nameless X-rays to the world on 28 December 1895. The picture of his wife's hand (115) was taken a week before he published his paper.

115, 116 Röntgen's first X-ray of a human hand—that of his wife, taken on 22 December 1895 (115). The ring she was wearing when the X-ray was taken stands out clearly on the ring finger. The vast improvement in the quality of X-ray pictures since Röntgen's pioneering efforts is clearly seen in the comparison between this picture and the modern X-ray of a hand (116). Minute changes in the layers of the bone, small erosions of its surface, and changes in its density can now be made out. From the appearances of bone and soft-tissue X-ray pictures, the radiologist is often able to suggest diagnoses involving more general disturbances of the body. For example, minor changes in the appearance of the bones may be the vital clue pointing to disease of the parathyroid or pituitary glands.

constitutes no less important an advance on the frontiers of medicine than the brilliant individual technical achievements which are given more prominence.

The conquest of the disease of past generations by associated social and scientific disciplines has enabled surgeons to concentrate on a whole new group of important diseases, in the forefront of which are the ravages caused by the rheumatic diseases on joints and the wreckage of limbs caused by the modern epidemic of accidents on the highways, in industry and at home. The virtual elimination of mass infectious disease has enabled a redeployment of effort both back to the original spheres of orthopedic surgery: the treatment of congenital abnormalities in infancy, such as clubfoot, dislocation of the hip, spinal curvature, etc. and into the realms of the completely new problems which are being created by the very excellence of the treatment of conditions which would previously have proved fatal. An example is the early treatment of infants suffering from meningocele (spina bifida), which saves the infant's life but often at the cost of presenting problems of formidable reconstructive surgery in these young children in later life.

Modern diagnostic techniques. One can hardly advance the treatment of any disease, whether by medical or surgical means, without an increase in the precision of diagnosis. This must, of course, precede any discussion of modern treatment.

The advent of diagnostic radiology (X-ray) was of the greatest significance in providing an important diagnostic weapon for the surgeon who has to deal with broken or diseased bones and joints. For the first 50 years after Röntgen's discovery surgeons were only too happy to accept a plain negative X-ray film. With these films it was possible to classify with a high degree of accuracy the various patterns of fracture which occur. Infections or tumors of bones and joints could be diagnosed with increasing precision and appropriate treatment initiated. The X-ray film was so valuable and represented such a great advance on previous clinical practice that a danger developed whereby surgeons were often led to 'treat the X-ray' rather than the injury or disease in a particular patient. There was a danger—and regretfully it still exists—that clinical acumen would be replaced by an X-ray examination. But the pitfalls are being recognized so that X-ray and other laboratory examinations are once more beginning to take their invaluable place as one factor in the diagnosis of a clinical problem.

The standard plain X-ray film is now considered appropriate only for routine and often preliminary investigation of a limb or spine. The advent of the image intensifier with a television screen projector now provides a far deeper understanding of the anatomy and physiology of joints in natural motion and enables us to study the abnormal mobility of joints which is not evident on plain X-ray films.

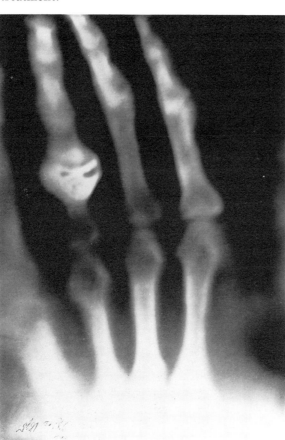

115

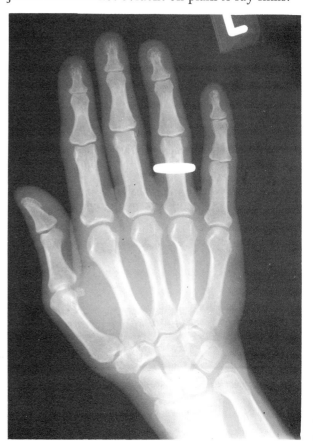

116

In the field of orthopedic surgery the concept of 'joint instability' is now becoming increasingly recognized as a not uncommon cause of pain and disability in patients previously considered to have no physical cause for their complaints 'because the X-ray film is normal'. Abnormal mobility at a joint is now recognized and for experimental purposes may be recorded by cine-radiography, a technique in its early stages of development at present, but through which a much more precise study of living, moving joints will be possible. It is now possible to inject a contrast medium directly into a joint. This consists of a harmless non-irritating fluid which is radio-opaque and, therefore, outlines the radiotranslucent lining membrane and cartilage of a joint. By this means various abnormalities may be detected which cannot be seen on plain radiographs. The use of the image intensifier and television screen facilitates this examination and the joint may be studied during movement. The contrast medium may on occasions be combined with sterile air so that a double contrast is obtained. In this way ruptures of a cartilage in the knee, or of tendons around the shoulder joint, or minor displacements or abnormalities of the hip in a newborn child, can often be accurately demonstrated. A similar technique known as myelography may be used in the spinal canal to verify the presence and the precise situation of an intervertebral disk protrusion or, less commonly, of a spinal tumor or congenital malformation of the spinal cord.

It is now possible to look directly into a knee joint by the technique of arthroscopy in which a telescope-like instrument is inserted into the joint distended with fluid so that its internal structure may be carefully scrutinized. This technique was pioneered by Watanabe in Japan and further developed in Canada and West Germany. It is still in its infancy but shows promise of becoming an added refinement in diagnostic technique for joint disease. Not only may the interior of the joint be examined, but precise photographs may also be taken of particular areas of interest and small specimens removed for laboratory examination.

Refined laboratory investigations of blood and urine now make it possible to diagnose a wide variety of skeletal disorders in childhood and adult life due to a variety of causes such as inborn errors of amino acid metabolism. Based on a more precise understanding of the mechanism of abnormal metabolism, the detection of such disease and its careful definition make it possible to treat or cure a variety of potentially crippling disorders of the skeleton. Some skeletal diseases—often rare—may also reveal themselves by the use of an electron microscope to study the precise cell structure with particular reference to chromosome abnormalities.

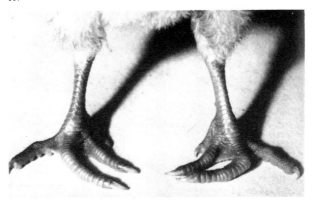

Congenital and developmental deformities.
Although a high proportion of orthopedic practice is concerned with the management of developmental deformities of limbs or spine, it is only in recent years that we have begun to understand the causes of these abnormalities. Previously they were considered mere 'accidents'—acts of God—not subject to scientific analysis and in no way preventable. The science of genetics has provided one explanation of several varieties of congenital malformation and parents may now be offered accurately based eugenic advice. The cause of many other congenital abnormalities remained shrouded in mystery until the Australians Gregg and Swan published their observations on the relationship between rubella (German measles) in pregnancy and the subsequent birth of a child suffering from a wide variety of developmental abnormalities. A fundamental advance in our understanding occurred. When Duraiswami, an Indian biologist working in the Department of Orthopedic Surgery at Liverpool was able regularly to reproduce congenital skeletal defects in young chicks by injecting insulin into the fertilized egg, the circle was complete. Until that time, abnormal genes were considered the cause of practically all congenital malformation. The work of Duraiswami has again revived, albeit in a modified form, the old argument between nature and nurture. He was able to produce in his chicks many deformities which simulated those seen in clinical work such as spina bifida, suppression of development of one or more vertebrae, and various deformities of limbs like clubfoot in the new born child, and some of these deformities were passed on to their progeny by the affected birds.

The size of the problem of congenital anomalies becomes evident when one considers the fact that it causes the death of approximately one-quarter of the human race either before or shortly after birth, and handicaps an appreciable proportion of the remaining population throughout their lives. The study of genetic factors which has made counselling of prospective parents a practical reality, combined with rapidly increasing studies of the effect of maternal environmental

117 Foot deformities in a chicken produced by the injection of insulin into the chick embryo, the demonstration made by the biologist Duraiswami referred to in the text. Although the cause of many congenital abnormalities remains unknown, a proportion can be attributed to external factors affecting the developing fetus. Two well-known examples of this are the results of the infection of the fetus by the rubella virus (German measles) contracted by the mother during the early part of pregnancy, and the tragic episode of deformities produced by the tranquilizing drug thalidomide. Duraiswami's demonstration finally established that external factors could produce deformities in this way. The search continues for toxic, infective and other avoidable factors which might affect the fetus in its uterine environment and thus be responsible for developmental malformations. At the same time, the prevention or early detection of errors of development due to defective genetic control within the fetus itself are increasingly susceptible to research and remedial action (see chapter 13).

factors, including the direct study of the amniotic fluid surrounding the developing infant in utero, now enables us to predict and possibly prevent the birth of crippled infants. We are already at a stage when this laboratory work has achieved some important practical results, such as the immunization of young girls against rubella prior to pregnancy and the avoidance of irradiation of the pelvis during early pregnancy, as well as the successful agreements amongst governments to abolish their testing of hydrogen bombs in the atmosphere which raised the level of background gamma-irradiation to dangerous proportions. Undoubtedly the search for further specifically harmful factors in the early weeks of pregnancy will increasingly disclose the precise etiology of many congenital malformations which are now the cause of so much family distress.

Surgery of muscles and tendons. Following the epidemics of poliomyelitis in the first half of this century, the surgery of paralysis of limbs by transferring healthy muscles to do the work of paralyzed muscles was refined. The knowledge gained at that time is now deployed in the treatment of paralysis resulting from other causes. The exact pattern of muscles which may be transferred—one to do the work of another—is now classified and understood. A person with a drop foot, for example, may now have a muscle transferred from the back of the leg to the front of the ankle which will enable him to raise his foot in walking. If the thumb is paralyzed and cannot grasp or pinch, an adjoining muscle may be 'borrowed' to carry out the important function of opposition of the thumb in pinching or grasping.

Lumbar spine—'Lumbago-sciatica'. From the layman's point of view no orthopedic problem concerns him more than backache. Low backache (commonly and usefully called 'lumbago') is possibly the commonest symptom bringing a patient to an orthopedic surgeon today. It is a symptom which is due to many causes and in the majority of cases it is a transient symptom, or there are long periods of remission between attacks. This is one reason why such an extraordinarily wide variety of empirical treatment is credited with success.

Although there are still large gaps in our knowledge of the causes and the consequent cure of low back and sciatic (leg) pain, it is true to say that in most cases we can now arrive at an accurate diagnosis and prescribe appropriate treatment. Only 50 years ago all the *uncommon* causes of low back pain were well known and carefully described; tuberculosis of the spine and primary or secondary tumors were recognized and accurately diagnosed, but there was little knowledge of the *common* causes of low back pain such as mechanical instability of the spine, stress or fatigue fractures and spondylolisthesis (the

118 It is sometimes necessary to confirm the diagnosis of an intervertebral disk protrusion (see illustration 119) or to demonstrate its extent. This picture shows one technique, where X-ray-opaque contrast medium has been injected around the spinal cord, which has then been X-rayed to give a frontal view. The break in the column of opaque material is due to its displacement in this region by a large disk protrusion, through which the X-rays pass unhindered.

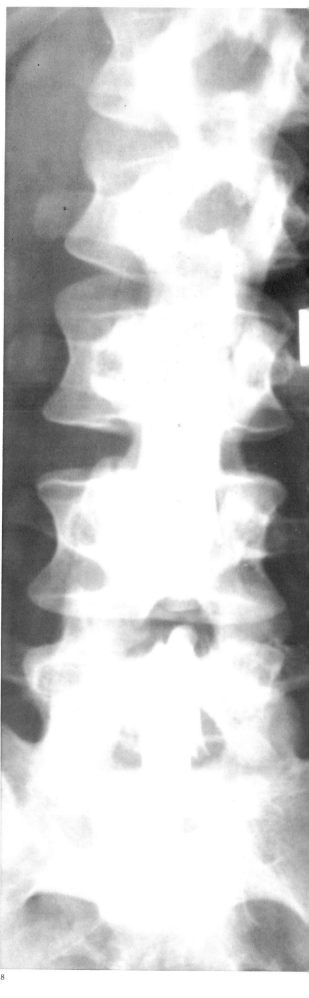

118

forward movement of one vertebra upon the other), and injuries or disease of the intervertebral disks. Because the common causes were not understood, treatment was always entirely empirical. The relief of low back pain by any sort of treatment was attributed to that particular treatment, rather than to the natural resolution of a condition which is often self-limiting. Sciatica (pain down the leg) associated with low back pain was considered to be a primary neuritis of the sciatic nerve and a fantastic array of treatments by leeches, cupping, and stretching of the sciatic nerve was used as recently as the 1930s.

It is easy to single out a number of landmarks which have revolutionized our diagnosis and treatment. Improved radiography with various special projections elucidated a number of important causes of lumbago. The original X-ray tube was not sufficiently powered to penetrate the heavy structures of the low back, but improved tubes and the invention of the Bucky diaphragm made it possible to obtain films of a reasonable diagnostic quality. The subsequent development of contrast myelography in X-ray examination added another important diagnostic aid. It was not, however, until a report in 1934 by Mixter and Barr that a complete and revolutionary advance in our understanding occurred. By 1937 there were already 40 cases of intervertebral disk protrusion in the lumbar region of the spine reported proved at operation at the Massachusetts General Hospital. Following this work a precise clinical syndrome was described consisting of a particular presentation of low back pain (lumbago) and associated sciatica due to intervertebral disk protrusion. The time had come when Mixter and Barr were able to say that lumbar intervertebral disk protrusions are not excessively rare and 'should be thought of in every case of back strain and sciatica'. The initial scepticism regarding the significance of disk protrusions was rapidly dissipated as surgeons gained personal experience. The considerable technical advances in the diagnosis and operative treatment of intervertebral disk protrusions now make it possible by careful analysis of the clinical findings, supplemented by radiological aids, to localize with great accuracy the precise site of the lesion in most cases and to proceed to its removal with safety and a remarkably high rate of satisfaction both to patient and surgeon. The relief of sciatic pain is in most cases dramatic and may be confidently anticipated.

Spinal curvature. American surgeons have been in the forefront of the surgical treatment of spinal curvature (scoliosis) in young persons. The accurate selection of patients who should be subjected to treatment was made possible by careful analysis of the natural history of the variety of patterns of curvature which may occur in a growing child. We are now able to say which curvature will become severe and require treatment and what form of treatment is appropriate. For many years treatment by surgical measures consisted of the correction of the curvature in an elaborate plaster-of-Paris cast and the subsequent fusion of the affected spinal segments. In 1962 Harrington of Houston reported a radical advance in the surgical management of scoliosis by using long metal rods embedded deep in the muscle by which he is able to 'jack out' the curvature on the concave side and 'jack in' the curvature on the convex side of the spine. Significant and rapid correction may be obtained in this way and is then combined with spinal fusion to maintain the correction.

The development of the artificial joint. The restoration of movement to a stiff joint has always presented a challenge to surgeons. To create a painless mobile joint has been a dream. Although there are many important medical and surgical techniques available for the relief of joint pain, the development of an artificial joint—in particular the replacement of the destroyed hip joint—has dominated the orthopedic surgical scene for the past two decades. It is at present beyond doubt the most dramatically beneficial procedure which it is possible to offer a crippled patient. Like all great discoveries it has, of course, a continuous story of partial achievement preceding the final breakthrough. For the first half of this century a variety of attempts were made to interpose material between two joint surfaces in order to improve its function and diminish pain. The history of these attempts is a truly international one: Kallio in Finland used specially prepared skin drawn over the head of the femur and lying between the head of the femur and the cup of the pelvis at the hip. Later sheets of fat or fascia, even gold foil, were tried by various American surgeons. Specially prepared glass molds were used. The advent of new materials enabled Smith-Peterson of Boston to design an operation based on the interposition of biologically inert material between the two parts of the joint. A mold of the new non-corrosive metal Vitallium was used and for many years gave excellent results. In the early 1950s the brothers Judet of Paris made a revolutionary advance. Not satisfied with interposing material between the two parts of the hip joint, they resected completely the diseased femoral head and replaced it with a new artificial head made of acrylic. The concept was sound but their method of fixation and—in particular—the choice of acrylic as the artificial substitute femoral head caused the operation to fail. The acrylic disintegrated and had to be removed. A few years later the American surgeons Moore and

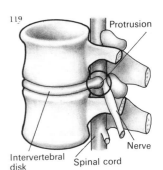

119 An abnormal intervertebral disk protrusion is the commonest cause of 'sciatica'. The intervertebral disks lie between the vertebrae, acting as a kind of cushion. Sometimes the soft center of the disk is extruded through the fibrous outer capsule and, by pressure on the nerves leaving the spinal cord, causes pain in the distribution of that nerve and may also lead to muscle wasting. The diagram shows the disk protrusion between two vertebrae, pressing on a nerve where it leaves the spinal cord.

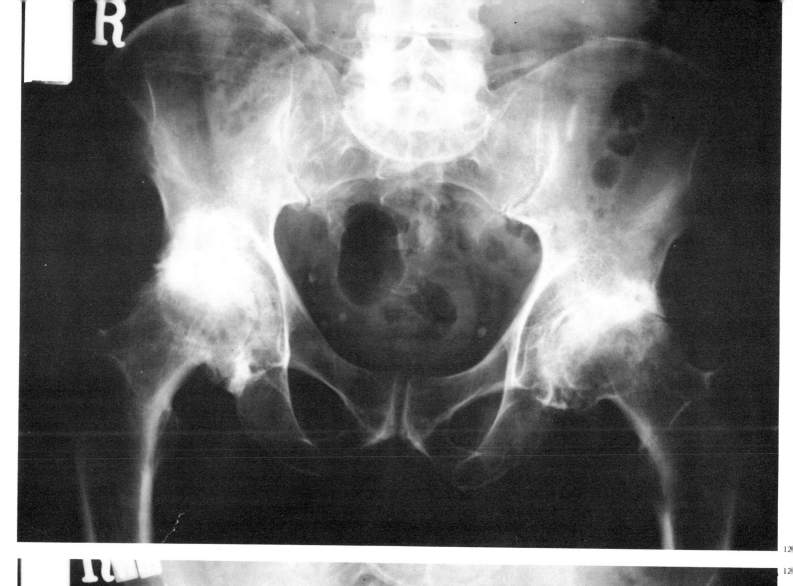

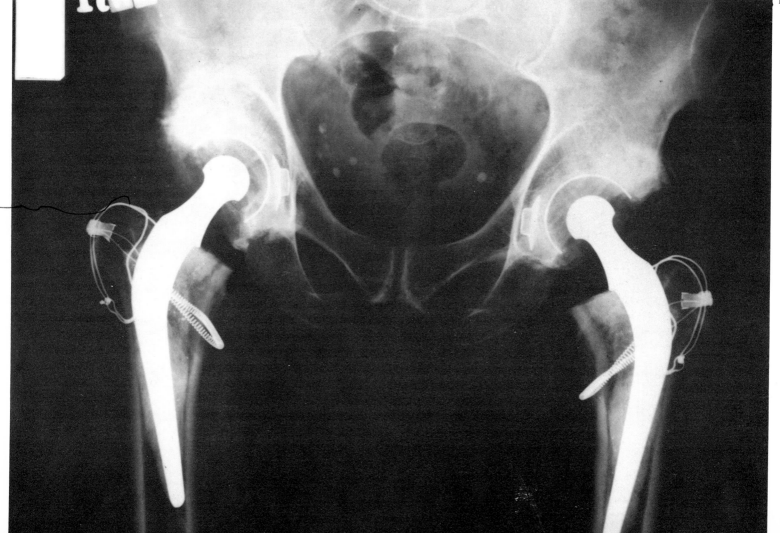

Thompson, using the Judet principle, achieved a notable advance when they replaced the resected femoral head by biologically inert metal placed within the shaft of the femur. This operation has stood the test of time in selected cases following fractures of the neck of the femur in normal joints but has been superseded in the treatment of arthritis of the hip joint when both sides of the joint are involved by disease. George McKee of Norwich decided to carry out a total replacement of the entire hip joint. His method consisted of seating a biologically inert metal cup within the acetabulum and using the Thompson type of artificial femoral head as the other component. This was a spectacular breakthrough but failed because the metal was unsuitable and there was no method of binding metal to bone. This was left to John Charnley of Manchester, who in 1960 reported a technique of binding the metal parts directly onto the bone by the use of plastic 'cement' made of methyl methacrylate (acrylic cement). Experience showed that the use of metal for both sides of the hip joint often led to unsatisfactory late results due to frictional debris which caused the metal parts to bind to each other. Charnley recommended that the upper part of the hip be replaced by a plastic substance and the lower part by metal. The standard operation now, with a few variations, is to use a high-density polyethylene cup in the acetabulum and a biologically inert cobalt-chrome metal femoral head. Both these parts are bound into their respective recipient bones by acrylic cement. This technique has now reached a stage of perfection when we may expect over 90 per cent of patients to be relieved of pain and have a greatly improved range of function of the hip joint. The early results amongst the severely handicapped patients is truly dramatic. How many years these new joints will last is not known, but the experience overall extends some 10 to 15 years and early results are brilliant for the hip joint, improving for the knee and rapidly developing in the non-weight-bearing joints like the elbow and shoulder.

Those who look for 'the triumphs of modern medicine' would do well to ponder on the thought that Theodore Gluck in 1891 replaced a diseased hip joint by an ivory ball and socket which was cemented and screwed into position. In principle this is the modern operation. Unfortunately for Gluck and the patients of his day the general level of technology had yet not reached the stage when he could use suitable plastics and metals, and his artificial hip was duly extruded. In 1938 Phillip Wiles in London, carried out a total hip replacement of both joints in a young person, but the stainless steel which he was obliged to use did not last many years.

The success of the contemporary operation of total hip replacement must be attributed not to the ingenuity of the modern surgeon alone, but in the first place to the state of the technological environment in which he works.

However excellent the surgical achievement of total hip or other joint replacement may be at the present time, it must nevertheless be said that it will probably turn out to be a transient phenomenon in the history of orthopedic surgery. After all, is not the ultimate aim of all surgery to eliminate the need for the surgeon? Important discoveries in the laboratory are just around the corner bringing an understanding of autoimmunity as a fundamental disease process responsible for rheumatoid arthritis, and possibly for other forms of arthritis, which now wrecks our joints which then have to be replaced (see chapter 8 and illustration 81). The basic properties of articular cartilage, in particular the enzymatic component of the degradation of articular cartilage which leads to joint destruction, are gradually being unravelled. A fuller understanding of the autoimmune process and the cause of articular cartilage destruction will no doubt in course of time remove a large volume of repair work from the orbit of the surgeon, just as the advent of a vaccine did to poliomyelitis. Not only will it be possible to prevent and control rheumatoid arthritis and the autoimmune ravages of joints, but the transfer of biological material, in particular total joints from dead donors, will be the order of the day. In the Soviet Union during the past several years considerable advance has been made in the transfer of total joints or parts of joints from the dead to the living. The method of freeze-drying tissue has made it possible to preserve skin, bone, cartilage or even whole joints until they are required. However, the all-important problem of immune rejection of the received tissue is not yet conquered. Its conquest is undoubtedly to hand and when this has been achieved there will follow a period when the evaluation of an artificial joint as against a biological donor joint will be necessary. Which of these will prove to be the most successful remains to be seen; but the prevention by medical treatment of arthritis in its early phase will certainly considerably diminish the occasion for their use.

Accident and fracture surgery. Death or injury by accident has replaced infectious disease as the epidemic of modern times. In Great Britain some 20,000 persons a year are killed by accidental injury; approximately one-third each on the highway, at work and at home. As a cause of major injury the danger on the highways of the western countries is exceeded only by a major war. What is particularly distressing is that road accidents kill more young people in the U.K. in each age group from 1 to 34 than any major disease or group of diseases. From 35 to 45 only

120, 121 Ageing of the cartilage surface of the hip joint is responsible for the pain and progressive immobilization which can be the distressing lot of many people in the later years of life. A combination of surgical expertise and engineering techniques has brought extraordinary relief and a new freedom of movement to many of these people. The upper X-ray shows the very roughened joint surface denoting the presence of severe osteoarthrosis affecting both hip joints and causing considerable pain and stiffness. The lower X-ray shows both joints after replacement by prostheses. The head of the femur has been removed and replaced by a metal head. The upper part of the joint—the socket (see illustration 125)—has also been replaced, in this case by a polyethylene cup (which is less opaque to X-rays than the metal part of the joint).

cancer and the diseases of the circulation are more lethal. Amongst older people domestic accidents are responsible for an increasing number of fatal injuries. Miners, foundrymen, factory and agricultural workers all pay a heavy price in death and disability.

In accident surgery many new advances have become apparent, but the most important requirement, the organization of a modern accident service, still lags behind the available technical and scientific skills. It is now recognized—but only too slowly being acted upon—that for the proper treatment of injured persons a concentration of facilities and skills is needed which can only be supplied in centralized accident centers attached to large hospitals. The impetus which surgeons have given successive Governments to encourage them to provide centralized accident centers is possibly the most important single advance which is being made in the modern management of the injured patient. It is of little value to have the most skilled surgeon available to receive the patient if he does not have all modern techniques available to him, such as the laboratory facilities for cross-matching immediately available blood, anesthesiologist, X-ray apparatus and technicians and immediate access to operating theaters. Ruscoe Clarke, notable surgeon to the Birmingham Accident Hospital, once stated: 'Accident surgery was the first surgery, it may well be the last.' It is a thought-provoking statement and the history of preventive medicine in orthopedic disease indicates that there is undoubtedly much truth in it. Many of the conditions now treated surgically will in course of time either be prevented or be treated by non-surgical methods, but the ravages caused by accidental injury will remain.

It is widely believed that great advances in accident surgery are occasioned by the circumstances and demands of war; that one of the few benefits of war is to advance surgery. A critical study however, does not—with few exceptions—bear this out. While it is true to say that a nation at war will give high priority to the development of surgery both in the armed forces and in the home countries, this impetus to surgery leads to *existing* knowledge becoming more widely disseminated and used. Techniques are more critically evaluated and the best techniques more rapidly deployed and made available. The atmosphere is, however, not conducive to the quiet thought which is required for scientific advance so that war seldom leads to any permanent improvement in surgical science or practice. The technique of blood transfusion and storage was greatly enhanced during the last war, but the fundamental scientific work of blood typing and matching was carried out in the years prior to the war. The war caused the

widespread deployment of this basic knowledge, with minor technical advances concerned with blood storage and carriage, but did not lead to any significant improvement in our understanding of blood transfusion. It was in peace time when studying the effects of highway accidents in Birmingham that Ruscoe Clarke and others were able to make important new discoveries concerned with fundamental knowledge of blood loss caused by accidental injury. It was also between wars that the British pathologist Sevitt and others advanced our knowledge of fat embolism as a cause of unexplained death following accident and that techniques were developed for detecting the globules of fat released at the site of fracture which subsequently become lodged in lungs, brain and kidney. Such advances, in what would seem to be the area where surgical understanding was most likely to be advanced by war, were made in times of peace. Similarly the technique of the internal fixation of a long bone by an intramedullary metal rod within the shaft of the bone is generally attributed to the work of the surgeon Kuntscher on injured soldiers in the German army. But the principles of this technique were initiated many years earlier, in time of peace, notably by Hey Groves of Bristol, and only failed at that time because the available metal was not of sufficient strength or suitable composition for the technique to succeed. There are two notable exceptions to the general thesis: Trueta during the Spanish Civil War developed a technique of treating the soft tissue components of a wound which represented an important advance in wound treatment and has stood the test of time, and also the surgery of peripheral nerves was greatly advanced in times of war. Peripheral nerves are particularly vulnerable to direct injury by penetrating high-velocity missiles. During World War II Seddon and his colleagues in the U.K. analyzed, classified and systematized the surgery of peripheral nerve injuries. Their work represented a great advance in fundamental surgical knowledge and continues both in principle and in practice today. The peripheral nerves are carefully dissected, freed and mobilized and then meticulously repaired by fine sutures of the surrounding nerve sheath or 'glued' together with a special biological substance prepared from blood clot. Very recently some Japanese surgeons have attempted the refinement of this technique by microsuture of the individual nerve bundles within the peripheral nerve sheath.

The development of suitable external splintage of a fractured limb has exercised the thought of surgeons through centuries and some form of hardening material using white of egg has been used for over a thousand years, its discovery accredited to Rhazes, an Arabian physician of the 9th century. Plaster of Paris was used from the

122 A fracture of the neck of the femur, the weight-bearing bone in the thigh, used to be tantamount to a death sentence. Not so much the injury itself, but the prolonged immobilization of the usually elderly patient led to lethal broncho-pneumonia or lung embolism. The scene changed radically when methods of rapid fixation of the broken bones were introduced, enabling the patient to be up and about within a few days of the accident. The engineering skill that goes hand in hand with modern ortho-pedic surgery is arrestingly demonstrated in this X-ray of a fractured hip-joint repaired with a pin and plate. A stout three-pronged pin is passed through, and a plate with a per-forated bracket at the upper end has been screwed into the shaft of the femur. Coupling pin and plate provides sufficient strength to carry the patient's weight.

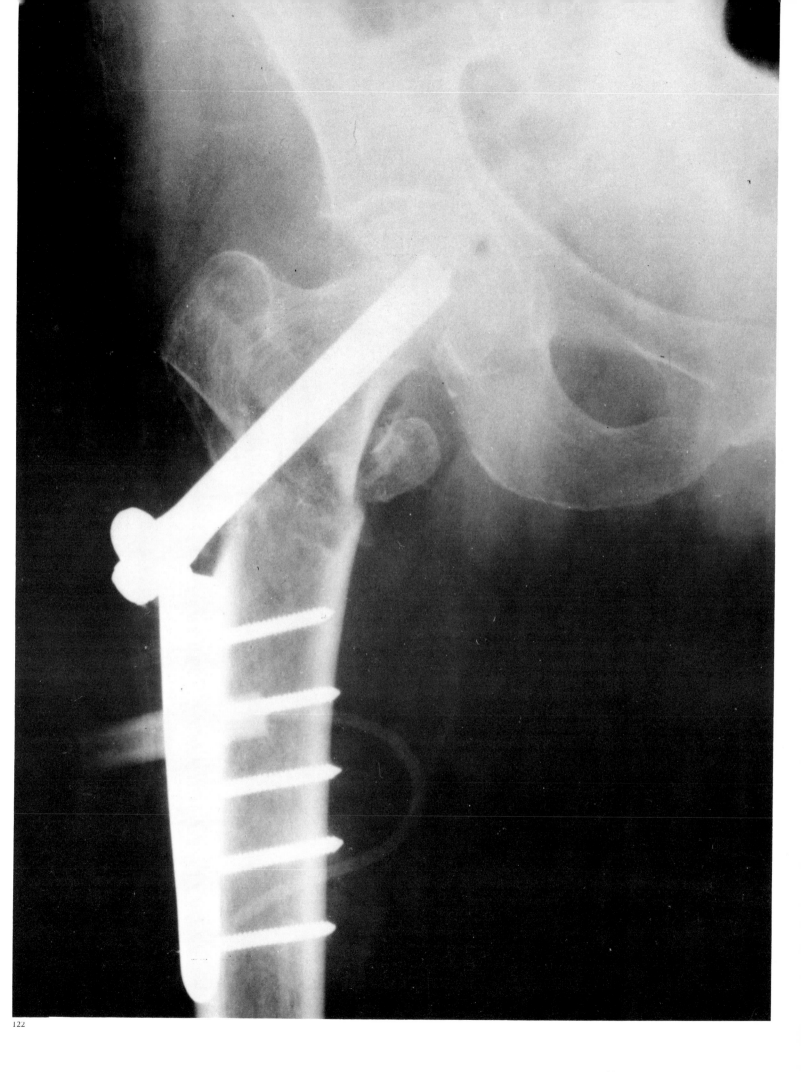

middle of the last century and popularized in America by Samuel John of New York who made the apparently simple but exceedingly important observation that the splint should be fitted to the limb and not the limb to the splint! Technical advances of manufacture now enable bandages impregnated with plaster of Paris to be presented to surgeons in an immediately usable form and greatly facilitate the technique of external splintage of a fractured bone.

At the present time there is an increasing tendency to use internal splintage for a fractured bone. Asepsis, anesthesia and modern metals which do not corrode within the tissues have tempted surgeons to deploy this technique very widely. In some cases it is a lifesaving procedure. Some 50 years ago an old person with a fractured hip had some 90 per cent chance of dying as a result of the immobility forced upon him by the fracture. By transfixing a fractured hip with an appropriate metal nail, doctors have dramatically reduced the death rate from this fracture during the past generation. Internal fixation for other fractures has a less dramatic result but is widely used to diminish the morbidity, pain, length of incapacity and final deformity of the limb. A fracture may be fixed with a simple screw of appropriate metal, by metal plates screwed to the shaft of the bone, or by intramedullary fixation by a long metal rod within the marrow cavity. Suitably chosen and firm internal splintage of a fractured bone has many advantages in many cases. The patient may lead a more normal life while awaiting the healing of the fracture and he is able to exercise the limb thereby preventing stiffness of the adjoining joints and wasting of the muscles. Innumerable techniques of internal fixation for various bones have been described. In principle two concepts are gaining ground at the present time: for a fracture of one of the major long bones—in particular a fracture of the femur—the suitable preparation of the marrow canal by power-reaming and the subsequent insertion of an accurately fitted intramedullary metal rod as developed and advocated by Kuntscher represents an important advance. A patient with a fracture of the shaft of the femur who might previously have had to lie in a hospital bed for three months or more and might not get back to his own work for a year can in this manner be dealt with in less than a quarter of this time. During the past few years Muller and his associates in Switzerland have brought the techniques of internal metal fixation to a high degree of perfection and have devised methods of maintaining compression between the ends of the fractured bones in order to improve the rigidity of fixation and—they claim—the speed of healing of the fracture. Although antibiotics make open positioning and fixation of fractured bones safer, there are nevertheless the obvious dangers of an occasional infection which may lead to a situation worse than that caused by the injury. It is for this reason that orthopedic surgeons select patients for internal fixation with some caution.

Experimental attempts are being made in animals to seek a form of plastic material which will bind the fractured bone together while permitting the new bone cells for the repair of the fracture to grow across and through the plastic material. Preliminary successes of such an experimental technique in Australia using sheep have unfortunately not yet been confirmed. It is in this general direction that the future treatment of fractured bones probably lies. Professor Brian MacFarland of Liverpool described his vision of the future in this way: 'The frequency of bone fractures will be unimportant because intramedullary fixation with thermostatic, homoplastic agents injected directly into the fracture site, cancellous in their form, set into the resilience and strength of steel, stimulating callus formation, and being resorbed in that process, will permit immediate weight-bearing in nearly every fracture.' It is a dream of perfection which must be striven towards.

The surgery of deformity, accident and repair advances on a broad front. Some of the advancing tentacles will no doubt shrivel and wither while others will develop and strengthen and some lead on to major triumphs of medical science. The idea of grafting one piece of bone to take the place of another has exercised surgeons for a hundred years. It was originated by the great French surgeon Ollier and further enhanced by Sir William Macewen of Glasgow in his brilliant monograph *The Growth of Bone* in 1912. The story of bone grafting is as exciting as a novel in which contending rivals, often men of passion and power, strove for mastery. The battle has not yet been resolved, but it has given rise to great advances in our understanding of how one piece of bone may be grafted upon another. The indications for the use of bone grafts are innumerable—to heal an ununited fracture, to replace bone lost by accident, or excised for disease. Recent advances in immunology now place complete success within our grasp. It is now known that the bone which is most suitable for transfer must have three well defined properties. The possibility of its immunological rejection can be reduced by freeze-drying; its capacity to induce the receiving host bone to provoke new bone (its induction potential) varies with the type of bone which is used; its reception and replacement by the host bone will depend upon its rapid resorption. In view of these criteria it is now known that the best bone for keeping in a bone 'bank' ready for use is that which has been freeze-dried, decalcified and cleared of its cellular debris. While it is obviously desirable to use the patient's own bone taken from one part and placed into another, this is not always possible and the ability to bank suitable bone in large quantities is a matter which lies in the forefront of surgery. Articular cartilage presents less problems in some ways but greater problems in others. Its immunological properties are probably not as important as those of whole bone but the method of its fixation onto a joint surface has not yet been mastered. A suitable 'biological glue' awaits discovery.

The ability to equalize a patient's leg length has appealed to orthopedic imagination for many years. Until 30 years ago the various operations consisted of either lengthening one leg or shortening the other. In 1932 a method of arresting the longitudinal growth of bone by destroying the growth-plate at the growing end of the bone was reported. The success of such an operation depends upon the calculation of the expected growth during the remaining years of the child's life. Errors have been diminished by the accurate studies of Abbot and Green of Boston. To overcome any possible dangers of miscalculation, Blount of Milwaukee devised metal staples to straddle the growth-plate which could be removed if necessary in course of time, when the bone would resume its normal growth. Various techniques of stimulating bone growth continue to be tried, but none successfully so except in the youngest of children.

The rapid advances in the chemistry of enzymes, vitamins and hormones as well as a fuller understanding of problems of immunity and auto-immunity have all considerably influenced the science and practice of orthopedic surgery. Conquest of degenerative joint disease by a deeper understanding of the auto-immune process and of the disordered biology of articular cartilage may reach the stage where joint operations are no longer required and if they are required the use of donor joints will be possible.

8 Rheumatism and Rehabilitation

Joints are formed wherever two or more bones of the body come into contact. Virtually all the movements of the body are dependent on the normal functioning of the joints—getting out of bed in the morning, eating a meal, walking in the street, or playing the piano. To provide for the considerable range of movement which many such activities require, the ends of the bones are modified in a particular way. For example, in most movable joints such as the knee and other so-called synovial joints, the bone ends are covered with cartilage and separated by a lubricant known as synovial fluid. The joint is enclosed in a strong fibrous capsule lined with a membrane which produces the lubricating fluid.

The range of movement possible at different joints depends upon a number of factors including the shape of the adjoining joint surfaces. Hinge joints like the small joints of the fingers allow only a small range of movement, while a ball-and-socket type of joint, such as the shoulder, enables movement to occur through numerous planes. The force to move a joint comes from muscles, which also combine with the tough ligaments attached to the bones to give joints their stability.

Gout. Of all the diseases which may affect the

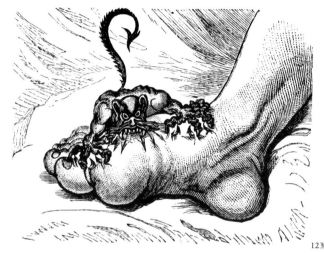

123

joints, this is the oldest established. The clinical features of gout were well known to the ancient Greeks, though it was the English physician Thomas Sydenham who first clearly differentiated it from other disorders in his famous *Treatise on the Gout* written in 1683. Sydenham himself was a sufferer from gout, which appears to have been a common disease at the time, chiefly affecting the upper classes. Among the famous historical figures afflicted with gout were Queen Anne, George III, William Pitt, Benjamin Franklin, Dr Samuel Johnson and Lord Nelson.

It was shown in the 19th century that there is an increased amount of uric acid in the blood of patients with gout, and gout itself was thought to be caused by the precipitation of crystals of sodium urate from a supersaturated solution. Despite minor modifications, this same theory is generally accepted today. The formation of sodium urate crystals in a joint can cause the intense pain, redness and swelling typical of acute gout. Most attacks start in the big toe, but other joints are susceptible. Sodium urate may also be deposited under the skin, in the cartilage

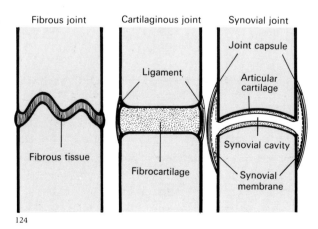

Fibrous joint   Cartilaginous joint   Synovial joint

Joint capsule

Ligament

Articular cartilage

Fibrous tissue

Fibrocartilage

Synovial cavity

Synovial membrane

124

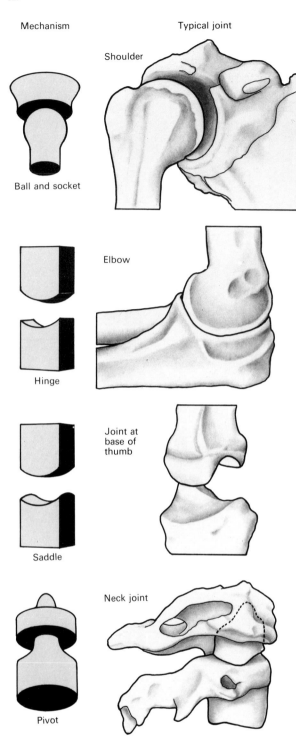

Mechanism

Typical joint

Shoulder

Ball and socket

Elbow

Hinge

Joint at
base of
thumb

Saddle

Neck joint

Pivot

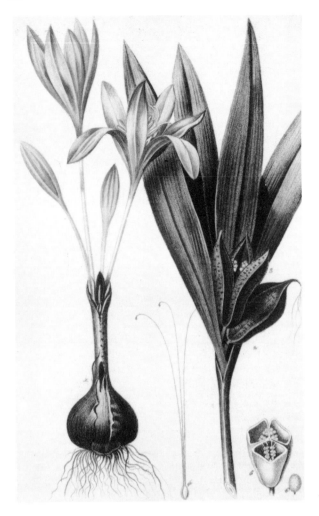

of the ear, and in the kidneys, where uric acid stones may be formed. Recurrent attacks of gout may produce chronic deformities of the joints, sometimes resembling rheumatoid arthritis.

Uric acid is formed as a breakdown product of purines, which are an essential component of cell nuclei. In gout there is often an increased production of purines leading to excessive formation of uric acid. The ability of the kidneys to excrete uric acid may also be impaired, causing a rise in the blood level. These abnormalities may be due to the presence of

other diseases, but in most cases of gout their cause is unknown. Since gout often runs in families, it has been postulated that there may be inherited defects in purine metabolism, predisposing to accumulation of uric acid. Some evidence for this has been discovered, including the absence of an enzyme involved in purine metabolism in cases of the Lesch-Nyhan syndrome, a rare childhood disorder, one of whose characteristics is gout. It is expected that further research will reveal other enzyme defects.

Many facts remain to be discovered about the factors which precipitate attacks of gout in those who are genetically predisposed to it. Excessive alcohol intake has long been known to play a part, and this may be partly accounted for by the fact that alcohol breakdown in the body causes an increase in lactic acid production, which in turn interferes with uric acid excretion by the kidney.

The treatment of acute attacks of gout was for a long time based on a substance known to the physicians of Byzantium, 1,500 years ago. This substance, colchicine, was extracted from the meadow saffron in 1814 and was the only satisfactory treatment for acute gout until the development of the modern anti-inflammatory agents phenylbutazone and indomethacin. These drugs often bring dramatic pain relief in a

125 This diagram shows a variety of types of synovial joint, illustrated by a diagram of their mechanism and a drawing of a typical example. The ball and socket joint allows movement in many different planes. A pivot joint allows rotation only. With a hinge joint movement is limited to one plane, while a saddle joint permits movement in two planes, but not rotation.

126 The acute attack of gout can be rapidly brought under control with colchicine, an extract of the autumn crocus or meadow saffron, *Colchicum autumnale*, shown here in an illustration from a medical herbal of 1814. The autumn crocus has been known since ancient times as a specific for the acute attack of gout. Its mode of action remains unknown, and its wide use is limited by its side-effects, such as colic and diarrhea. Other anti-inflammatory drugs such as phenylbutazone are equally effective in controlling the acute attack of gout. The drugs mentioned earlier (123) are used to achieve long-term control of the condition.

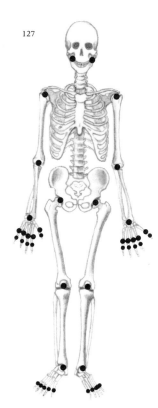

127 A diagram of the skeleton indicating the joints commonly affected in the arthritis of rheumatoid disease. The degree of involvement ranges from troublesome inflammation or stiffness of a few joints to a devastating, crippling disease which destroys most of the joints of the body and also affects many other systems, causing grave and chronic reduction of health which may even be lethal. Although the cause of rheumatoid disease remains unknown, modern treatment has rescued many victims from a life of chronic pain, immobility and invalidism. This has been achieved by a carefully balanced mixture of anti-inflammatory drugs and physio-therapy, sometimes aided by gold injections which mysteriously seem to subdue the disease process.

matter of hours. The treatment of chronic gout is aimed at reducing the raised level of uric acid in the blood, to prevent further acute attacks. Two types of drug are used; those such as probenecid and sulfinpyrazone which act on the kidney to increase the excretion of uric acid, and allopurinol, more recently discovered, which has a specific blocking action on an enzyme involved in the formation of uric acid, thus decreasing the amount produced. All these drugs have had a considerable effect in reducing pain and suffering among the victims of gout.

Rheumatoid arthritis. Gout causes inflammation in the joints. Many other joint disorders are inflammatory: that is, they are characterized by pain, swelling, redness and warmth of the affected joints. The most common disorder of this kind is rheumatoid arthritis which affects about one per cent of men and three per cent of women. In contrast to osteoarthrosis, it appears to be largely a disease of modern times. There is some evidence that it was described by Hippocrates, but before the 19th century it was not clearly distinguished from gout and other types of 'rheumatism'. Nevertheless some famous historical figures, including Christopher Columbus and Mary Queen of Scots, may have suffered from it.

The illness is most common in the 30 to 50 age group and usually begins rather quietly, with the gradual onset of pain, stiffness and swelling particularly in the small joints of the hands, wrists and feet, and spreading to involve the larger joints. Sometimes the onset is more acute,

with severe joint pains, fever and weight loss. Usually the disease runs a fluctuating course of remissions and exacerbations, and in many people it settles down, leaving little or no residual disability. Repeated episodes of inflammation, however, cause damage to the joints, producing characteristic deformities, and about ten per cent of those who are ill enough to require hospitalization at the onset may end up crippled by the disease. Unfortunately there is no way of identifying this group, and distinguishing them from the 60 per cent who remain economically and socially independent ten years after the onset.

Rheumatoid arthritis is sometimes referred to more generally as rheumatoid disease, because it has effects on other parts of the body as well as on the joints. It may cause inflammation in the blood vessels, eyes, salivary glands, heart and lungs. Nodules form under the skin of some patients, particularly over bony pressure points such as the elbows, and anemia is yet another complication, quite commonly seen.

A great deal of research is being carried out into the causes of rheumatoid arthritis. Much is already known about the progression of the disease and about methods of interfering with the pathological processes involved.

A popular theory for many years was that rheumatoid arthritis was caused by an infection. Areas of sepsis were sought and were held responsible for the continuing disease. Many patients had their teeth or tonsils removed to eradicate such 'focal sepsis', but this line of

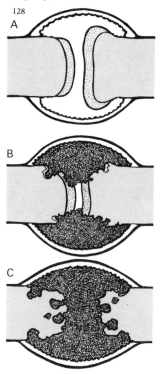

128
A

B

C

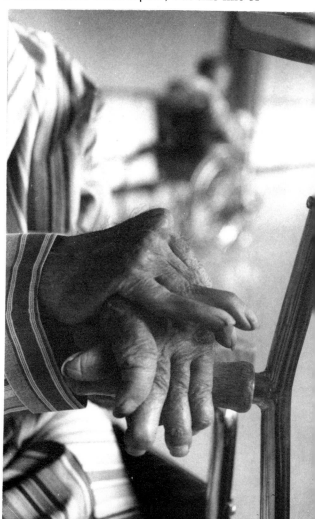

129

treatment has been abandoned. The search for some infective agent in rheumatoid arthritis goes on, however, and recently some groups of scientists claimed they had found certain microorganisms in the joints of sufferers. Other researchers have been unable to substantiate these claims, and a considerable controversy exists as to whether any organisms found are the cause of the disease, or are merely secondary invaders of an already damaged joint.

Whatever the initial cause of rheumatoid arthritis, many doctors believe the disease to be self-perpetuating once it has started. The mechanism can be explained in terms of the body's reaction to a foreign substance: when a foreign substance (antigen) is injected into the body, antibodies are produced which effectively neutralize it and allow the white blood cells to destroy it. This is part of the body's defense against infection, and a similar process is involved in the rejection of transplanted organs. The process depends upon the recognition by the body that certain substances are 'foreign' to it, and therefore it must also have a means of identifying its own proteins as 'self'. In certain circumstances the mechanism goes awry: proteins of the body are not recognized as 'self' and antibodies are formed against them. Diseases that result from such an immunological mistake are known as 'autoimmune', and there is evidence for the existence of autoimmunity in rheumatoid arthritis. (See illustration 81.)

In the 1930s Cecil, Nichols and Stainsby found that blood from patients with rheumatoid arthritis was able to cause certain bacteria to clump together. It was discovered later that this reaction was due to certain substances in the blood, now known as rheumatoid factors, which enhance its normal antibacterial activity. Waaler and Rose in the 1940s developed a special test for detecting these factors. Rheumatoid factors have been shown to be antibodies directed not against bacteria or other foreign substances, but against a constituent of the body itself—a particular protein which has been altered in some way. Moreover, in rheumatoid arthritis large numbers of plasma cells—the cells that form antibodies—are found in the synovial membrane of affected joints producing rheumatoid factor.

Now, all this does not mean that rheumatoid factor is the *cause* of rheumatoid arthritis; indeed, it is found in some people who do not suffer from arthritis. Nevertheless, there is good evidence that rheumatoid factor and other auto-antibodies present in the joints can perpetuate the inflammatory process. The theory goes like this: suppose the rheumatoid factor combines with some unknown antigen within the joint. Then white blood cells leave the bloodstream and enter the joint fluid to engulf the antigen-antibody complex. While in the joint, the white cells release enzymes from small particles, known as lysosomes, which they contain. It is these lysosomal enzymes that are responsible for the inflammation and tissue damage.

This hypothesis does not say what initiating factor makes the joint tissues antigenic. The most generally accepted view, at the moment, is that a microorganism may infect the joint initially, setting up an inflammatory reaction. In those people who are in some way genetically predisposed, the inflammation causes an alteration in proteins present in the joint, making them *appear* foreign and thus inducing the production of antibodies against them, with the consequences previously described. The fact that areas other than joints are sometimes involved in the rheumatoid process could be partly explained by the travelling of antigen-antibody complexes via the bloodstream around the body.

When the exact cause of rheumatoid arthritis is discovered, treatment will no doubt be aimed at eliminating the cause. Meanwhile most of the treatments available are directed towards relief of pain, preservation of function, and prevention of deformity. They cannot reverse the effects of the already established disease, although they may slow down or stop any further progression.

In acute flare-ups of arthritis strict rest is a useful way to get the inflammation to settle down and to avoid straining the ligaments and tendons around the joints, which are important for joint stability and which may already have been weakened by the inflammatory process. In addition, drugs to relieve pain may be required at all stages of the disease. The most effective, used by many patients, are those that combine anti-inflammatory activity with pain relief, such as aspirin and the newer drugs phenylbutazone and indomethacin. Because of their specific effects on inflammation they damp down the early morning stiffness which is often so incapacitating. But these drugs do not alter the natural history of the disease, they merely make its effects tolerable while spontaneous remission is awaited.

In some cases further measures must be taken, including treatment with antimalarial agents such as chloroquine, or injections with gold compounds. Both types of treatment can be very successful in establishing remissions, but both have serious side-effects and are only to be used under strict medical control. The same is true of the corticosteroid group of drugs, based on cortisone and hydrocortisone, the naturally occurring hormones produced by the adrenal glands (see chapter 3).

These drugs are certainly extremely powerful anti-inflammatory agents which can provide striking relief of symptoms. Unfortunately, in the early years of treatment unnecessarily large doses were used and the result was an array of

128 This diagram shows stages in the evolution of rheumatoid arthritis. This is essentially a disease of the synovial membrane which lines and lubricates many joints, and it is a thickening and inflammation of this membrane (A) which may be the first, and is sometimes the only, manifestation of the disease. As it progresses an ominous sign is the growth of inflammatory tissue from the synovial membrane into the structures of the joints themselves, shown here as destruction of the joint cartilage and even erosion of the underlying bone (B). An advanced stage of this destruction is shown in (C), where the articulating bone ends have been totally disorganized. The joint may become replaced with scar tissue which unites and obliterates what was once a mobile joint.

129 The results of rheumatoid disease graphically depicted in the distorted hands of an elderly victim. It is not only the joints that show the severe effects of the disease: there is also wasting of all the other structures of the hand. This is partly the result of disuse, but it is also accounted for by the involvement of the muscles of the hand in the rheumatoid disease itself. The elbow crutch which is also visible in the picture is one of many devices which assist the disabled rheumatoid patient (see also illustration 136).

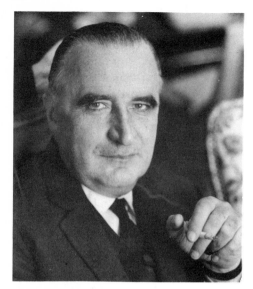
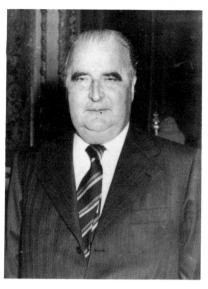

130, 131 An apparently miraculous cure for rheumatoid arthritis, introduced in the late 1940s, was cortisone, a natural product of the adrenal glands. Many synthetic modifications of the adrenal steroids have subsequently been produced in the laboratory. These powerful anti-inflammatory drugs, however, though often conferring great benefits, were soon found to have side-effects, all unwanted and some serious. One of these, 'mooning' of the face due to salt and water retention by the body and abnormal deposition of fat, is evident in these two photographs of the former French President Georges Pompidou, the later one taken in January 1974 after he had been receiving steroid therapy for what was reputed to be a serious blood disorder. Adrenal steroids may also provoke osteoporosis (thinning of the bones), diabetes, high blood pressure, and suppression of the body's reaction to infection and stress. (This last side-effect is taken advantage of when adrenal steroids are given to transplant patients (see chapter 11) where the major problem today is the rejection of the 'foreign' tissue.) Nevertheless, carefully used and with appropriate safeguards, this series of drugs can confer great benefit and, under certain circumstances, may be life-saving. The advantages and problems of their use illustrates well the fine balance that must sometimes be struck between costs and benefits in modern medicine.

132 A rare cause of backache, ankylosing spondylitis, is illustrated in this X-ray photograph. The supple ligaments which normally permit but constrain movements of the individual vertebrae become inflamed and are finally converted to bone themselves. Careful inspection of the X-ray will reveal bridges of bone linking the normally independent vertebral bodies. In the lower part of the picture a dense central vertical spear of abnormal bone may be seen through the vertebral bodies,

unpleasant and dangerous side-effects, without much more than a temporary effect on the disease. The production of a moon-face, bruising, thinning of the bones, peptic ulceration, liability to infection and suppression of the activity of the patient's own adrenals are all hazards of steroid treatment which discourage prescription of these drugs except in low dosage to the few cases where nothing else will do. Injection of steroids directly into joints, however, is very useful as an intermittent treatment in some patients.

The exact mode of action of all these drugs is uncertain, but one effect common to nearly all is a stabilization of the lysosomal membrane, preventing the release of the tissue-damaging enzymes. In the belief that rheumatoid arthritis may be an autoimmune disease, other forms of treatment have been tried which have a more fundamental effect on immunological mechanisms. These are the cytotoxic (cell-killing) or immunosuppressive agents, much used in transplantation patients for decreasing the body's immune response and thereby preventing graft rejection. Several of these have been used in rheumatoid arthritis with encouraging results. Another new drug with a different mode of action is penicillamine. It appears to reduce the amount of rheumatoid factor present, and has been shown to have a beneficial effect on rheumatoid arthritis. But all these modern drugs have major side-effects and are not yet included in the standard treatment of arthritis.

Physical treatments are of great value in rheumatoid arthritis. Splints may help to rest inflamed joints and together with suitable postural advice may prevent joint deformity. Application of wet or dry heat directly or by the various types of radiation may improve blood flow in affected areas, relieve muscle spasm and allow the use of therapeutic exercises to preserve the range of joint movement and build up muscle power. Hydrotherapy, the use of exercises in a heated pool, is based on one of the oldest ideas in

physical treatment, derived from the increasing popularity of spas in the 18th century. The principle is that of Archimedes, namely that a body immersed in water becomes lighter by an amount equal to the weight of fluid it displaces. In practice this means that a man of 132 pounds weighs only six pounds under water, a considerable reduction in the effect of gravity. If the water is warmed, movement of stiff and painful joints becomes easier. The use of all these types of treatment has to be carefully controlled and supervised, as excessive activity can increase the symptoms and cause a deterioration of the arthritic state.

The surgeon's role. Orthopedic surgeons play a small but increasingly important part in the management of rheumatoid arthritis, and a wide range of operations has been devised for different stages of the disease. As the disease process originates in the synovial membrane, a logical approach is an attempt to remove this membrane early on. This operation, synovectomy, has been carried out for many years and frequently appears to have been successful in arresting the disease. In other cases it has not been so successful, perhaps because of the difficulty of removing the whole synovium, which tends to regrow rapidly from fragments left behind. Synovectomy is most appropriate to the knee and some of the small joints of the hands, and is only applicable in early arthritis where little or no joint damage has occurred.

Another type of operation sometimes used in more advanced disease is that of osteotomy, in which a wedge of bone is removed so that the joint surfaces can be brought into better alignment. If a joint is severely damaged, painful and unstable, a satisfactory operation may be that of arthrodesis, in which the joint is permanently stiffened. Naturally this is to be avoided if at all possible, but it may be the best solution, particularly for the knee, and it has the significant advantage of providing complete pain relief.

The biggest advance in joint surgery, however, has come with the development of arthroplasty—the creation of artificial joints. In the simplest type of artificial joint the bone ends are removed, and the bones are merely allowed to move freely in relation to each other, held in position by the muscles and ligaments. This is a satisfactory pain-relieving operation for the joints in the balls of the feet, and has also been used for the elbow and the hip, although in the latter situation some stability is inevitably lost. If stability is to be retained, it is necessary to preserve some sort of articulating joint. An early way of doing this in the hip was by placing a molded cup between the head of the hip bone (the 'ball') and the pelvis (the 'socket'). This worked well in many cases, but had too many disadvantages to be really useful in rheumatoid arthritis.

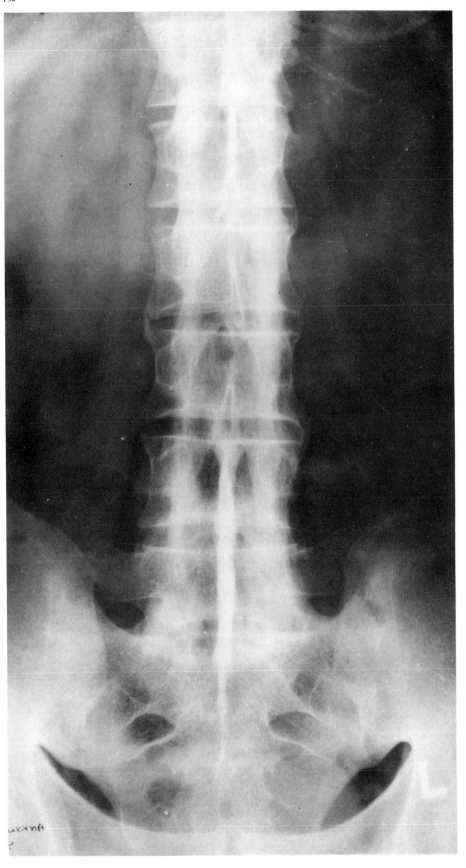

These snags have now been overcome by the total hip replacement, pioneered by British surgeons in the late 1950s (see chapter 7).

But the hand presents a special problem for surgeons. Patients are often most conscious of deformities of the fingers, but an operation is never carried out for deformity alone, the keynote being preservation of function. It is useless to restore to normal the shape of hands affected by rheumatoid arthritis if their ability to function efficiently is jeopardized. Hand surgery is a specialized field, and is only undertaken after most careful consideration. Useful procedures include synovectomy, fusion of unstable joints, tendon repairs and transplants, releasing tightened muscles, and arthroplasty with or without artificial joints. Several such artificial joints have been made, one of the simplest being composed of a single flexible rod of silicone rubber. The technique for performing the operation is improving all the time, and some surgeons will now replace finger joints in the out-patient department, although this is far from being a universal practice at present.

Ankylosing spondylitis. This is another inflammatory joint disease of unknown cause. Evidence of this disease has been found in skeletons up to 4,000 years old, though the first clear written description appeared in 1695. Unlike rheumatoid arthritis it mainly affects men and involves the joints of the spine, which tend to stiffen up gradually as the disease progresses. Ankylosing spondylitis usually starts with low back pain and stiffness and, although an uncommon disease in the general population, it is nevertheless a significant cause of these symptoms in young men. In one U.S. Army hospital during the Second World War, ankylosing spondylitis was found to be the cause in 18 per cent of soldiers admitted with chronic backache. The disease is often self limiting but in some patients it progresses to cause complete fusion of the spine with a stooping posture, restricted spinal movement and chest expansion. In the worst cases patients used to be virtually bent double, but this can always be avoided with modern methods of treatment. Up to a third of patients may have arthritis in the limb joints, rather similar to rheumatoid arthritis, but rheumatoid factor is not found in the blood. In addition to their joint problems some patients have inflammatory changes affecting the eyes and heart.

X-ray treatment was once popular and provided considerable relief. The X-rays were directed at the spine and it is now known that the large doses used could affect the bone marrow in the vertebrae, and in some cases cause leukemia. This treatment has largely given way to the use of anti-inflammatory drugs. The mainstay of treatment, however, is exercise to maintain spinal mobility and a good posture. Short periods of intensive physiotherapy and hydrotherapy may be beneficial, but postural exercises which can be carried out at home are generally the best guarantee against deformity. In a few cases orthopedic operations are required. With good treatment 80 to 90 per cent of patients are able to

fusing their rearward spinous projections, normally linked only by mobile ligaments. Interest in the causation of this condition has been stimulated by the recent demonstration that 95 per cent of patients with ankylosing spondylitis have inherited the same tissue type, HLA-B27 (see page 140).

hydrotherapy. Formerly the waters were thought to have some special healing properties, either as a result of their temperature or thanks to their mineral content. Thus arose the partly therapeutic, partly fashionable popularity of such places as Bath and Baden Baden. Illustration 133 shows elegantly attired bathers relaxing in the beneficial waters at Leuk in Switzerland about 1873. Modern hydrotherapy (134) is based on the supportive properties of the water which allows patients to exercise painful joints relieved of the effects of gravity. This is only one of the many forms of physical medicine which have played so important a role in the relief and rehabilitation of patients with joint, bone, muscle and even nerve disease. Passive and active movement, the retraining of weakened muscle, the provision of ingeniously designed devices and, above all, the active, optimistic approach to treatment, have maintained in active and productive life many who, a generation ago, would have been consigned, demoralized, to the sick-bed.

remain in full-time employment.

The cause of ankylosing spondylitis is unknown, but recent research has provided very strong evidence for a genetic predisposition in those affected by the disease.

Joints may be involved in certain infectious diseases. In some of the viral illnesses such as infective hepatitis and German measles, there may be a transient inflammation of the synovial membrane of the finger joints. And some bacterial diseases, including tuberculosis and brucellosis, may cause considerable joint damage. Treatment here is directed at eliminating the causative organism.

Diseases of connective tissue. Another group of diseases, sometimes referred to as the diffuse connective tissue disorders, may be related to rheumatoid arthritis, although the joint symptoms are less severe and are but one part of the disease. One of these, systemic lupus erythematosus, has aroused great interest among immunologists. Although joint pains and a typical skin rash are the usual features, there may be involvement of the blood, lungs, heart,

nervous system and kidneys. The disease is very variable in its course in different individuals. The evidence for an immunological disturbance is that blood tests reveal the presence of a wide range of auto-antibodies, the most characteristic of which are directed at components of the nuclei of the patient's own cells.

It is suggested that these antibodies can form 'immune complexes' with the nuclear antigens, and that these complexes lodge in the small blood vessels, especially in the kidney. One of the proteins in the blood known as complement becomes attached to the complexes, and is able to initiate the inflammatory process. As in rheumatoid arthritis the cause of the disease is unknown, but there is some evidence from studies both on humans and on mice that a chronic viral infection may be the primary event. The disease is potentially a serious one, and may result in kidney failure. The outlook has been considerably improved by the use of large doses of steroids, and early evaluation of immunosuppressive agents suggests that they will have an increasingly important role in treatment.

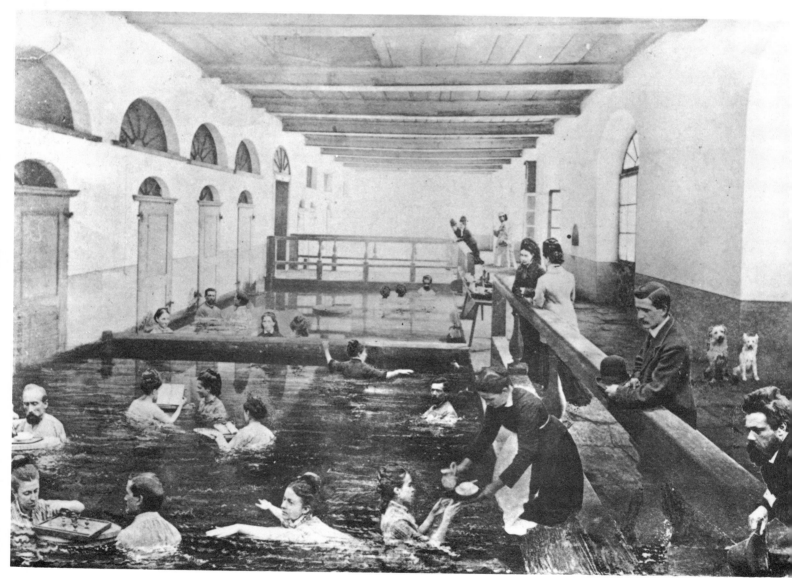

133

Rheumatic fever. This is one disease whose cause is a little better understood. It was probably known to Hippocrates, but at that time all arthritic diseases were considered to be variants of gout. The term 'rheumatism' to describe an illness separate from gout was first used by Guillaume de Baillou (1538-1616), but it was due to the writings of Thomas Sydenham in 1675 that rheumatic fever was firmly established as a distinct entity. It attacks mainly children and adolescents, and is seen as a fever and migratory arthritis, often accompanied by a characteristic rash and inflammation of the heart muscle and valves. The latter is the most serious aspect, and may produce permanent damage. Attacks of rheumatic fever are always preceded by an infection of the throat with a particular type of streptococcus, but this is not thought to be the direct cause of the disease. Rather the streptococcus is believed to share common antigens with the human heart, so that antibodies produced against the bacterium can attack the patient's own tissues. There is considerable evidence for this theory, but it is not a complete explanation as many people are exposed to streptococcal infection without developing rheumatic fever. There may be some genetic basis for different individuals' reactions to the organism.

Over the last 100 years there has been a dramatic reduction in illness and death due to rheumatic fever in developed countries, as the disease has decreased both in incidence and in severity. This improvement has resulted through social rather than medical measures—the elimination of poverty and overcrowding, and the introduction of better housing and public health provisions. Since the discovery of sulfonamides and penicillin, prompt and specific treatment for streptococcal sore throats has been easy and this has further reduced the incidence of rheumatic fever. Treatment of the established disease has changed little in recent times, the mainstays being rest and aspirin therapy, although the worst consequences of heart valve damage are now amenable to the refined techniques of cardiac surgery.

As rheumatic fever has declined in importance, so another cause of arthritis in children has claimed more attention. This is juvenile rheumatoid arthritis, or Still's disease, first described in the 19th century. It often begins with pain and swelling in the joints, fever and a rash, and unlike rheumatic fever it may produce joint damage as well as stunting of growth. Treatment includes anti-inflammatory drugs (though steroids can cause more growth retardation), suitable exercises and splints, and surgery when necessary. The disease is chronic so full emphasis must be placed on social support and continuation of education in a special school if

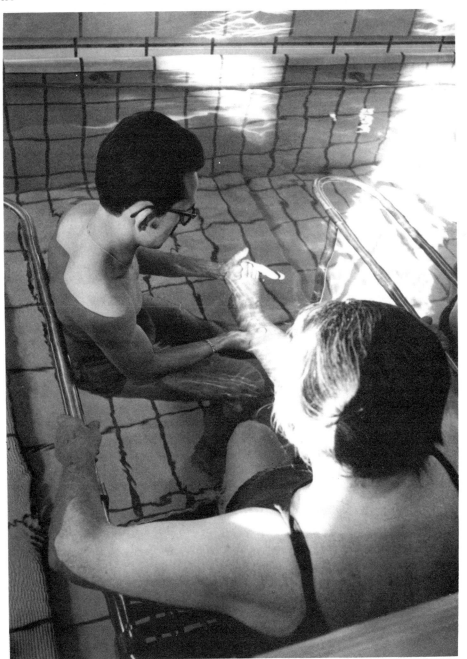

necessary. With good treatment, most sufferers are able to lead normal adult lives.

Osteoarthrosis. In view of the vast amount of work performed by the joints in a lifetime, it is not surprising that they are subject to wear and tear. Normally, the body tissues have considerable powers of regeneration, but as ageing takes place the rate of degeneration exceeds the rate of repair, and in the joints this is reflected in degenerative joint disease, or osteoarthrosis.

Man has always been subject to osteoarthrosis. It has been seen in the skeletons of Egyptian mummies and even as far back as Java man, half a million years ago. Today it is widespread and X-ray surveys have shown that about half of all adults are subject to osteoarthrosis in some degree. Over the age of 65, the prevalence rises to more than 95 per cent. Fortunately, X-ray changes are not always reflected in symptoms, and most people with some degree of radiological abnormality are perfectly well and symptom-free. Nevertheless when the large weight-bearing joints such as the hips show severe changes on X-ray, the patient is usually in pain and there may be considerable disability.

Other factors apart from ageing are important in the causation of osteoarthrosis, including congenital malformation of the joints, previous damage due to injury or arthritis, and excessive strain due to obesity or occupational overuse. One survey showed osteoarthrosis of the knees to be five times more common in coal miners than in office staff. Nevertheless osteoarthrosis often occurs in the absence of any of these predisposing factors, and there is some evidence that heredity may play a part in this group.

The changes that affect the cartilage early in the development of osteoarthrosis are the subject of considerable investigation and controversy, for only by preventing or reversing these early changes could osteoarthrosis be conquered. Once the cartilage has worn away and the bone ends are exposed, the process cannot be effectively eradicated, but pain and disability can be considerably limited by pain-relieving drugs, muscle-strengthening exercises, and sometimes surgical operations.

Degenerative changes may also occur in the spine. The vertebrae, which make up the spinal column, are separated from one another by intervertebral disks. These normally act as shock absorbers, smoothing out the jolts sustained by the spine during daily life. When degenerative changes occur in these disks they lose their elasticity and become thinner. The mechanics of the spinal column are altered, so that it is less able to cope with the stresses to which it is subjected, putting extra strain on the muscles and ligaments which normally give it stability. In addition the spaces between the vertebrae may become narrowed, leading to alterations in the surfaces of the vertebrae and changes in the contours of the bone. All these changes may cause chronic or recurrent pain, which is particularly disabling when it affects the lower part of the back—one of the major causes of loss of time from work. Pain in this region of the spine is often referred to popularly as lumbago. Similar changes may occur in the neck, a process referred to as cervical spondylosis.

Occasionally, the central pulp of the degenerating intervertebral disc may be squeezed out from between two vertebrae. This 'slipped disk' often follows sudden strain and may be acutely painful. It is by no means confined to the middle-aged, occurring often in young, fit people, particularly those in strenuous occupations. In the low back, a slipped disk may cause 'sciatica' by pressure on one of the nerve roots leaving the spinal cord, causing pain spreading down the back of the leg. The symptoms usually settle with rest on a hard surface and pain-relieving drugs, allowing healing to occur. This may be followed up by use of a corset, and suitable postural exercises. Some patients are helped by manipulation. In a few cases where there is persistent pain, or pressure on nerve roots, an operation may be required to remove the protruding part of the disk, and sometimes to fuse the affected vertebrae together.

Diseases of bone. Bone is not an inert substance, but is continuously remodelled throughout life, a balance being maintained between bone formation and resorption. The latter process predominates from the age of 30 onwards, so that the bones become thinner due to loss of protein and mineral content. In certain situations this thinning is more marked and may be detected on X-ray as osteoporosis. The bones are weaker and more subject to stress, fractures are more common, and the vertebrae become compressed—which explains the loss of height so frequent among the elderly. A vertebra may collapse completely, resulting in considerable back pain. No treatment is entirely satisfactory, but analgesics, exercise, anabolic hormones and calcium supplements all have a part to play.

Paget's disease, first described by the British physician Sir James Paget in the 19th century, is a condition in which the rates of bone formation and resorption are grossly accelerated in the affected areas, and the bone architecture is completely distorted. Bone involved in the process becomes softened and expanded, and the weight-bearing bones of the legs become bowed. The disease may be symptomless, but sometimes causes severe pain. In recent years there has been rapid advance in the search for a cure for Paget's disease, and work is currently in progress on several agents which appear to be effective additions to the symptomatic treatment at present available. These are the cytotoxic substance mithramycin; calcitonin, a hormone produced by the thyroid gland; and the diphosphonates.

In osteomalacia the defect is a widespread demineralization of bone, usually due to a deficiency of vitamin D and reflected in bone pain, tenderness and muscle weakness, with difficulty in walking. In children vitamin D deficiency causes rickets. Although almost eradicated by good nutrition it is still a problem in the poorer countries, particularly when exposure to sunlight is inadequate and the skin cannot act as an alternative source of vitamin D. These conditions can be cured with vitamin D and calcium.

Over-enthusiastic treatment with vitamin D is avoided as excessive dosage increases the level of calcium in the blood. This can produce unpleasant symptoms and may result in kidney damage.

Another type of bone disorder is caused by overactivity of the parathyroid glands. These glands produce a hormone which can deplete the bones of calcium, and cause diffuse rheumatic pains. Treatment is in the hands of the surgeon, as removal of the parathyroid tumor—the usual cause of overactivity—will relieve the symptoms.

The soft tissues. Rheumatic symptoms may arise neither from the bones, nor from the joints, but from the surrounding tissues, including the joint capsule, ligaments and tendons. Aches and pains originating from these structures are referred to as soft tissue rheumatism. This is a common complaint, accounting for about one-third of days lost from work due to rheumatic disease. The causes of soft tissue rheumatism are poorly understood, though a number of factors such as unaccustomed exercise, occupational overuse, injury, postural strain, exposure to damp and cold conditions and even anxiety may be involved. One common condition is fibrositis, in which pain and stiffness are felt in localized areas usually on the back of the neck, shoulders, and lower back. There may be areas of acute local tenderness (trigger points) in these areas, probably due to muscle spasm. The patients are otherwise well, with no evidence of the weight loss or general ill health which may accompany other rheumatic diseases. Treatment consists essentially of reassurance as to the good outcome of the complaint, along with suitable analgesics, heat and massage, and occasionally injections of local anesthetic and steroids. Underlying psychological problems may also need attention.

Soft tissue rheumatism may be localized to a specific joint. The shoulder is often affected after an injury, and symptoms may range from varying degrees of pain to the complete loss of movement known as a frozen shoulder. The symptoms may arise from inflammatory changes in the joint capsule or tendons of the muscles moving the shoulder, or sometimes from deposition of calcium in the tendons. Heat, local injections and gentle exercises may all be helpful in treatment.

Pain may occur around the elbow joint due to injury to the tendons attaching the muscles that flex and extend the wrist, the well-known golfer's and tennis elbow. Like those other occupational hazards, housemaid's and clergyman's knee, they usually respond well to steroid injections.

The correct diagnosis of soft tissue rheumatism is of considerable importance, because the majority of conditions are benign and often curable, and they must be distinguished from the chronic diseases such as rheumatoid arthritis which may sometimes begin in similar ways. Another point to note is that skeletal pain is often of non-skeletal origin. Pain in the shoulder, for example, may be referred from the heart or the gall bladder, or may even be due to a spreading lung cancer. Full investigations may therefore need to be carried out in difficult diagnostic cases, for in soft tissue rheumatism the results are almost always normal.

An exception is the condition known as polymyalgia rheumatica in which elderly people are afflicted with aching and stiffness in the muscles around the shoulders and hips. This is characteristically worse in the morning, and often so severe that the victims have great difficulty in getting out of bed. The exact cause is unknown, but in a proportion of cases there is an associated inflammation of cerebral arteries which can occasionally cause blindness. The abnormal test in this condition is a consistently raised erythrocyte sedimentation rate. It has been found that relatively small doses of steroids of the cortisone type produce a dramatic effect, relieving symptoms usually within 48 hours, and safeguarding eyesight, so that early diagnosis of this not uncommon problem is of paramount importance.

Rehabilitation. At all stages in the chronic rheumatic diseases a major aim is to return the patient to a useful role in society. This is accomplished by rehabilitation, which is the result of an integrated approach based on the team work and special individual skills of doctors, nurses, physiotherapists, occupational therapists, social workers and other trained personnel. The importance of this to the community is clearly shown by the size of the problem. The National Health Survey in the United States in 1957-9 indicated that nearly 11 million people suffered from arthritis and rheumatism, of whom a quarter were definitely limited in their activities, and ten per cent were grossly disabled and incapable of work. In Great Britain, of 300 million working days lost annually because of sickness, arthritis and rheumatism account for one tenth. Because of their tendency to cripple without killing, the rheumatic diseases are the most important diseases in socio-economic terms. Rehabilitation is applicable not just to rheumatic disease, but to all conditions capable of causing disability. Eight per cent of the population over the age of 16 are thought to suffer from some kind of disability which interferes with their lives to a greater or lesser extent. In addition to rheumatic disease, there are some more common disorders which are neurological in origin. These include cerebral palsy, muscular dystrophy and spina bifida in children, paralysis of limbs due to strokes and spinal injuries, and multiple sclerosis. Past sufferers from poliomyelitis may require help in rehabilitation centers, though new cases are now a rarity in the advanced countries. Another important group of patients are those with orthopedic problems, particularly following war, industrial or road traffic injury, or amputation of

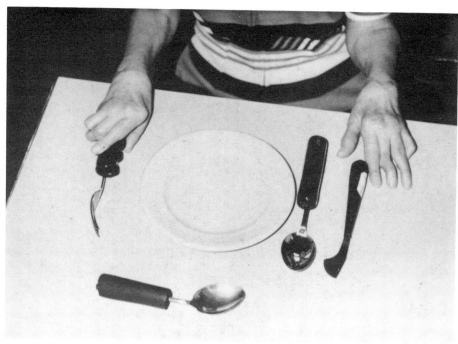

and could lead to further joint damage. Within this framework, the physiotherapist works to increase muscle strength and joint mobility, and to prevent deformities where possible. Functional re-education helps to maintain overall mobility and the ability to perform specific tasks despite paralyzed muscles and deformed joints. An important technique for disabled patients to master is movement from one site to another, for example from bed to wheelchair to toilet. For certain types of ailment the work of the physiotherapist is supplemented by that of the remedial gymnast who specializes in more intensive exercise and other measures for the alleviation of specific problems, which may be carried out in groups in a gymnasium. The occupational therapist has come a long way from her original role as the provider of diversional activities to relieve the tedium of a hospital existence. Tasks such as basket weaving may be provided to develop hand function, as well as to stimulate the patient's interest, though the main consideration will be given to perfecting the performance of the activities required for daily life. Occupational therapy departments contain model kitchens, bathrooms and other facilities to enable the patients to prepare for their return to the domestic environment. In addition, assessments of the situation in the patient's own home are carried out.

A wide variety of aids and equipment is available to make the best use of the residual function of disabled patients, and technical departments are attached to occupational therapy units to develop and modify such equipment. Dressing aids include special devices for doing up buttons, the use of Velcro instead of buttons, and long-handled shoehorns. Long-handled combs and razors can be provided for patients with limited upper limb movement, and cutlery with specially thick handles for those with a poor grip. Bathing may be made possible by the use of a handrail, a bath seat, and a non-slip mat. The use of a toilet may be facilitated for those with restricted hip movement by providing a rail and a raised seat. Similarly a high stool may make a considerable difference to a housewife's ability to work in the kitchen, as may the use of trolleys, a split-level oven, and replacement of water taps with levers. Gadgets are available for patients who have difficulty in bending to pick up objects from the floor. Crutches of different types can be designed for patients with individual problems. Chairs with 'ejector' seats may be useful for those who are unable to stand up unaided. Tip-up beds have been produced, and electric hoists can be installed for patients unable to climb stairs. Wheelchairs may be required for patients with poor lower limb function. The occupational therapist will be able to advise on the necessary modifications to the patient's

135, 136 The problems of the patient with chronic rheumatoid arthritis are not necessarily due to pain, but may be a consequence of disordered function. A patient with a poor grip, for instance, finds every-day activities difficult or even impossible. The patient in illustration 135 is unable to use ordinary cutlery, but the simple expedient of increasing the size of the handles has solved the problem. Simple gadgetry of this kind can greatly ease the practical difficulties of activities like eating, and a variety of devices is shown in the drawing.

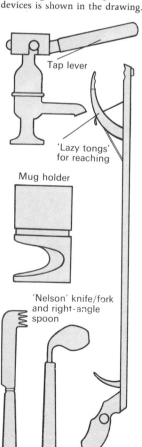

Tap lever

'Lazy tongs' for reaching

Mug holder

'Nelson' knife/fork and right-angle spoon

136

limbs, or with congenital limb defects, as occurred in the thalidomide tragedy. Rehabilitation is also an intrinsic part of the treatment of geriatric and psychiatric patients. The techniques of rehabilitation in individual diseases may differ, but the basic principles are the same.

The first step is the assessment of the patient's condition, from several points of view. The physician's role in outline is to diagnose the disease, initiate and supervise treatment, and evaluate the patient's response to it. An appraisal of the severity of the disease and the likely outcome are important factors in deciding on the suitability of various rehabilitation procedures.

The physiotherapist can assess the patient's muscle power, and range of movement or limitation at individual joints. A functional assessment is of key importance and is carried out by the occupational therapist. It is essential to know the degree of independence of the patient in performing everyday activities such as washing, bathing, dressing, feeding and going to the toilet. The social worker can fill in the details about the patient's social and domestic situation, together with difficulties encountered at work. In some cases a psychiatric assessment is also needed. In this way a complete picture of the patient's difficulties may be built up, together with some idea of his capacity for improvement and of the sort of life he will be able to lead in the future. The goals set for him must be realistic, understood and accepted by the patient, and at all times his family must be brought into the discussion and encouraged to help.

Rehabilitation takes place within a setting of continuing medical care. During a flare-up of rheumatoid arthritis, the physician will know for example that certain exercises are too strenuous home. Some limited work training may also be carried out in the occupational therapy department.

Another type of aid is the artificial limb for amputees usually produced in special limb-fitting centers. Artificially powered upper limbs have been utilized in the treatment of children with congenital limb defects.

The organization of rehabilitation services varies greatly from country to country. Some services are provided by hospitals, some by local and central government, and some by voluntary agencies. Often the impetus for the development of rehabilitation services has been provided by the need to retrain disabled soldiers after wartime. This has led to a recognition of the needs of the disabled as a whole, both in the provision of medical services, and, through industrial rehabilitation, in the re-adaptation of those recovering from illness or injury to suitable work. Further progress depends upon the whole community realizing its obligation towards the disabled. This means that not only must patients and their families be made more aware of the help available from existing services, but more must be done to adapt the environment to the needs of the disabled. Planners and architects should be involved to ensure that public buildings and shopping centers in future are designed to allow their full utilization by the disabled. How many cinemas or theatres at the present time are able to be used by people confined to wheelchairs?

Only by a complete re-appraisal of our attitudes to this situation can we ensure that those afflicted with chronic and disabling disease can live full

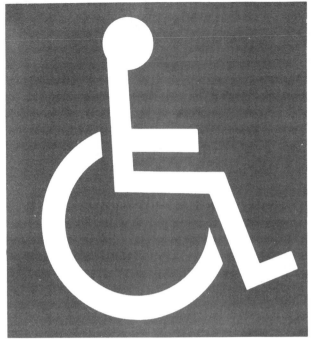

137 One of the features of society today is the provision of special facilities for disabled people confined to wheelchairs. This symbol is used in public buildings to indicate or identify such facilities as special lavatories with wide doors to accommodate wheelchairs, or access ramps where otherwise steps would present an insuperable obstacle. Part of the process of rehabilitation is the provision of devices and simple additional assistance such as fixed wall rails, bed hoists, and ramps inside the patient's home, modifications which may be undertaken by skilled teams of workers before the patient is discharged from hospital. These activities, often pioneered by voluntary charitable bodies and then undertaken on a regular basis by established social agencies, are part of the wide concern that society is showing for the disabled in the community. Much remains to be done to extend this process: for instance, many theaters remain inaccessible to the disabled.

and creative lives in the wider community, and that their disabilities do not become the insuperable handicaps which for many in the past have meant permanent institutionalization.

Here, as elsewhere, medicine's triumphs are not confined to the laboratory or medical clinic, but extend out into society, involving first the ancillary professions, then the provision of new implements and methods for patients and instruction in their use, and encompassing even the incorporation of a simple wheelchair ramp in a public building. To the disabled patient, it is triumphs in these spheres that mean most.

9 Brain, Mind and Nervous System

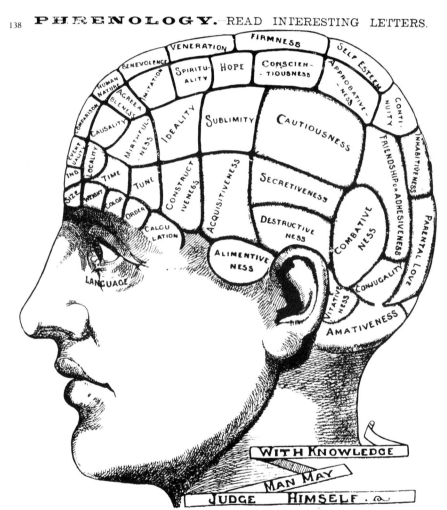

138

138 The dawning consciousness that many intellectual and emotional faculties had physical origins in the brain, 'the organ of the mind', is represented in the phrenological head of 1893 illustrated here. It was thought that prominences and deficiencies in the overlying skull pointed to corresponding 'bumps' and 'hollows' in the underlying characteristic, thought to be literally located

The brain and the spinal cord constitute the central nervous system from which nerves pass to all parts of the body. The whole of the nervous system, but especially the central portion, has many qualities which distinguish it from all other organs of the body. It represents the most highly specialized tissue in the body in which virtually all functions have been sacrificed for the development of just one; namely, the

transmission of messages by means of electrical impulses generated by complex chemical changes. All living cells have a small electrical potential across their membrane or outer surface and this property provides the basis for impulses that travel along the nerves and across the junctions between nerves that are present in hundreds of millions in the brain. For the perfection of this activity, nerve cells have sacrificed almost all powers of reproduction and of defence against noxious agents. Once the cells have reached a certain degree of maturation they are virtually incapable of repair, though the end fibers that form the peripheral nerves are capable of some regrowth.

Along with this high specialization goes a need for great constancy of temperature and chemical environment. The brain, for example, shows signs of oxygen lack earlier than almost any other organ, and it can be irreversibly damaged by a lack of the essential energy-producing substances within about a minute.

The brain also differs from the rest of the organs of the body in another important way, which will be mentioned only briefly now and elaborated later. This difference is that its functions are acquired as a result of learning and experience from birth, rather than being inborn mechanisms more or less unaffected by the environment. It follows from this that there are tremendous individual differences between brains, and indeed most of the science of psychology rests upon the study of such individual differences.

In this chapter the term 'brain' will be used loosely to refer to that organ which can be seen inside the skull; which can be directly stimulated electrically at operation and influenced by drugs; and which can be examined at post-mortem. The term 'mind' will be used when referring to

112

the functioning of the brain as manifested in thought, feelings and behavior—so that the word 'mind' has a psychological connotation and includes the result of self-observation and introspection as reported to others as well as direct observation of behavior. The resemblances and differences between the brain and the mind have been elaborated by philosophers at great length. Here all that need be said is that most doctors interested in psychological medicine have to accept an uneasy dualism. Most of us recognize, however, that there must be some theoretical 'rapprochement' between mental states and physical events of the brain, if we are to understand them fully. The uneasy dualism is reflected in the two very different specialities interested in the brain and the mind, namely neurology and psychiatry respectively. Both these disciplines have profited greatly from the advances of scientific medicine in the last hundred years, though these advances have resulted in very little closer contact between the ways of thinking of the two specialities. It is still convenient therefore to consider the respective contributions of neurology and psychiatry rather separately, however deplorable this might be in theory.

The brain as a physical organ is prone to the same kinds of disorders as other organs, so that malformations, infections, injuries and degenerations can afflict it with resulting profound changes in function. The effects of severe physical damage can be devastating and permanent because of the brain's lack of powers of regeneration, as already mentioned. The brain and spinal cord are well protected from physical trauma by the skull and bony spinal column, but this very protection carries its own danger in that space-occupying disorders, such as tumors and hemorrhages, can squeeze the rest of the brain as they form because of the inflexibility of its coverings. Thus, even further damage can result over and above the effects of the actual destruction of brain by the growth or clot itself.

The effects of increased intra-cranial pressure constitute neurosurgical emergencies, and the perfecting of the techniques of brain surgery to deal with these in the last 40 years has resulted in the saving of many lives.

The neurosurgeon must know his way round to the nearest millimeter in some parts of the brain if vital functions are not to be irreparably damaged. Many ingenious techniques have been devised to show up possible deformities of brain shape as a result of tumors or hemorrhages, so that the neurosurgeon can accurately open up the skull and get to the diseased area of the brain with the least possible damage to the normal tissues around. A simple method that has been known for some time is the injection of air or oxygen into the spaces in the brain, which then show up in X-rays, since X-rays go through the air more easily than through the brain tissues. A fluid opaque to X-rays, similar to that which is used for the investigation of the gastro-intestinal tract, is also sometimes used for spinal cord lesions. The contrast medium can also be used by

139

in the brain according to the map drawn on the surface of the head. The localization of function which does in fact exist within the brain in no way resembles what is suggested here.

139 This diagram, conceived by the great Canadian neuro-surgeon Wilder Penfield (1891-1976), shows the actual localization of motor and sensory function in the brain cortex and indicates the disproportionate area given to the mouth, face and hand, compared with the rest of the body. The numbered sections of the surface cortex relate to the different parts of the body as follows: 1, toes; 2, ankle; 3, knee; 4, hip; 5, trunk; 6, shoulder; 7, elbow; 8, wrist; 9, hand; 10, little finger; 11, ring finger; 12, middle finger; 13, index finger; 14, thumb; 15, neck; 16, brow; 17, eyelid and eyeball; 18, face; 19, lips; 20, jaw; 21, tongue; 22, swallowing.

140-2 The real topography of the brain is represented in these drawings, showing the view from above and below and a vertical section seen from the side. The complex, infolded convolutions of the brain surface, the cerebrum, give it a very large total area, and it is this that distinguishes man from his nearest relations in the animal kingdom. Below the cerebrum lies the cerebellum, responsible for the integration and smoothing of muscular and reflex activity. Lying in front of this is the bulge of the mid-brain, where ascending and descending fibers joining the brain and spinal cord are collected together in bundles. In the view from below, the cut ends of the important cranial nerves can be seen clearly. Most striking, perhaps, is the large size of the optic nerves, an indication of man's heavy dependence on vision.

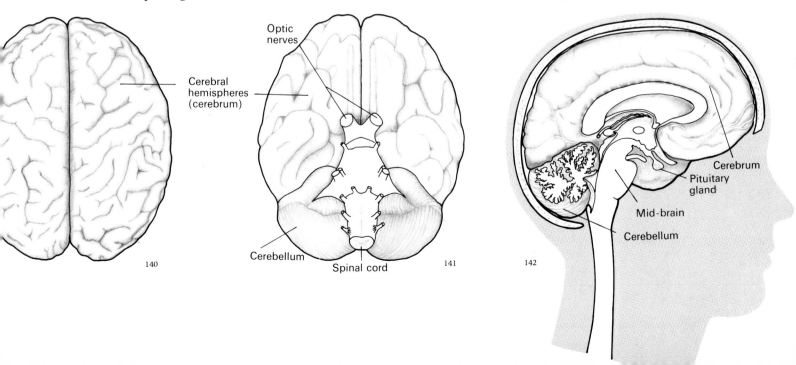

Optic nerves

Cerebral hemispheres (cerebrum)

Cerebellum

Spinal cord

Cerebrum

Pituitary gland

Mid-brain

Cerebellum

140   141   142

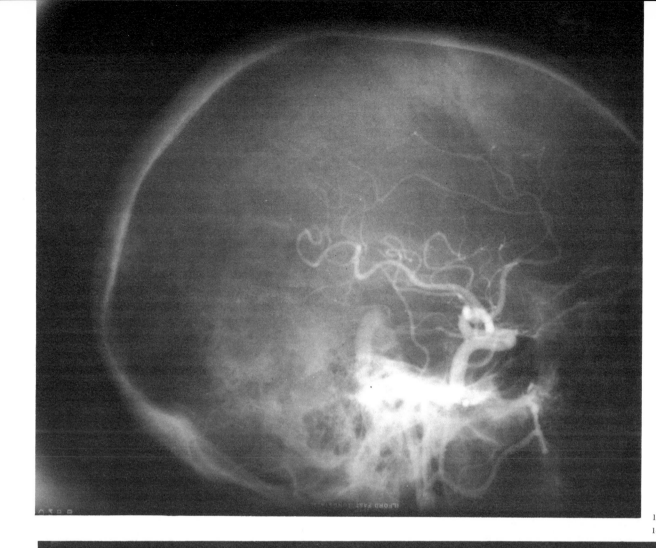

143, 144 A great advance in the diagnosis and treatment of disease of the brain and its blood supply came with the ability to inject a solution opaque to X-rays into the carotid artery, which feeds the head, and to take a rapid succession of X-ray photographs of the solution as it traverses the brain. The normal carotid angiogram (143) shows the carotid artery, coiled as it enters through the base of the skull, and rapidly dividing into long, convoluted branches coursing over the surface or into the substance of the brain tissue. A few seconds later, the radio-opaque solution passes more widely out of the main arteries into the tissues and 144 is another carotid angiogram (in a patient) showing the general opacification as the solution passes through the finer vessels. However, at the front of this general opacity can be seen a sharply circumscribed area with a greater flow. This has outlined the abnormal circulation in a brain tumor, in this case a meningioma. This tumor, growing from the surface covering of the brain and encroaching on the brain substance beneath, produces a variety of symptoms depending upon the function of the area of underlying brain concerned. Its detection and removal can totally restore to normal a person who had previously been grossly incapacitated.

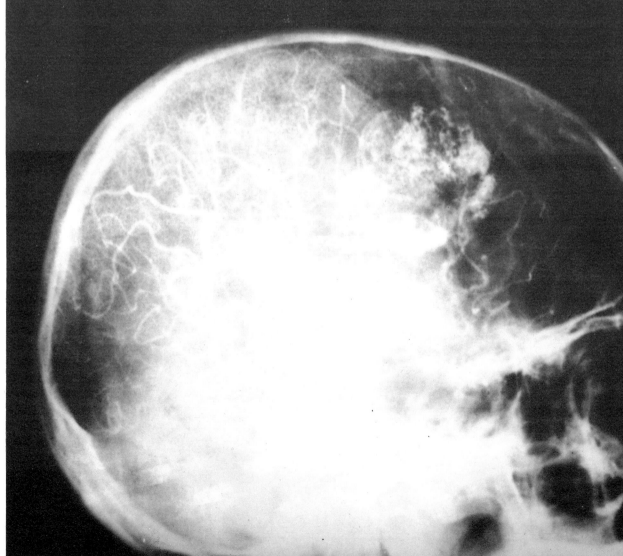

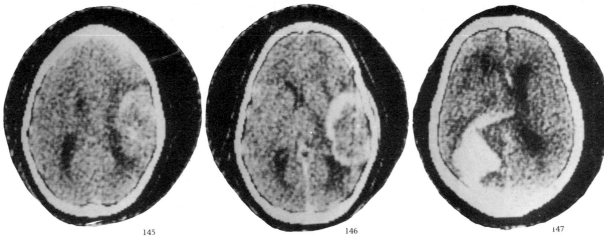

145   146   147

injection into the arteries supplying the brain, so that rapid serial X-rays will show up the fine structure of the arteries and then the veins in various parts of the brain. Both these procedures are not entirely without risk and these days two more recent techniques are usually tried first. In one, a short acting radioactive substance is injected, the radioactivity of which is then picked up by a special gamma scanner. Abnormal tissues such as tumors will pick up the radioactive substance at a different rate from normal brain and the latter may be deformed by the growth so the pattern of radioactivity is asymmetrical or distorted. Shifting of the brain from one side to the other can also be demonstrated using an ultrasonic technique, which is not very accurate but is perfectly safe and easy to apply so that it is a useful screening test. An even newer technique, embodied in the EMI scanner, may completely revolutionize diagnosis of abnormalities within the skull (see illustrations 145-7).

The management of strokes is an area to which neurosurgeons have made significant contributions in the last few years. A stroke is one example of the effects of a sudden interference with the blood supply to particular areas of the brain. Those parts of the brain which are connected with the control of movements of the limbs are specially liable to the effects of disease of the arteries. The arteries can be blocked by thrombosis, that is, a clot; or sometimes by an embolus, that is to say a small clot which starts off, usually from disease in the heart, wander up the main arteries, and lodges at the end of a vessel in the brain; or, thirdly, the arteries or veins may actually burst and blood pour out, sometimes over the covering of the brain or, more seriously, plowing into the actual brain substance. It has been known for some time that these hemorrhages most commonly occur because of weaknesses in the walls of the arteries, which balloon out, causing aneurysms. The arteries containing these aneurysms can be clipped off in cases where the rest of the circulation is good enough to take over the

supply of the area of the brain involved. When an embolus is the cause of a stroke, it usually arises from atherosclerotic arteries in the neck. Further episodes can often be prevented by surgery of the diseased arteries.

As well as surgery, the patient also needs an active program of rehabilitation. It has been realized that, even in the case of middle-aged persons, considerable degrees of improvement in function can occur if the limbs are kept moving and patients are actively taught to make the movements that they seem temporarily to have forgotten how to organize in their brains. The various diseases that affect the arteries of the

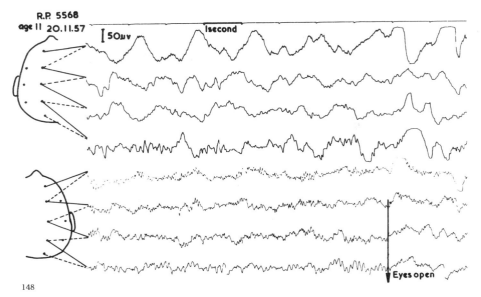

148

brain are usually part of general arterial disease and the measures used to deal with high blood pressure, described in chapter 4, are often applicable to patients suspected of having serious cerebrovascular disease.

Another useful technique for analyzing brain function is the electroencephalograph which records the minute electrical changes produced by the brain. The potential differences produced by neurons are exceedingly small and for a long time scientists were sceptical that anything could be recorded through the intact skull. However, millions of nerve cells seem to synchronize their

148 An electroencephalogram. As the electrode diagram shows, the first four channels of recording are from the left side of the head from front to back, and the second four from the right side front to back. Channels 4 and 8, from the posterior part of the head, show the normal so-called alpha rhythm of about 10 cycles per second that is interrupted at eye opening. There is an asymmetry in the front part with irregular slow activity on the left side which other investigations showed to be due to an abscess in this part of the head.

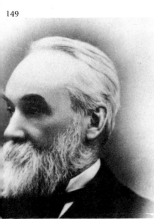

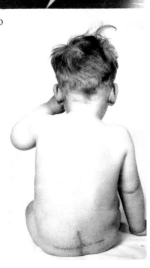

149 John Hughlings Jackson (1835-1911), one of the fathers of modern neurology. Following the spurious maps of the phren- ologists, the scientific study of localization of function within the brain is usually considered to start with Paul Broca (1824- 80). Hughlings Jackson's later clinical studies, especially of people with epilepsy (until then neglected by most neurologists and psychiatrists) led him to propound theories of the local- ization of function which continued to inspire observation and experiment for many years afterwards and were sub- stantially confirmed only com- paratively recently by the work of neurosurgeons like Wilder Penfield (see illustration 139).

activities so that a difference in electrical potential, sufficiently large to be picked up by electrodes on the head, is generated. The electrical activity of the brain is very complicated, but it has only a rather limited number of ways of showing abnormalities. The most important occur in the disorders associated with epilepsy.

This is a common symptom, especially in children, and like so many symptoms, such as cough or fever, it can have a variety of causes from the trivial to the serious. Electroencephalography has greatly helped in sorting out the different sorts of epilepsy, but in other ways it has been somewhat disappointing as a method of investigation. As already mentioned, only the synchronous activity of a large number of cells can be picked up through the intact skull—which is about as far away from a fine analysis of what is going on as a microphone suspended from an airplane above a big city would be for trying to unravel the workings of a commercial firm.

So far only the ways of investigation and treating gross structural changes have been mentioned, but the condition of Parkinsonism illustrates a new development that may have far-reaching consequences. Parkinsonism is sometimes known as 'the shaking palsy' as the sufferers show characteristic tremors of the limbs at rest, with alterations in gait and facial appearance that are diagnostic of the condition. Even in the heyday of the neuropathological study of the brain at post-mortem, the essential lesion was for a long time missed, and in fact it had a brief vogue as a purely psychological disorder. Then it became a curiosity of pathological anatomy, related to the death of certain cells at the base of the brain whose function seemed to have an inverse relationship to other unaffected areas. For a while, therefore, surgeons attempted to make new and further lesions in the brain in the hope of restoring the balance between the damaged areas. In recent years, however, there has been a wholly new approach, to understand which it is necessary to go back to describe briefly more about the functioning of nerve cells.

As already mentioned, the nerve cell is specialized for the transmission of a message or, more accurately, the transmission of an electrical charge which is capable of causing another neuron to fire or, if firing, stop firing. The passage of this electrical charge is accompanied by minute chemical changes, much as the production of currents from an electric battery is accompanied by a chemical change—so that it is a moot point whether one can describe the source of energy as electrical or chemical, since it is really both. Certain fairly simple substances have been known to be specially related to this electrical charge. Two of them—adrenalin and

acetyl-choline—have been known for a long time, but it has been suspected that there were other chemical transmitters in the central nervous system that were probably related chemically to acetyl-choline but slightly different. One of these, dopamine, has now been more or less accurately identified, and it was then shown to be especially deficient in those parts of the brain which are affected by Parkinsonism. Recently, it has been shown that feeding large doses of a precursor of this drug (L-dopa) to these patients resulted in a dramatic improvement of many of the symptoms (dopamine itself cannot be introduced into the brain). Even some of the psychological symptoms sometimes associated with Parkinsonism which are the result of a chronic virus infection of the brain, known as encephalitis lethargica, were temporarily relieved.

Mental handicap is another area where the most interesting advances in recent years have been in the field of neurochemistry. Mental handicap is now the currently accepted term for what was for a while called 'mental subnormality' and before that 'mental deficiency'. As each term gathers an aura of opprobrium around it, so neutral words have to be devised for the unfortunate group of people who are born with, or acquire early in life, such damaged brains that they are unable to function at a level of intelligence that is needed for our civilization. Everyone has a general idea of what is meant by intelligence, but the assessment of the psychological functions that compound it is often by methods that seem remote from education and the social skills in which intelligence is conventionally regarded as operating.

Mental handicap can be broadly divided into two great groups of causes. There are children suffering for the most part from the most serious forms of handicap, who usually have obvious damage to their brains that that can be seen, for example, at post-mortem. There is a much larger group of mainly moderately subnormal children whose brains seem to have no such obvious damage but who, nevertheless, function in society at well below the average level. This latter group will be discussed further below, as it is the former types of disorder where some interesting technical advances have been made in the last few years.

Children may acquire serious brain damage as a result of physical trauma, for example head injury, or of infections such as meningitis. An abnormal birth is particularly liable to produce damage, as a result of either the unwise use of forceps or the prolonged squeezing of the baby's head in a long difficult labor, leading to the blood supply to the brain being nearly cut off for so long that irreversible anoxic damage occurs.

In addition to these causes, it is now recognized that various events in utero can also impair the nutrition of the brain so that it grows in the wrong way. Genetic factors may also at times contribute to malformation, though these are at the present time regarded as less important than they used to be. Several inborn errors of metabolism affecting cerebral function have now been identified. In the case of phenylketonuria, described in chapter 3, a special diet if started within days of birth can eliminate the symptoms of subnormality. The diet, however, is very difficult to maintain, and there is still some doubt about the extent of recovery of function as not enough of these children have been followed long enough into adult life. It should be stressed that the condition of phenylketonuria is very rare indeed, so that this dietary control makes a negligible difference to the problem of treating mental handicap as a whole. However, the theoretical implications are of great interest and, as so often happens, the pathological condition can be used as a sort of natural experiment to investigate the metabolic pathways underlying many cerebral functions.

As a less happy example of the application of medical skill in the area of subnormality, the case of spina bifida should be mentioned. This is a congenital malformation which mainly affects the spinal cord rather than the brain. The spinal cord is formed very early in fetal life from a tube of cells that begins as an open plate and only slowly closes up. If the tube is not properly closed, then the nerve cells will remain open and the skin, bone and muscle that normally cover the cord also do not grow properly. As a result, parts of the central nervous system are exposed and after birth will rapidly get infected, leading to death of the infant unless complicated surgical procedures are embarked upon. In the last few years, a number of these infants have been operated on so that they are able to live several more years rather than just weeks or months.

However, it is now being realized that this reconstructive surgery often leaves children who are permanently disabled physically, and often subnormal too because of secondary brain damage, so that their lives are a misery to those who have to look after them. A profound ethical problem therefore arises acutely when one of these children is born. There are only a few days in which to decide the probability of surgery being of value, or whether the infant is likely to be always so damaged that it is wiser not to pursue active treatment at this stage but to allow the infant to die soon, as it inevitably would have done up to the recent past. (See chapter 13.)

It is probable that at birth the human brain has more or less as many cells as it will ever have, but the connections between the cells are still relatively undeveloped, especially in certain parts of the brain. The whole organ shows a rather curious, lop-sided evolution. Some parts of it, particularly those which seem to be connected with feelings and with the nervous control of certain bodily functions, such as heart rate, movements of the stomach and intestines, and so on, have undergone comparatively little change in the course of evolution from our near neighbors in the animal world, like monkeys. On the other hand, other parts, especially the so-called cerebral cortex— the part of the brain which is nearest to its outer surface—have undergone a tremendous change in what is a comparatively short time evolutionarily speaking. The factors that make for the development of the connections between the cells of the newest parts of the brain are generally supposed to be a mixture of inborn genetic tendencies and environmental experiences. Until quite recently, the latter were thought to be relatively unimportant, but in view of some ingenious experiments on the development of the brains of animals, such as cats, it now seems

150 Defective closure of the brain and spinal cord—the neural tube—results in the condition often known as spina bifida, which may vary in extent from a tiny bulge at the lower end of the spinal cord to large and crippling neural tube defects. Surgery can repair the protrusion of cord, nerves and covering membranes, as in the case of the boy shown here, who has been successfully operated on, but usually can do little if there is also serious disturbance of nervous transmission to the pelvis and lower limbs. So severe is the disability that, if it can be detected during fetal life, it is regarded as good grounds for a therapeutic abortion in some countries. The technique of amniocentesis, the withdrawal of small quantities of the fluid which surrounds the developing fetus (see chapter 12), now enables us to pick up tell-tale chemical clues to the existence of this defect. The child shown here was not amongst the most severely affected and could be expected to lead a perfectly normal life.

151, 151a Recent research in animals has begun to discover how some of the connections between brain cells are built up in infancy in response to experience of the environment. The individual cells in the areas of the brain associated with vision, whose minute electrical activity can be measured experimentally with implanted microelectrodes, do not simply respond to stimuli in one spot of the visual field, like a speck of rare earth on a television screen responding to the scanning 'eye' of the TV camera: particular groups of cells are specialized in recognizing particular aggregates of visual stimuli denoting, say, movement in a particular direction, or characteristic shapes. The two cats pictured here were brought up in visual environments designed to exclude all stimuli except vertical and horizontal lines respectively. They were kept in the dark, except for periods spent in these striped cylinders, where they also wore ruffs so they would not see their own bodies. Later it was found that the neurons in the visual cortex of each cat 'fired' selectively in favor of light bars oriented nearest to the orientation it had experienced. These artificial and extreme laboratory experiments are far removed from the variety of visual experience to which animals and humans are exposed in their formative years. Even so, they may be the beginning of a path leading to an understanding of the physiological brain processes associated with memory and learning in man. They may also have clinical relevance, providing insight into the causes of developmental disorders (such as squint) in human babies.

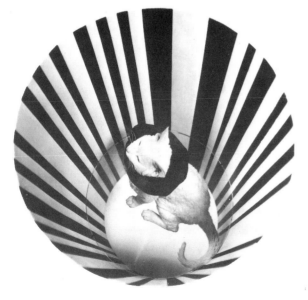

151

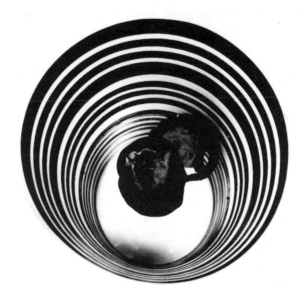

151a

probable that environmental experiences may determine the richness and direction of many of the neuron connections. If confirmed, this observation will be of profound importance, both theoretically and practically. It has always been a mystery how the brain changes during the psychological processes of learning. In fact, one of the famous investigators in this area concluded from his study of rats' brains that 'learning is impossible'! We see here, of course, a particular example of the nature-nurture conflict that has grumbled on in biology and medicine for a long period, and needs no more elaboration here at the present time. The fact is that people's minds vary enormously as regards thinking capacity, the expression of the feelings, and almost all psychological functions. These differences must in some way be reflected in physical differences in the brain that have so far eluded us. In practice, a constant reference back to possible underlying neurophysiological mechanism in brain functions is quite unnecessary in our understanding and management of many psychological disorders, and still less in our appreciation of normal development and individual difference.

Everyday observation, as well as sophisticated medical and psychiatric investigation, confirm the fact that the mind is capable of profoundly influencing many bodily functions. The acute changes are obvious to everyone who has had a sudden fright, when the heart races, there is a cold sweat, a desire to pass water, perhaps involuntary movements at one end or the other of the intestinal tract leading to vomiting or diarrhea, and many other symptoms. There are individual differences in the reactions of patients to painful or alarming stimuli, that can be related to personality characteristics measured by particular tests. People are also notoriously variable in their response to drugs, of which alcohol is easily the best known. Furthermore, a drug may affect the same person in different ways at different times, depending on the mood and social environment—again something which is a matter of everyday observation with alcoholic drinks.

Since it is probable that the direction and intensity of many of these responses are 'learned', that is to say the result of environmental experiences rather than inborn tendencies, it follows that the study of many psychological states, both normal and abnormal, can be understood only from the point of view of the life history of that particular person. For example, what makes one person frightened of spiders and another of heights? It is clearly a matter of particular experiences. It is still an open question whether there is such a thing as a 'constitutional' tendency to some general psychophysiological instability that may manifest itself in one or

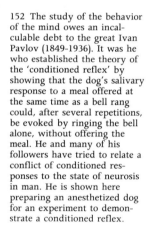

152 The study of the behavior of the mind owes an incalculable debt to the great Ivan Pavlov (1849-1936). It was he who established the theory of the 'conditioned reflex' by showing that the dog's salivary response to a meal offered at the same time as a bell rang could, after several repetitions, be evoked by ringing the bell alone, without offering the meal. He and many of his followers have tried to relate a conflict of conditioned responses to the state of neurosis in man. He is shown here preparing an anesthetized dog for an experiment to demonstrate a conditioned reflex.

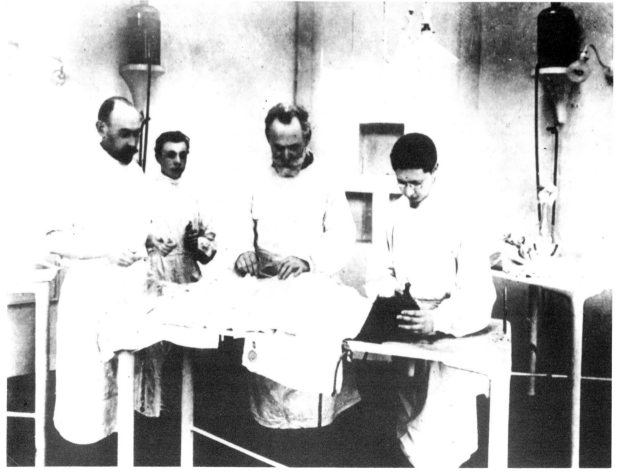

152

other of the types of disorders.

In spite of all this uncertainty, the trade in drugs that influence mental processes is far greater than in any other branch of pharmacology. What Aldous Huxley calls 'Noah's epoch-making discovery' of the fermentation of grape juice was the start of the search for tranquility, stimulation, ecstasy, or other mental states that has had a big new twist in recent years. Yet, in spite of the millions of dollars, Swiss francs and pounds (not to mention other currencies) poured into psychopharmacology, as it is called, the fact remains that all the important drugs were either already known to the ancients or have been discovered quite by accident. There should be an obvious relationship between our understanding of the chemistry of the brain, as referred to in the discussion of Parkinsonism, and our knowledge of drugs acting on brain functions, but so far the two areas of investigations have hardly cross-fertilized each other at all.

As an example we may take the phenothiazine series of drugs which have been known for more than 20 years. They have an important, if limited, role in the management of acute mental disorders and a more limited role in the management of certain chronic ones.

A common psychiatric emergency is that produced by the person who becomes acutely excited and unmanageable in his home or in a hospital ward. Various psychotic conditions may produce such a state—mania, schizophrenia and drug effects are the three most common—and such patients must often be admitted on a temporarily compulsory basis. Formerly strong sedative drugs such as morphine, the barbiturates and chloral hydrate were needed to calm the patient, who was thus more or less anesthetized. Drugs such as chlorpromazine (thorazine), however, calm the patient with little or no impairment of consciousness so that his cooperation with treatment can be established sooner. (In passing, it should be noted that even in this acute 'medical' situation the attitudes and actions of the psychiatric staff are very important. Nurses' long-suffering tolerance, understanding and sympathy can help the patient to control himself and reduce the duration of disturbance and the amount of drug needed to control it.)

In recent years a further technical advance in the use of these drugs for chronic mental disorders has been made by the introduction of long-acting preparations so that the drugs' calming effects can last two weeks or more. Patients who would not co-operate with taking drugs for as little as once or twice a day can now be successfully managed as out-patients in the community rather than having to be in hospital for little more reason than to get the drugs. Alongside these practical advances a mountain of theory about the causes of mental disorders has

been built upon the molehill of hard fact relating to the mode of action of these drugs, which has hardly been connected at all to any biochemical, genetic or other possible physical cause of these psychoses. However, these drugs were introduced into common psychiatric practice in most countries in the western world, round about the same time as the whole nature of the mental hospital changed under the influence of group psychological methods. It has therefore been extraordinarily difficult to tease out the relative importance of the drug and the change in attitudes of the caring staff to the management of patients with chronic psychiatric disorders. There is no doubt of the effectiveness of these drugs in acute mental states, so that few patients, for example, need to remain on compulsory orders in hospital for more than a few days. The effects of the drugs also wear off rapidly when stopped, and with one possible exception they seem quite devoid of long-term irreversible damaging effect.

In only one psychiatric condition does there seem to be some glimmering of 'rapprochement' between the psychological and the physiological, and this is the current mental disorder sometimes known as 'manic-depressive psychosis'. This relates to a heterogeneous collection of patients whose only common factor is a tendency to mood swings. Many patients have only dips down in their mood to depression occurring every few months or years. Some also go up into over-excitement or mania. Characteristically, in between the attacks the patients are quite normal, though some may remain fairly chronically on the high or low side of activity perhaps for years. It seems probable that

GALVANISM in PICCADILLY

153 Galvanism was another early approximation to the understanding of the connection between mind and matter in the brain, perhaps even more absurd than phrenology. The word 'galvanism' is its useful metaphorical legacy in our language. The newly discovered electrical force was credited with quasi-magical powers. From a 'little black box' of the time a practitioner is shown here administering a flow of Galvanism which, it seems, is exciting lively new thoughts in the mind of the patient. This situation also illustrates very well the enormous power of suggestion in medicine, the Galvanism here acting as a rather special sort of placebo (see chapter 15).

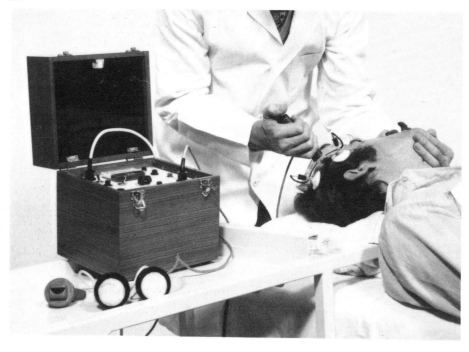

154 The physical treatment of major psychiatric disorder finds its most dramatic expression in the use of electroconvulsive therapy in the treatment of severe depressive illness. A brief pulse of electricity (at normal household voltage but involving a low current flow) is discharged between electrodes placed across the head. As the electricity traverses the brain it triggers a convulsive seizure. Nowadays the convulsion is virtually abolished by pre-treatment of the patient with muscle relaxing drugs, and unconsciousness is induced with a rapidly-acting anesthetic. A further improvement in technique is shown here, where, by appropriate placing of the electrodes, the current is passed through only one half of the brain. After a course of four to twelve such treatments, separated by intervals of a few days, there is usually a most dramatic lightening of mood, removing the very real risk of suicide. Although memory of recent events is diminished by the shock, this largely re-establishes itself over the next few hours and little or no irrecoverable loss occurs.

155 Group therapy represented on the stage in the play *Captain Oates' Left Sock* by John Antrobus at London's Royal Court Theatre. The actors portray the moods of anxiety, preoccupation and despair which characterize emotional disorders, perhaps no more prevalent than before, but certainly more frequently recognized in contemporary society. The interaction of disturbed people with each other in groups is used as a method of psychotherapy partly because of its inherent value as a method, partly because of the limited resources available for treatment on a 'one to one' therapist to patient basis.

chemical transmitter substances, closely related to dopamine, already mentioned in connection with Parkinsonism, are present in excessive or diminished amounts in certain parts of the center of the brain and that this could account for the symptoms, though it is still unclear why these substances should be present in abnormal amounts.

The so-called antidepressant drugs are known to affect the metabolism of such compounds (and many others). They are useful in treatment of patients with depressive symptoms though there are still too many unaccountable failures. In these latter cases recourse is usually had to the older treatment of electric shock therapy. This treatment is a good example of 'serendipity'. The story starts with the incorrect observation of the rarity of schizophrenic symptoms in patients with epilepsy, from which by false logic it was decided there could be some biological antagonism between these conditions, and that therefore convulsions might improve the psychosis. The induction of convulsions by rapid injection of certain drugs turned out in fact to be much more effective in depression than in schizophrenia. The technique was then made more humane by the use of electrical currents which produce an instant amnesia, rather than chemicals to induce the fit. The further refinement of doing the whole treatment under the influence of a combined injection of short-acting anesthetic and muscle relaxant drugs (to prevent fracture from the violence of convulsive movements) has perfected the present simple and not unpleasant procedure that is relatively free of side-effects. In spite of many biochemical, physiological and psychological investigations, especially in the early enthusiastic years of the use of the treatment, its mode of action remains essentially unknown.

It is also curious how little cross-fertilization there has been between the study of the psychiatric associations of naturally-occurring epilepsy and the therapeutic effects of induced convulsions.

Nevertheless, we shall hopefully get better control of these patients suffering from violent mood swings with drugs affecting the metabolism of the naturally-occurring substances related to them. Meanwhile, by what can be regarded as little more than a fluke, it has been established that a very simple chemical, a salt of lithium, can diminish the violence of the mood swings in some patients.

This observation is stimulating further biochemical investigations but it is obvious that the opportunities for study are limited. No animal analog to a manic-depressive illness has yet been discovered or invented, and quite clearly repeated sampling of the chemistry of the brain cannot be carried out in intact human beings.

These advances seem to be more successful than parallel investigations into the chemistry of schizophrenia, which is a much more chronic and disabling mental disorder.

The study of schizophrenia leads once again to the heart of the nature and nurture controversy with strongly held opinions, by lay people as well as experts, on the relative importance of biochemical on one side and experiential factors on the other in the production of this serious illness. So-called psychoses of this kind used to be fairly sharply distinguished from neuroses—the anxiety, obsessions, hysteria, phobias, which consistute a great bulk of the minor psychiatric disorders seen more in general practice than in specialized psychiatric hospitals. These latter disorders were regarded as more or less purely environmental in origin and treated accordingly. However, the great split between the genetically or organically caused psychoses and the environmentally or psychogenically caused neuroses has largely broken down to the benefit of the treatment of both groups. On the one hand there is now clear evidence of psychological environmental events precipitating, for example, relapse of schizophrenia. On the other hand, non-specific genetic tendencies towards both neurotic and psychotic behavior are recognized (though these are less highly regarded than formerly). The differences between one type of disorder and another within these two classes are essentially descriptive and not causal.

The revolution in patient care produced by the application of group psychological methods has already been alluded to, but now needs more elaboration. During the Second World War psychiatrists were few in number and faced with tremendous problems of treating large numbers of men with mental disorders. This provided the stimulus for systematic study of group rather than individual methods of helping people. The theoretical ideas behind much of this research stemmed largely from Freud, and they rest fundamentally upon the assumption that there is some psychic energy that may vary from person to person and from time to time in the same person. This energy or drive has to find its expression, if not in natural activity then by diversions into certain types of symptoms. Freud was an observer of genius, and his descriptions of the origins of many mental disorders remain the major cornerstone of contemporary psychiatry. This is in spite of the fact that any theory which presupposes psychic energy is more or less scientifically untenable. Biologists have long ago given up any notion of vital energy distinguishing living matter from non-living matter. There is no reason at all to assume that psychic energy is likely to be exempted from the general scientific principle that energy is essentially a construct rather than something which can be observed directly. Yet in spite of this theoretical weakness, dynamic theories of behavior have come to stay— at least for the foreseeable future of psychotherapy. Amongst other things, they provide the patient and the therapist with a common language that enables persons to make sense of their own lives. Communication is the essence of psychological treatment, whether occurring in the individual situation with one therapist and one patient, or in a group situation of many patients together with one therapist or several.

It should not however be thought that Freudian theory has been the only significant advance in psychology relevant to mental disorder in the past quarter of a century. Allusion has already been made to the problem of learning in relationship to brain and mind function. There are many types of learning theory, some of which have become influential in the treatment of certain limited forms of mental disorder, in particular those so-called phobias in which a patient has a specific fear of a particular object or situation.

The significance of the broadening of the theoretical bases of psychiatry is not just that more conditions may be treatable by psychological methods, but that a coherent body of theory and practice is being built up to cover all psychological treatments. For example, the learning and practice elements in dynamic psychotherapy are now being recognized, as are the 'transference' (i.e. doctor-patient personal interaction) factors in apparently 'objective' behavioral therapy. The medical models of disease are increasingly seen to be inappropriate to most psychiatric disorders. They are being replaced by models based on psychological, and to a lesser extent sociological, theories. For example, the social characteristics of the wards of psychiatric hospitals greatly influence their

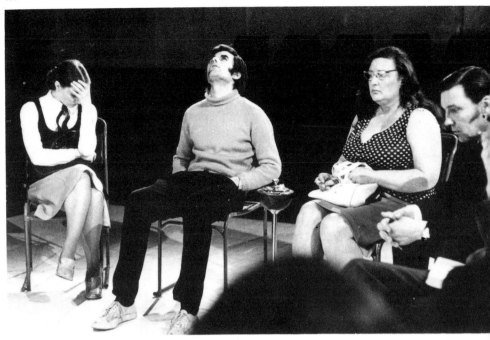

therapeutic value. The old-fashioned hierarchical way of working was copied from medical and surgical practice where it is for the most part still appropriate (though increasingly coming under fire). It is inappropriate to physically active patients who, for example, use their beds only to sleep in and not for treatment. Therapy *is* the social interactions between themselves and with the staff of all varieties, whether doctors, nurses, occupational theraptists or psychologists. The term 'therapeutic community' aptly epitomizes the changing attitudes that have probably been more influential over a wider range of psychological conditions than all the psychotropic drugs. It is worth noting in passing that this revolution in psychiatric practice largely came about through the exertions of busy consultant psychiatrists in ordinary mental hospitals of forbidding architecture, solidity and geographical remoteness. Academic psychiatrists played virtually no part, while academic psychologists and sociologists looked down their noses at this applied and practical stuff which seemed as much unworthy of their notice as engineering was to physicists in Victorian times!

The effect of these changes has been to improve the standing of psychiatry as a scientific discipline so that it seems no longer just a poor relation of neuropathology. At the same time, however, it has meant that the concept of mental disorder, understood as a disturbance of interpersonal relationships, has extended widely outside the conventional medical framework and into education, penology and social work. It would take too long to describe all the changes in attitudes and practice in all these fields, but some reference to child psychiatry, especially with regard to mental handicap, will

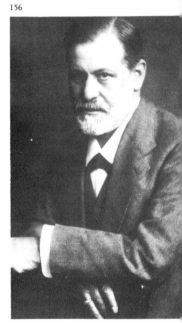

156 Sigmund Freud (1856-1939). Freud's contribution to the understanding of normal and disordered human psychology was in many ways the turning point in man's understanding of himself. Though it was based upon a rather selected and circum-scribed group of people, Freud's analysis of the role of instinct-ive drives and of the painfully built control mechanisms ex-plained much that had been studiously ignored by earlier, more idealistic or romantic psychologists. It was perhaps his appreciation of sexuality in the very young which most disturbed the public opinion of his time, though much of the criticism levelled against him was ill-informed. It is clear that no single school of thought is able to explain the complexity of human thought and behavior. Pure Freudianism is little practised, though Freudian theory remains influential.

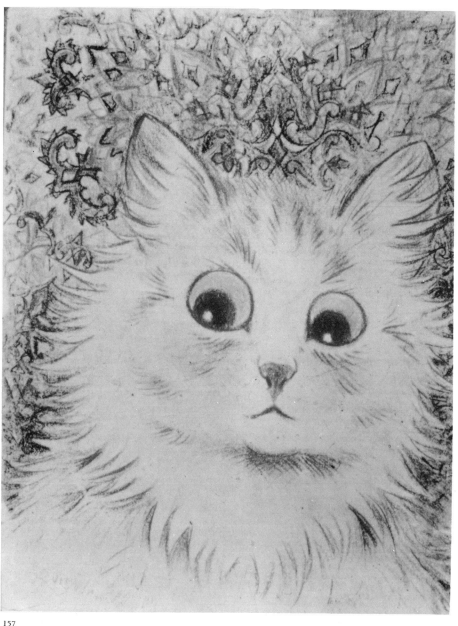

illustrate the effects of changing perspectives.

As already mentioned, there are two main groups of handicapped children: there are those already discussed who are severely subnormal and have gross brain damage, and there are those who are usually less severely retarded and have no obvious disease of the brain. These two groups contrast in many ways; for example the former, rather rare, children occur sporadically in all social classes, and their occurrence seems for the most part unrelated to psychological environmental factors. In contrast, the group that is for the most part mildly subnormal is often called 'subcultural' because such children are seen much more often in families of the lower social classes, who also show evidence of social disorganization; for example, poor parental standards of care, unstable job record, unsatisfactory housing conditions, overcrowding, large families, etc. The parents' own past history suggests that they themselves come from deprived surroundings. A high proportion of them went to

special schools by reason of being educationally subnormal or otherwise handicapped. It is therefore easy to see that such families were often regarded as evidence of 'poor stock' with mainly hereditary tendencies to low intelligence and social inadequacy. The pendulum has now swung in the opposite direction and it has been assumed that most of the disabilities can be traced to adverse social circumstances. There is no doubt that better provision of all social services — education, housing, medicine, etc. — does improve the performance of such disadvantaged children. The medical contribution consists in identifying possible factors like malnutrition and chronic physical disease, which are still very important in less developed countries. The psychiatric contribution consists in further study of how this so-called cycle of deprivation can be broken by helping deprived parents to become more human and effective parents. Close study of these families shows that often it is not so much formal low intelligence that makes them bad parents but their own clamant emotional needs, preventing them from providing the necessary consistency and stability of physical care and social training and tolerating the emotional demands of small children.

The care of small children of pre-school age is at the present moment a no man's land where pediatric clinics, health visitors, family physicians, all may be involved but without the clear line of responsibility that, for example, rests on the school medical service once the child is old enough. In no area is it more clearly seen that medicine is a part of the social services. It must be seen to function effectively within that whole.

In the last chapter reference was made to some of the human, social and emotional factors involved in the management of patients, especially those with chronic illnesses. The special neuropsychiatric contribution to understanding these problems consists in, first, helping the physician to sort out to what extent brain function may be interfered with by medical illness, thereby reducing the adaptability of the impaired organism. For example, patients with high blood pressure, even without an obvious stroke as well, may show some degree of impaired mental functioning or dementia. Numerous drugs affect functioning of the nervous system and may produce impairment in concentration, difficulties in thinking, irritability, apathy and a whole range of possible changes extending to frank confusion with disturbance of consciousness. Many of the drugs affecting the nervous system are slowly cumulative so that these effects may not be apparent for some weeks and can easily be missed.

However, even more important than the organic effects on personality are the psychological influences on patients' tolerance of

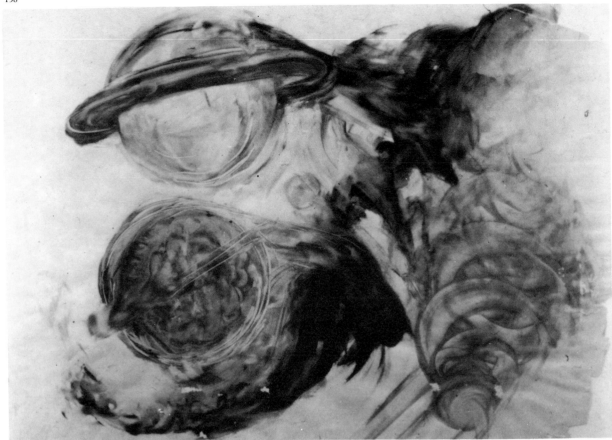

physical disease and their attitudes to the physicians trying to help them. It is a commonplace of medical teaching that one must treat the patient and not the disease. In an extreme form this implies, for example, that doctors may on occasion have to decide when a terminal illness can no longer be effectively reversed. Sometimes doctors have to take such decisions alone, for example when the patient is too ill to understand what is going on and there are no responsible relatives around. More often, one hopes that, as it has been well said, doctors make decisions *with* and not *for* their patients. Every doctor has to learn to make elementary assessments of the personalities of those with whom he has to deal. Family physicians, above all, usually learn to know their patients as people very well. Specialists in particular diseases, working from a hospital base, tend to have a more cross-sectional view of the condition they are treating and therefore of the patient. Treating the patient rather than the disease also requires some self-understanding, as had already been mentioned in relationship to the important factors in psychotherapy.

At the same time it is important not to forget that medicine is also a social service. At times doctors have to ask themselves for whose benefit are their skills being deployed—is it for the patient or the State? Does the patient really need what he seems to want, or at any rate demand? Family physicians particularly are well aware of the way in which patients may use minor

physical disorders or symptoms to obtain the doctor's help in some family crisis or social situation. On the other hand, what benefits to the State are provided by medicine and the social services? Who will decide on the priorities between specialities—for example, whether to spend money on psychiatry or geriatrics? As well as possible decisions that need to be taken about scarce resources within medicine itself, there are also difficult decisions to be made on priorities between medicine and other social services; for example, is money to be spent on better hospitals or better schools? When the British health service was founded 25 years ago, it was naively assumed that the better deployment of resources would result in such improvement in general health that the cost of the service might actually diminish. In practice, the cost is soaring and shows no signs of levelling off. In the case of diseases of the brain, one perhaps sees more clearly than anywhere else the limitations of so-called 'maintenance medicine'; that is to say, the support by artificial means of a failing organ function. In the case of dialysis for kidney disorder the advantages are usually fairly clear, but a prosthesis for the brain has a Frankenstein quality about it. The psychiatrist's role must thus, inevitably, be defined by what society wants, perhaps more clearly than for any other branch of medicine.

157, 158 'Great wits are sure to madness near allied', in Dryden's words, and the artistic productions of psychotic patients, especially of schizophrenics, interest psychiatrists, art critics and historians alike. A distinction can be made between the mad artist and the madman who paints. The former communicates with others whose understanding of 'reality' (whatever that is) is thereby enhanced, while the latter merely fills his private world with his own esoteric symbols. The picture of a cat (157) is from a famous series of paintings by Louis Wain, showing a progressive stylization and disintegration as the artist became more and more psychotic. The contemporary painting by a schizophrenic above (158), showing whirling planetary orbs, exemplifies a characteristic preoccupation with cosmic themes and events. From the therapeutic point of view, paintings and other artistic productions of psychotic patients can sometimes be used to help them to come to terms with their illness.

10 Vision and Hearing

159 The eye is the most highly specialized organ of special sense which man possesses. This sectional diagram displays its important components. To the left is the tough but crystal-clear cornea, separated from the lens by a fluid cushion, the aqueous humor, and the iris diaphragm, the aperture of which is seen as the pupil. The shape of the lens, determining the focus of the image of the outside world on the retina, is controlled by the ciliary muscle which encircles it. The wall of the eyeball is lined by the retina, a fine but densely packed layer of light-sensitive cells, along with their nerve fibers which conduct the light-evoked electrical impulses through to the optic nerve and thence into the brain.

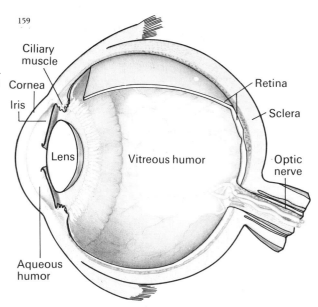

159

Ciliary muscle

Cornea

Iris

Lens

Vitreous humor

Retina

Sclera

Optic nerve

Aqueous humor

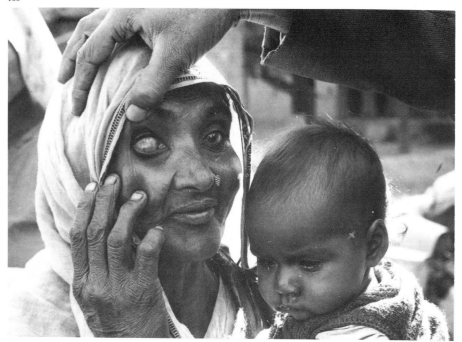

160

The eyes

To the ancient the eye was the gateway to the soul, the recipient of the Sun-God's emanations and the transducer of his evil thoughts. Blindness was the penalty for impiety or sexual lapse, and even if it occasionally offered wisdom as its recompense, any attempt at treatment was counted as an interference with God's proper judgement. So an army of blind beggars abounded, beneath any social stratum, rejected as lepers, and abandoned to their wretched fate.

Two eye diseases dominated their nosology: for, of the three injurious humors that were held to seep forwards from the brain, one evidently simply passed out through the nose, the second passed out as the catarrh of an 'ophthalmia', and the third oozed over the front of the lens to form a whitish film across the pupil, known as a 'hypochyma', or 'cataract'. From prehistory until the recent century eye doctors were primarily concerned with treating these two latter disorders—the damaging ophthalmia, usually provoked by the trachoma chlamidium, and the insidious blindness caused by a 'cataract'.

Trachoma is an infection of the surface of the eye that infiltrates the cornea and erodes the sight; and throughout history it seems to have been endemic in the Middle East, since special forceps for plucking out the ingrowing lashes which result from the inflammation were even found in the pyramids of the seventh dynasty of Egypt. Since then it has constantly been the camp-follower of invading armies—of the Greeks whom Cyrus led into Persia, then of the marauding armies of Islam, who carried the blinding contagion as far as Spain and South China, of the returning Crusaders who brought it back again to Western Europe, as did the returning armies of Napoleon from the Levant, and finally of the returning armies of Allenby during the First World War. The attack on trachoma in recent decades has been on a heroic scale, backed by W.H.O. and countless research units. Thirty years ago it was responsible (at any rate, in part) for about 30 per cent of the world's blind. Now, like tuberculosis, it is receding into the role of a minor, if widespread, nuisance, thanks to the clearance of any secondary infection by an increasing array of antibiotics, to a world-wide understanding of hygiene, and to the recent isolation of the chlamidium itself.

Cataract. The history of cataract is even more impressive. In most old people the lens of the eye, which lies just behind the pupil, becomes greyish and less transparent, and in some of them this change progresses till the eye is virtually blind. Clearance of this obstructed pupil, by inserting a needle at the corneal margin which then knocks the opaque lens backwards onto the floor of the eyeball, was indeed the first of all true surgical operations, since it was practised at least by 3000 B.C. in both Egypt and the Himalayas. This rather crude operation of 'couching' the cataract is still being performed in outlying parts of India and Africa, by a technique which has barely altered in over 5,000 years. In 1742 Daviel discovered that one could open the eyeball and extract the opaque nucleus of the cataractous lens, rather than leave it, often damagingly, within the eyeball; and slowly his improved method became accepted (although seven years later the arch-charlatan, Chevalier Taylor, removed the cataracts of both Bach and Handel by the old couching technique, and succeeded in blinding them both). Since then instruments and techniques have steadily improved. Thus in 1773 Sharpe, an English doctor, learned how he could evacuate the entire lens, after incising the eyeball, by pressing below the cornea with his thumb-nail. Colonel Smith, a pioneer in the Indian Medical Service, then invented forceps which could safely lift the whole lens out of the eye; and in 1960 the Polish surgeon Krwawicz perfected a freezing probe which could pull the whole lens out, without relying only on a grip on its tenuous capsule. Still more recently a 'phako-emulsifier'—which breaks up the lens and so allows it to be sucked out by a wide-bore needle—has been introduced. But we have yet to discover the exact factors which render the ageing lens opaque and, although spurious 'cataract-cures' are widespread, there is still no known method of preventing or delaying the progress of these senile opacities.

Glaucoma is second only to cataract in western countries as a cause of blindness. The part of the eye in front of the lens contains a watery fluid, the aqueous humor, and if for any reason this fluid is secreted faster than it is reabsorbed, the

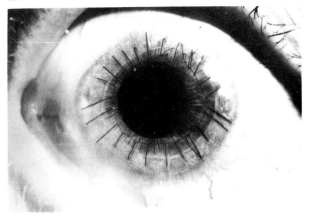

161

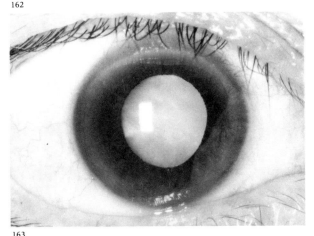

162

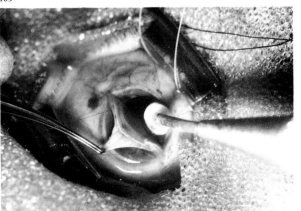

163

160 A dramatic improvement in the vision of people affected with trachoma, like the woman shown opposite, has been the development of corneal grafting. The white, opaque cornea effectively blocks light from entering an eye which may be otherwise quite healthy. This is the late, 'burnt-out' stage of the disease, the earlier manifestations of which are probably present in the small child whose eyes show tell-tale evidence of chronic inflammation and increased secretions. This is largely a disease of subtropical regions in areas where standards of public hygiene are generally low.

161 The restoration of the gift of sight must be considered amongst the highest of the benefits that modern surgery has offered to mankind. The replacement of a circular area of the opaque cornea with a graft taken from a donor eye is demarcated by the line of fine radial stitches which holds the graft in place.

162, 163 The lens of the eye maintains its crystal clarity by the operation of complex bio-chemical mechanisms. If these are disturbed by disease, opacification of the lens, or 'cataract', may rapidly develop (162). A more slowly progressing opacity is often seen in elderly people without any known cause. Blindness caused by cataract may be relieved by the removal of the opaque lens, its optical function being replaced by an appropriately shaped spectacle lens. 163 shows an operation for cataract where the opaque lens is being removed from within the eye through an incision made along the margin of the cornea, using a 'cryoprobe' to which the lens adheres by freezing. A crude form of this operation has been practised since prehistory.

pressure rises and glaucoma develops. The increased pressure constricts the flow of blood and the retinal tissue starts to die.

Understanding of the eye and its disorders lagged well behind that of our other organs, and until the seventeenth century the lens was still thought to be the essential organ of sight (rather than the retina) and to lie in the very center of the eyeball, rather than forward in contact with the iris. Until that time there had been a vague separation of the two major forms of blindness. The first was known variously as 'gutta opaqua' (since the pupil appeared grey) or 'hypochyma' because it was thought that this derived from a whitish humor, which had spilled down in front of the centrally-placed lens; this became a 'suffusio' in Latin, and was finally re-hellenized as 'cataract'. The second form of blindness was labelled 'gutta serena' (since the pupil remained

164, 167 Photographic technology has made great contributions to the understanding and treatment of eye disease. The retinal camera, which is specially adapted to illuminate and photograph the interior of the eye (164), makes a permanent photographic record of the delicate structures and blood vessels deep within the eye. The photograph opposite taken with a retinal camera (167) shows the retina with its blood vessels emerging from the optic disk, the point where the optic nerve and blood vessels perforate the eyeball.

165 An important development of retinal photography is illustrated here. The fine detail of the retinal blood vessels has been made to stand out by the injection of fluorescein into the circulation. As this passes through the eye, retinal photographs are taken under blue light and through an amber filter. This suppresses all light other than that at wavelengths

164

clear); and since, in such cases, the interior of the eye sometimes appeared bluish-green, they added the term 'glaucosis', or later 'glaucoma'. The latter was paradoxically attributed to damage of the lens itself, for it was again only in the seventeenth century that Richard Banister, an English oculist, noticed that these eyeballs also seemed very hard when felt through the upper lids. The acute form of glaucoma, in which there is a greenish-blue haze obscuring the iris and pupil, follows a strangulation of the fluid outlets from the eye, and is painful and prostrating, and rapidly leads to blindness if the pressure is unrelieved. To the Arabian Sams-ad-din it was styled 'migraine of the eye' or 'headache of the pupil'. It was not until 1857 that Friedrich Von Graefe, Professor of Ophthalmology at Berlin, discovered a way of relieving it by opening the eye and removing a sector of the obstructing iris; and by 1875 it was found that physostigmine, extracted from the South Indian calabar bean,

would contract the pupil, and this could sometimes abort the attack. After the Second World War came the drug acetazolamide, which would further help by inhibiting the secretion of aqueous humor, and still later came the 'osmotic' softeners, for a half-tumbler of 'antifreeze' (glycerol) will suck fluid out of a strangulated eyeball, even when the physostigmines and acetazolamides have failed.

In the 'simple' form of glaucoma the increase of intra-ocular pressure is insidious, and the gradual extinction of sight is not immediately obvious since it first affects the more remote parts of the field of vision. Thus the condition is as readily overlooked by the doctor as by the patient, unless he happens to spot that the increased pressure is distorting the eyeball at its weakest point (where the optic nerve leaves it) when checking the interior of the eyeball with his ophthalmoscope, or, knowing that there is glaucoma in the family, persuades himself that the eyeball does not indent very easily to the fingers. Glaucoma is the more dangerous, not only because it is easily missed, but because the damage already done is irrecoverable; yet it can simply be arrested, and, as with most diseases, this is more easily achieved in the early stages than when it is far advanced. Again it was found that the juice of the calabar bean had a controlling effect on the eye pressure (although the mechanism of this control is less understood) and physostigmine drops and acetazolamide tablets, two or three times a day, will usually contain the pressure and arrest the damage. If not, a little drainage vent can be fashioned surgically, which will let the pent-up aqueous humor escape.

The gradual evolution of an efficient way of inhibiting trachoma, clearing a cataract, and arresting a glaucoma, follows the familiar patterns of medical and surgical advances elsewhere, with

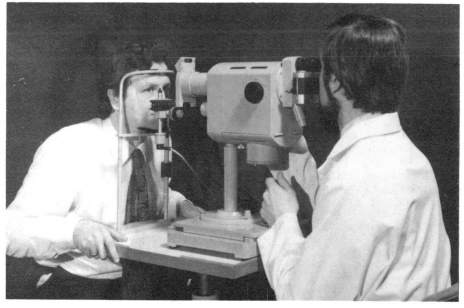

emitted by the activated fluorescein. This normal eye shows the fine terminal branching of the retinal arteries and the absence of blood vessels in the macular area, the region of the retina which is used for finely discriminating central vision. It also shows the 'streaming' of the blood as it returns on the venous side of the circulation, the fluorescein hugging the walls of the veins and leaving a central dark column of blood without the dye (top right and bottom right corners of picture).

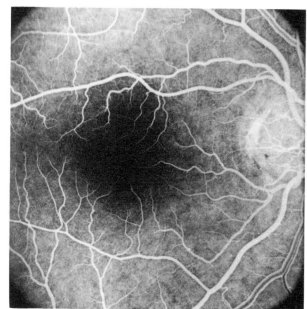

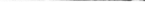
165

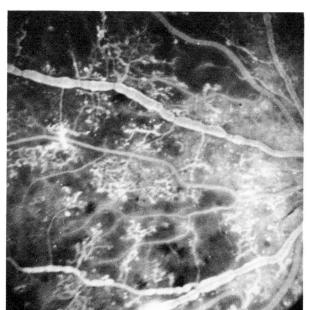
166

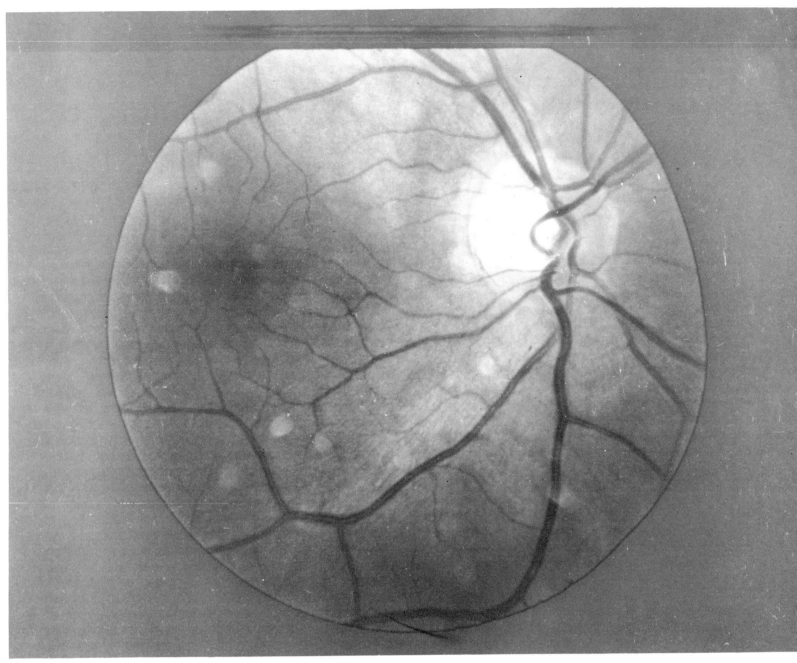

167

the stage-by-stage perfection of a standard technique. Two other blinding eye disorders have yielded to more dramatic surgical control in recent years—retinal detachment and corneal scarring.

Retinal detachment. The retina is a gossamer-like sheet containing the light-sensitive rods and cones and lining the inner surface of the eyeball. To the latter it is very loosely attached, and if it is torn by injury or just through being stretched (as in short-sighted eyes), it readily falls forwards into the vitreous cavity, and its cells progressively die through separation from their nutrient bed. Until the First World War it was so irremediable that one professor had declared that 'anyone who attempts to treat a retinal detachment is either a knave or a fool'. Nowadays over 90 per cent of detached retinas can be replaced. First the Frenchman Gonin tried to adhere the retina back

onto the choroid by inserting chemical irritants, then by applying thermocautery to the overlying scleral (outer) wall of the eyeball; later electrolysis was used, and finally the application of a freezing probe (which coagulates and renders 'tacky' the underlying choroid, but does not destroy the cells of the sclera in the process). Before the Second World War it became apparent that scarring within or in front of the retina often prevents it from falling back against the wall of the eyeball, so the latter must be indented in order to reach it, and kept indented by inserting a 'plomb', as of silicone sponge, or more simply by encircling the equator of the eyeball with a tight strap. Meanwhile a more direct and novel approach had been suggested by Meyer-Schwickerath in Germany: he, under direct observation through an ophthalmoscope, was able to cause a localized coagulation

166 This abnormal fluorescein retinal angiogram illustrates the great disorganization of the finest blood vessels in the retina of a diabetic patient. It also shows the sausaging or segmentation of normally smooth venous channels and the network of abnormal new vessels growing into the retina and into the cavity of the eye. Retinal disease of this sort, due to diabetes, is now one of the commonest causes of blindness among middle-aged people in advanced countries.

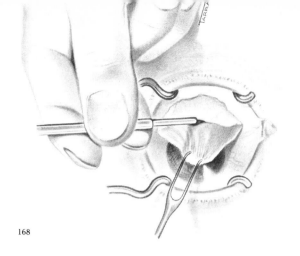

168

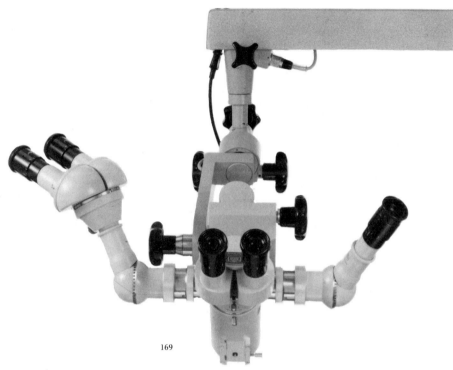

169

168 A rise in pressure within the eye can seriously damage the function of the retina and optic nerve, leading to blindness. Sclerectomy, removal of a small portion of the sclera, in this picture by use of a circular trephine, allows the aqueous to escape beneath the flap of conjunctiva, which is seen lifted forward on a hook during the operation, but is subsequently sewn back in place.

169 Microsurgery of the eye and ear is performed with the help of the operating microscope shown here. The operator uses the main binocular eyepieces at the center. Assistants have binocular or monocular access to the same image (left and right respectively). The protruding controls regulate the position and focus of the instrument. In some modifications these can be operated by foot control, leaving the surgeon's hands free. Magnification up to eighty fold can be achieved with systems of this sort. The operator views the eye or ear along the path of the illumination provided by the instrument itself.

of the choroid around any retinal tear, before the retina had become too separated, by directing through the pupil an intense beam of ordinary light. This was the fore-runner of the laser, which has as yet only a limited use in rectifying detachments. Retinal surgery is still in its adolescence, and new methods of investigation and microscopic techniques are constantly being elaborated.

Corneal scarring. The cornea, the window of the eyeball, is exposed and vulnerable. So scarring of the cornea after injury or ulceration is common, and still accounts for a quarter of the blind in most underdeveloped countries. Trachoma is endemic in many of these areas and is primarily responsible, but in addition there may be a miscellany of infections such as gonorrhea, measles, and smallpox; and when these are combined with a lack of vitamin A (which so often coexists, and which alone can cause the infant's cornea to melt away), a dense opacity is left covering the whole central area of both corneas, and a child is blinded for life.

Over the last century the whole scene has

changed. First, in 1881, the incidence of gonococcal ophthalmia in the new-born (contracted from the infected maternal birth passages) was dramatically curtailed by Credé's introduction of his prophylactic silver nitrate drops (reducing the incidence from over 10 per cent of births to under a half per cent); and these were soon being inserted as a routine into the eyes of all the available new-born babies. Nowadays, in advanced countries, these prophylactic drops are generally omitted, as the infection can so readily be eradicated by antibiotic and sulfonamide treatment before there is any material damage to the cornea. The widespread availability of effective antibiotics has indeed altered the picture of most forms of corneal ulcer, in combating the secondary infection which did most of the ultimate damage; and keratomalacia (from lack of vitamin A) readily yields to massive doses of vitamins, if these can be given in time.

Even so, there are many areas where treatment is available too late, if at all, and corneal scarring is still a common cause of blindness; and for these the grafting of a disc of healthy cornea to replace the scar may dramatically restore the sight.

Corneal grafting is, in essence, a far older story than detachment surgery, since a technique had been proposed in the eighteenth century by de Quengsy. This was elaborated by Erasmus Darwin, who added the suggestion that the corneal scar should be excised with a trephine 'the size of a small crow-quill'. The first successful graft was in fact done on a pet gazelle by Samuel Bigger, while he was a prisoner of the Egyptians in the wake of the Napoleonic wars; and in the succeeding decades several spirited but disastrous attempts were made to replace the scarred human cornea by disks of glass, or of cornea taken from various animals. By the end of the last century, proper antisepsis and anesthesia had transformed the scene, and the first successful human graft was achieved in 1905 by Zirm in the small Moravian town of Olmutz; but the failure-rate was so high that even in the 1930s the number of grafts done in London can barely have exceeded six a year.

At the close of the Second World War corneal surgery at last came into its own. Ultra-fine needles and suture materials (such as 'virgin silk', extracted by Cesarian section from the virgin silkworm, and even finer synthetic fibers) allowed direct edge-to-edge suturing, and rendered obsolete the old straddling sutures and splints which had formerly sought to hold the graft in place. Antibiotics kept the graft clean, and steroids countered the antibody reaction which usually spelled rejection of the graft (and still does, in about every sixth case). The supply of fresh donor material has been eased by the establishment of 'eye banks' and, since such corneas lose their viability in a few days, a technique for deep-freezing corneas was established in London which can preserve their viability indefinitely, at the temperature of liquid nitrogen. Nowadays interest has shifted to methods of obtaining a clear window in those corneas which are too seriously scarred to permit a normal graft to remain transparent, using acrylic inlays, with elaborate methods of retaining these in place (as by embedding the acrylic cylinder in a ring of dentine from the root of a canine tooth, which has been excised from the same patient—an 'osteo-odonto-keratoprosthesis'), and of seeking to alter the refraction of the eye, either by inserting between the corneal layers an acrylic lenticulus, or by sculpturing the cornea, after freezing an excised corneal segment until it is solid—a 'kerato-mileusis'. Attempts to extend the areas of grafting beyond the central disk of cornea have also had a very limited success, but there is little chance that it will ever be possible to graft in a new retina or a whole eyeball.

Of the many other eye disorders which our advancing knowledge and techniques have helped to resolve, two further groups are worth mentioning, partly because they have become problems only in those more developed countries where all these 'advances' are being achieved.

A squint (a deviation of the visual axes) is normal among most animals, since their eyes are usually directed sideways, and are thus grossly divergent. Only among the primates, who, along with the birds, have the added refinements of color vision and stereoscopy, are the eyes constantly kept straight. This capacity is learned during the first few months after birth, as a reflex action which soon becomes conditioned and unconscious. The common form of squint (the convergent, 'concomitant' squint of small children) is usually precipitated when this habit is still imperfectly established, and some emotional disturbance (such as parental antagonism, or the arrival of a new and competing baby) upsets the child's self-control—hence the greater frequency of squint in our sophisticated societies. The essential treatment lies in preventing the in-turned eye from becoming poor-sighted from disuse, since the sight can only be recovered if this 'lazy eye' is quickly forced into action, usually by covering up the master eye, so allowing full binocular vision to be established. Surgery to the external muscles may be required, to place the eyes in correct alignment. But the refinements of full binocular function and the intricacies of squint therapy are so complex that the subspeciality of 'strabology', with its supporting professional body of 'orthoptists', has become a major component of the ophthalmological world.

Refractive errors. In contrast to squints, the

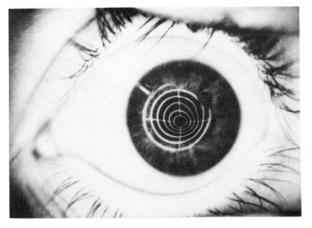

170

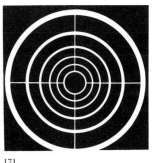

171

refractive errors have always been with us, irrespective of our primitive or sophisticated state, and humans have always had about the same proportion of long- or short-sighted eyes, or eyeballs that are slightly flattened ('astigmatism') or just focus less well because of age ('presbyopia'). These refractive errors simply provide the retina with a less well focused image, and appropriate convex or concave lenses can then improve the sharpness of the picture. Although spectacles were officially invented in 1317, until the turn of this century they were virtually restricted to simple pebble lenses, which helped the elderly presbyope to read and which were purchased from street-vendors' trays. Now nearly half the population of the U.S.A. wear spectacles, a tribute to commercial acumen and efficient salesmanship rather than any genuine need. The eyes themselves can never be damaged by not wearing spectacles or even by wearing the wrong ones; and they are justified only if they clarify the view (or, occasionally, ease an eye fatigue) sufficiently to justify their nuisance value. However, this same commercial enterprise has produced lens shapes, patterns and tints which the more sensitive wearers may appreciate, not to mention contact lenses, which are an immense help to the very rare patient with a distorted cornea and a cosmetic convenience to the legions of short-sighted who dislike being seen in glasses.

The blind. In all forms of eye disease the advances in treatment during the last decades have been impressive. But there still remain over four million blind in the world, and the social problem of blindness is always with us. Until the eighteenth century the blind were rejected as beggars, whom society ignored, and who were generally assumed to be wholly irremediable; and when, in 1749, Diderot started an inquiry into their capacities with suggestions for their emancipation, he was imprisoned for three months at Vincennes. By 1784 Haüy had founded an 'institute for the young blind', first in France, then in Russia and finally in Berlin; and in Liverpool two blind men succeeded in creating

170, 171 An ingenious method of locating abnormalities of the surface of the cornea is the recording of the deformation of a light image projected upon it with a device known as a kerato-scope. Deformity and obliteration of the upper left quadrant of the target image on the surface of the eye is clearly visible by comparison with the normal projected image. Deformity of the cornea may seriously distort the visual image. Correction can often be achieved by the provision of a suitably-shaped contact lens, but surgery may be required.

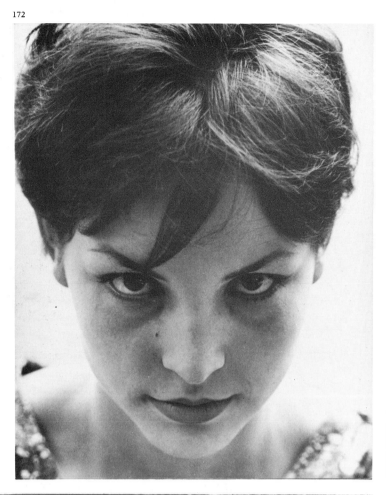

172

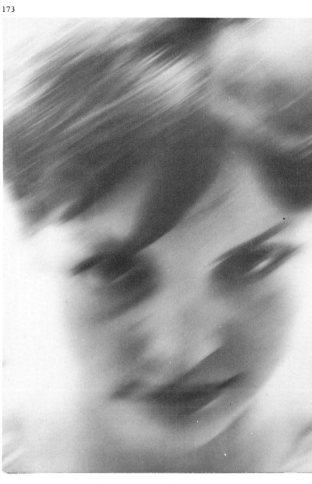

173

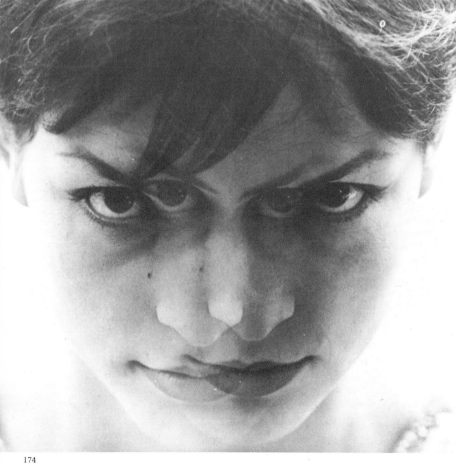

174

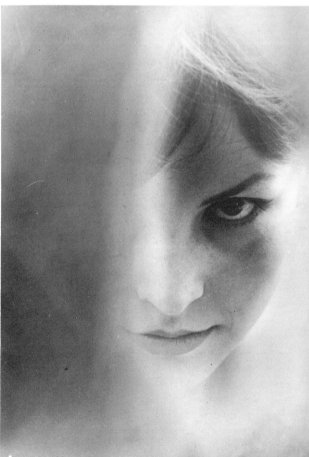

175

the first English blind institute in 1791. Haüy also was the first to emboss letters on paper so that the blind could read, and in 1826 Louis Braille, who became blind at the age of three, and had been a pupil and later a professor in Haüy's institute, perfected his script of embossed dots which has remained the standard ever since. Since the turn of the century inventions to ease the daily life of the blind and add to their fulfilment have been pouring in. In England there are now over 2,000 'talking books' available on cassettes (the recorders are provided free to all on the partially-sighted register) and there are three weekly magazines, thirteen monthly magazines, four two-monthly magazines and seven quarterly magazines embossed in braille, covering most of the specialist interests, and more are constantly becoming available.

The ear

The organs of hearing are not only extremely delicate, but are also exposed to infection because of their proximity to the nose and throat. Altogether the vulnerability of these organs results in a very large number of people suffering from a degree of deafness sufficient to make their lives difficult, and to affect their place in society. The picture, however, is far from gloomy and over the past 20 years advances so remarkable have been made in the treatment of deafness that otology has become unrecognizable from what it was before this period.

Advances in the understanding of disorders of hearing have been dependent on the accurate description of the ear's anatomy and physiology, and our knowledge of the extraordinarily delicate mechanical processes which conduct sound waves from the outer ear to the auditory nerve serves to remind us of medicine's purely descriptive achievements in many other areas.

It has been traditional to describe the ear as being divided into three parts, and indeed these parts are so separate both anatomically and from the point of view of function that they must continue to be considered separately.

The external or outer ear consists only of the pinna and canal which leads to the other structures in the skull. The pinna certainly has a role to play as it directs sound towards the canal and is of some help in allowing the position of a source of sound to be localized, but it is only rarely that abnormalities of the external ear are responsible for deafness.

The ear canal or external meatus ends blindly where a membrane lies stretched across its path. This is a strong structure held tense by a fibrous ring at its circumference. It is called the tympanic membrane or ear drum and vibrates when sound waves reach it through the ear canal. The tympanic membrane separates the outside air

from a cavity in the temporal bone of the skull. This space is known as the tympanic cavity and lying within it is a little bone which, because of its shape and mode of action, has long been called the malleus or hammer. It moves when the membrane vibrates in response to sound and transmits these vibrations to a second bone. This is called the incus or anvil, and in its turn it sets in motion the third tiny ossicle which is called the stapes because of its remarkably stirrup-like shape. Altogether this is a very complex mechanism for the transmission of sound, and indeed in some animals such as birds it is replaced by a single ossicle. On the other hand it offers a delicate system of levers which transfers the vibrations received on the relatively wide surface area of the tympanic membrane to the much smaller one of the footplate of the stapes.

This last ossicle transmits its movement to a small opening in the inner wall of the middle ear. It leads to what we call the inner ear, and is known as the oval window. There is another opening called the round window between the middle and the inner ear, closed off by a thin membrane only; and yet a third opening, which this time leads to the outside air through a narrow channel, the Eustachian tube, which

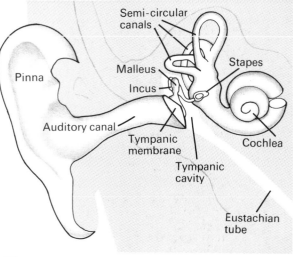

Semi-circular canals
Stapes
Malleus
Pinna
Incus
Auditory canal
Tympanic membrane
Tympanic cavity
Cochlea
Eustachian tube

177

opens in the nasopharynx in the throat at the back of the nose. This tube is very important as it allows air to pass in and out of the middle ear and so keeps it at atmospheric pressure.

The inner ear is another cavity in the temporal bone deeper than the middle ear. Its shape is very complex, consisting of one part which is shaped into a spiral very similar to a snail-shell, and another part from which three little semi-circular canals emerge at right angles to each other. Because of its complexity, the inner ear cavity is referred to as the bony labyrinth. It is filled with a fluid called the perilymph which is chemically very similar to the cerebro-spinal fluid which bathes the brain. In this cavity,

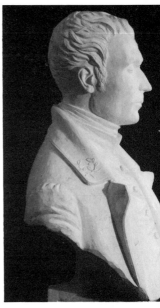

172-5 For those blessed with normal vision it is not easy to imagine the distortion of images produced by eye disorder. Simple aberrations of the focusing mechanisms of the eye, the corneal curvature and the fine focus of the lens, may give the effect represented by the blurring and twisting of the attractive face (173) seen with normal vision in 172. Disease of the retina will cause partial areas of blindness with windows of normal vision (175). Even slight loss of the co-ordinated movements of the two eyes may break down the single image normally perceived into the double image–diplopia–shown in 174. Modern technology in the correction of the muscle control of the eye, or surgery for localized disease of the retina, or the correction of refractive errors of the eye with spectacles or contact lenses, can greatly improve vision.

176 Louis Braille (1809-52), blinded in an accident at the age of 3, developed the now universally used system of lettering and numbering for the blind named after him. He used different combinations of raised dots, perhaps derived from the upholstery nails which his father employed to teach his son to read. This fingertip code has made literature, mathematics and even musical notation available to the blind. This general approach is used now in Asia and Africa as well as in Europe and America and, although modifications have been devised, it remains standard. Blind people using braille have become successful computer programmers.

177 This diagram shows the principal components of the ear, whose mechanisms are described in detail in the accompanying text.

surrounded by the perilymph, also lies a sac, which shapes itself to the semi-circular canals and the snail-like cochlea and includes two other balloon-like swellings, the utricle and the saccule. This thin-walled sac is called the membranous labyrinth and the fluid which fills it is called endolymph. The endolymph has a different chemical and physical constitution from the perilymph and this leads to an electrical difference across the membrane. These differences are very important in all sense organs because the nerve impulse which a sensory stimulus produces is often generated by changes in the electrical state of these surfaces.

The membranous labyrinth contains two sense organs, that of balance and that of hearing. The organ of balance consists of sensory cells in the endings of the semi-circular canals and in certain areas of the saccule and utricle. These are stimulated by the currents in the fluids brought about by movements of the head.

The organ of hearing, known as the organ of Corti, consists of a long series of cells placed along the coils of the cochlea. These sensory cells are stimulated by the vibratory movements in the fluids set up at the oval window. These, as previously described, are the direct result of movements in the tympanic membrane and ossicular chain brought about by sound vibrations. The impulses from the sense organs of hearing and balance are conveyed to the brain by the auditory nerve.

Congenital deafness. Children who are born deaf create a special problem in that a child who has never heard speech cannot learn to speak. It was because of this that in the past those who were born deaf were called deaf-mutes. We have ceased to use this term today because it has been realized that muteness is only a result of the deafness and not an extra disability. Furthermore, an understanding of the problem, together with the development of electronic means of amplification of sound, has brought about completely new methods for teaching deaf children. By dint of skill and patience, specialist teachers are now able to get many of these children to speak intelligibly. Of course there are many degrees of deafness, and the very severely afflicted have a smaller chance, but there must remain very few children indeed who can truly be called mute.

Probably the majority of congenitally deaf children used to be the result of either German measles (rubella) contracted early during pregnancy or blood incompatibility between mother and child (the rhesus baby; see chapter 5). Nowadays parents have learned to welcome opportunities for their daughters to get over German measles early in life and the new vaccine against rubella should reduce the number of mothers at risk even further. Rhesus

incompatibility is now also under control with readily available blood transfusion of the new-born so that today the majority of child deafness is probably hereditary in origin.

All these children are deaf because of poor development of the inner ear and nerve of hearing. No surgery can cure them, but there are some cases where very difficult and complicated operations may be helpful. These are children where the ear canal and middle ear structures have not developed and can be reconstructed to some extent, but in order for this to be worthwhile the inner ear and nerve must be normal. Among these is the tragic group of children, whose mothers took the drug Thalidomide during pregnancy.

Otosclerosis is a particularly important cause of deafness because of its peculiar nature. It is also relatively common among people of working age. It is due to the fixation of the stapes bone in the middle ear. Layers of bone mount up around its edges making it so solidly fixed that it cannot transmit the vibrations of sound from the rest of the ossicular chain to the inner ear. The condition is hereditary, indeed it is inherited as a dominant character because the child of an otosclerotic parent has a 1 in 2 chance of becoming deaf. It is also hormone-dependent—it tends to get worse during pregnancy and may vary in intensity with the menstrual cycle. The deterioration is a marked feature of the disease and in the past has led to the tragic situation of a young woman in her early twenties becoming more severely deaf with each pregnancy. When we consider that there were no adequate hearing aids virtually until after the Second World War, we can see their plight was quite disastrous.

The surgical treatment of otosclerosis has been one of the victories of medical history. Starting in the last century with the courageous attempts by two Frenchmen, Petit and Miot, to mobilize the ossicle (by gaslight with little magnification), treatment progressed and finally, after many other pioneering operations, John Shea in America perfected the one now in use—stapedectomy. The stapes is completely removed and replaced by a piston of teflon or stainless steel or by a wire prosthesis. Although problems may occur in every operation, the results in the vast majority of these patients are highly satisfactory.

Chronic infections of the middle ear. These patients form the other great group of people deafened by inadequate transmission of the sound vibrations by the ossicular chain. They include all those with discharging ears and perforated ear drums. Often some of their ossicles, in particular the incus, are eroded so that there is a loss of continuity in the chain.

Although the majority of chronic middle ear infections are unpleasant and disabling, but not

178 Magnification has changed surgery of the ear beyond recognition over the past two decades. Surgery can now bring relief to many patients with what was previously regarded as incurable deafness. This photograph shows an ear operation with the operating microscope in progress.

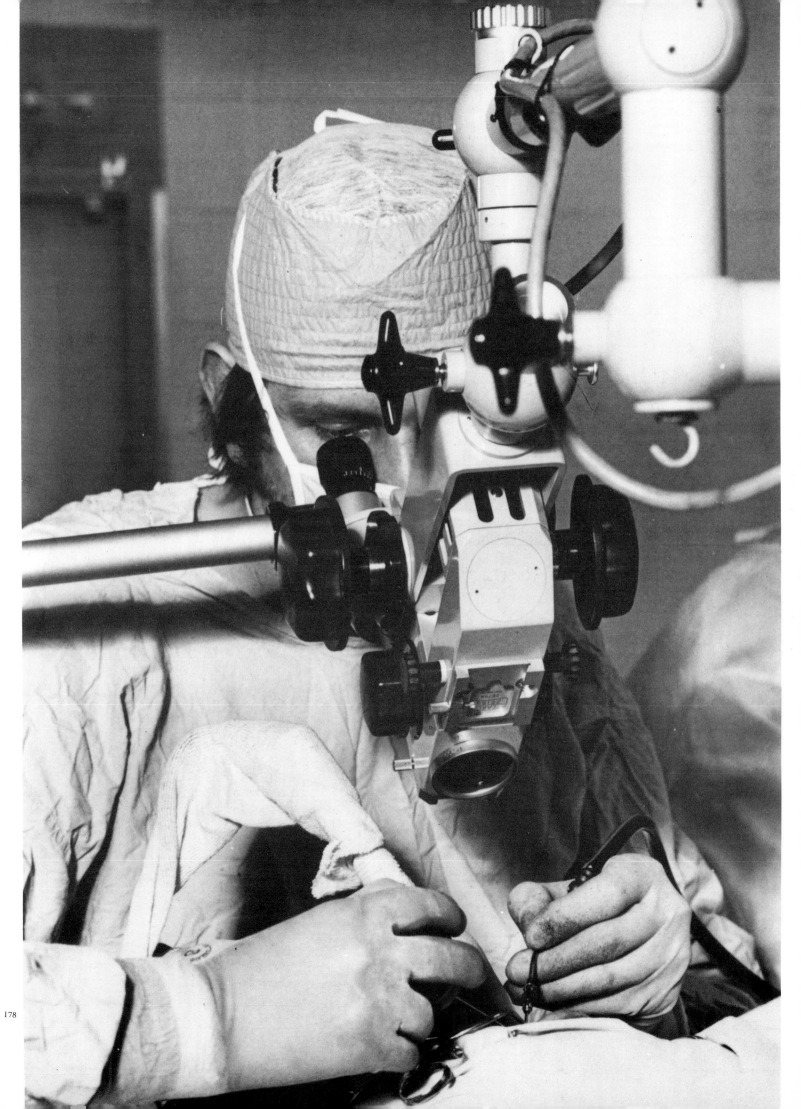

dangerous, there are some which, if left untreated, can cause serious, even fatal, illness.

As the result of the demands of otosclerosis surgery an array of instruments for fine work has been developed, the most important of which is the operating microscope. Furthermore, ear surgeons have learned new skills and these have now come to be applied to the chronic infections. It is now possible to graft new ear drum heads using membranes taken from the surface of the muscles above the ear. These grafting operations are now very successful and techniques are such that it is rare to see a graft that does not take. Closing perforations in this way not only allows people to go swimming but prevents further infections from getting into the ear.

Improving the hearing here is a more difficult proposition than in otosclerosis as so much depends on how much damage has been done by past infection. If the middle ear is filled with scar-tissue, for instance, the chances of a great improvement in hearing are poor. Nevertheless a large number of patients are greatly helped by the surgeon's techniques which now involve refashioning ossicles or often replacing them by new ones taken from cadavers.

Neuro-sensory deafness. At present when deafness is due to poor function of the inner ear or the nerve of hearing there are no medical or surgical means of treating it.

The advances that have been made concern prevention. We have learned that loud sounds will damage hearing irreversibly. Although industry has recognized this more and more, young pop fans seem not to be aware of this problem. Many drugs, including some antibiotics like streptomycin, injure the auditory nerve and can cause deafness and have to be used with care. Even simple drugs like aspirin can damage the hearing if taken in large quantities.

A great deal of research in neuro-sensory deafness is now in progress and those in this field feel hopeful that it will not be too long before advances can be made here as well as in middle ear deafness.

Our understanding of hearing disorders is intimately related to our ability to measure hearing accurately. Originally, hearing tests consisted of asking the patient if he could hear soft sounds like the tick of a watch held close to, or at an increasing distance from, the ear. The whispered or spoken voice was used in a similar way, but of course these methods were imprecise. Pure tone audiometry, where electronically generated signals of different frequencies are presented to the patient at varying amplifications, was a great advance, but such methods are subjective and demand the cooperation and understanding of the patient. The past fifteen years have seen increasing efforts made to develop new, objective hearing tests, such as that known as evoked response audiometry. In this the sound perceived by the ear is picked up as an electrical response from the auditory cortex cells of the brain by way of sensitive electrodes applied to the scalp. These signals can be sorted out from the other electrical activity of the brain by using an averaging computer. Considerable progress has been made and more can be expected.

Hearing aids. Where medicine and surgery cannot assist the deaf patient, reliance has to be placed on hearing aids. Improvements in performance and reductions in size, which can minimize the deaf patient's discomfort and self-consciousness, have brought great benefits. The cupped hand of ancient man led to the Victorian ear trumpet. Today this has almost completely given way to the electric hearing aid. Transistors, the miniaturization of components, and the mercury cell, have made it possible progressively to decrease the size of the hearing aid to a point where microphone, amplifier, receiver, battery and controls can all be packed into an instrument hidden behind or even within the ear. Developing technology can be expected to produce even greater wonders. The only limiting factor is the behavior of the deafened ear when exposed to amplified sound.

11 The Kidney and Organ Transplantation

In the past, doctors have had to watch their patients die from incurable diseases affecting vital organs. When only one part of the body was diseased the question naturally arose: why not give the dying man a new organ to provide the missing body functions? Until the 1960s the answer to this question was clear: no matter how great the need for a grafted organ, the usual behavior of the recipient towards such a valuable gift was to destroy it by a process called immunological rejection (see chapter 5).

This biological reaction, suicidal in this context, has, therefore, been the focus of research for many scientists. Much has been learned, and now methods of holding graft rejection in check have been developed. This chapter will summarize such work and explain the present position of organ grafting, concentrating particularly on kidney transplantation since most progress has been made with this organ.

The functions of the kidney. Although the kidney is very compact with a clear-cut overall

179, 180 The delicate and intricate functioning of the kidney, man's chief organ of excretion, has been investigated with great success in this century. The blood vessels in the diagram of the whole kidney (179) convey blood to and from the kidney by way of renal artery and renal vein respectively. The urine, a solution of waste products and salts in water, is excreted by way of the ureter. The two main processes of the kidney which take place in the nephron, the functional unit of the kidney, are illustrated, greatly enlarged, in 180. The fluid contents of the blood are filtered under high pressure at the glomerulus, a fine knot of tiny blood capillaries surrounded by a hollow capsule. The second process is that of selective reabsorption (and some further excretion) which occurs as the glomerular filtrate passes through the tubular portion of the nephron. It is on the function of tubular reabsorption that diuretics have their effect. If sodium reabsorption in the tubule is reduced, increased amounts of salt and water are excreted and the patient's undue accumulation of these is corrected. The renal tubule has a variety of functions at different points along its course. Diuretics with a specific site of action have been developed which can act more or less selectively upon these specific functions, lessening the risk of unwanted depletion of other salts. The kidney also has an endocrine function, the secretion of renin, which tends to raise low blood pressure arising from undue salt and water depletion by promoting sodium retention. Another effect, the constriction of small blood vessels, may contribute to high blood pressure in kidney disease.

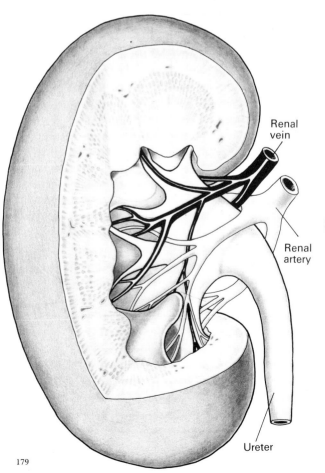

Renal vein

Renal artery

Ureter

179

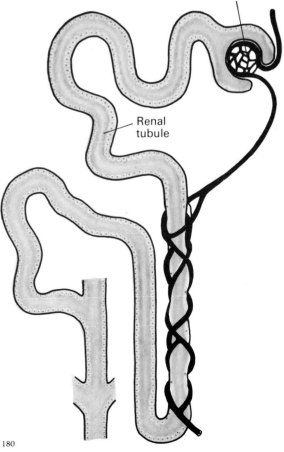

Glomerulus

Renal tubule

180

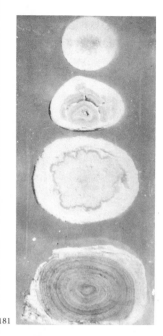

181

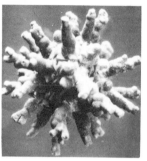

182

structure, microscopic examination shows it to consist of about a million functional units called nephrons. Each nephron consists of a blood filter, called the glomerulus, and a complex tubular duct opening out into the main kidney duct or ureter, which carries the final fluid—urine—from the kidney into the bladder where it is stored until voided. The initial filtrate leaving the glomerulus is blood without its cells and protein. Down the tubule goes this fluid—water with a variety of salts and waste products of the body dissolved in it. Many of the salts and most of the water are needed by the body, so they are reabsorbed from the tubule of the nephron back into the bloodstream, leaving only excess water and waste products to be excreted as urine. There is a large reserve of nephrons so that health can be maintained perfectly when one kidney is removed. The nephrons in the remaining kidney compensate by enlarging.

In order to fulfil these complicated procedures of filtration and selective reabsorption, the kidney

181 The formation of stones in the urinary tract is a major problem in hot climates and, to a lesser extent, in temperate conditions, due to the problem of maintaining salts in solution in a concentrated urine. Often forming around a tiny nucleus of organic material, 'stones' made of calcium phosphate or chalky material may accumulate in the urinary pathway. Forming in the kidney, they may pass into and obstruct the narrow ureter which drains into the bladder, causing severe pain and arrest of renal function on the affected side. The photograph shows the laminated appearance of these stones cut across after removal.

182, 183 Urinary stones may grow to considerable size and take up grotesque shapes if they form within the bladder or the main collecting sac of the kidney. The type of branched stone shown here, taken from the bladder, may also form in the pelvis of the kidney. In the X-ray picture (183) a 'staghorn calculus' of this kind has totally filled the pelvis of the right kidney. When this happens, the function of the affected kidney is destroyed. Modern surgical techniques have made it possible to remove small stones through the urinary pathways themselves, by grasping them and crushing them so that they can be passed as a fine powder. Larger stones require appropriate surgical incision and repair.

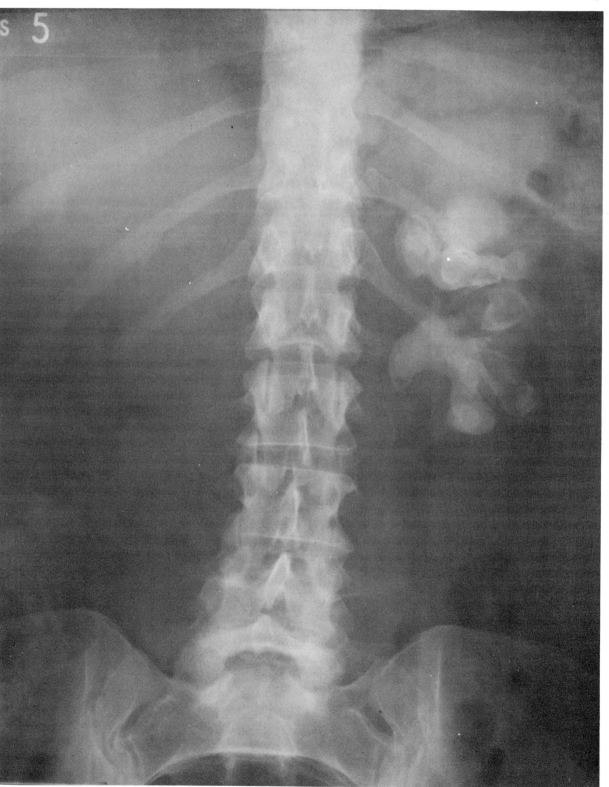

183

requires a very luxurious blood supply. A large artery brings blood rich in oxygen and other substances necessary to provide energy for the kidney, and the blood returns to the heart through the renal vein.

There are only three main connections of the kidney—the artery, vein and ureter—so if these three tubular structures are severed, the kidney can be removed. Successful grafting requires a technique for rejoining the vessels and ureter to the recipient, so that the kidney can function. In practice the most satisfactory position for a grafted kidney is in the lower abdomen above the groin. The vessels of the kidney are joined to the recipient's pelvic blood vessels and the ureter is implanted in the bladder. While the kidney is removed from a blood supply it suffers damage, and if it is left at body temperature for more than an hour the damage becomes irreversible. But if the kidney is chilled, the speed of damage is slowed so that it may withstand up to 12 hours without blood. For longer periods of kidney preservation a complicated apparatus has been developed to provide the organ with an artificial circulation of cooled fluid containing oxygen. In this apparatus kidneys can be kept in good condition for two days, although banking of organs for long periods has not so far been achieved.

The artificial kidney. Since most of the functions of the kidney are known, their substitution by artificial means would appear to be a reasonable objective, and it has been achieved by a process called dialysis. It works like this: if blood is put into a cellophane bag and the bag immersed in

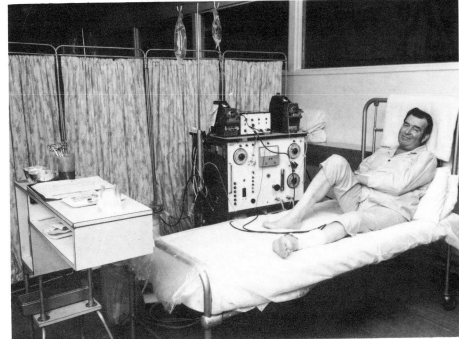

184 A patient undergoing renal dialysis in hospital. The patient is connected via an arterio-venous shunt in his left leg to one variety of the artificial kidney machine. The patient's blood is pumped into the machine by his own heart. A pump in the machine returns the blood to the patient's vein after it has passed through the dialysis capsule, a plastic chamber containing a circular coil of semi-permeable membrane across which the excretory products pass, just visible at the foot of the bed. A second pump adds heparin, contained in one of the plastic bottles, to the circulating blood to prevent clotting; the second bottle contains saline which may need to be added to the circulating blood. The patient will spend three periods of 10 hours each week in this way and will remain in hospital for about 6 weeks learning how to dialyse for himself at home later.

185 This diagram shows the position of the transplanted kidney in relation to the patient's own kidneys, and emphasizes the comparative simplicity of the kidney's connections which surgically makes the kidney the easiest organ to graft.

water, then the salts and waste products will pass through the cellophane from the blood into the water. Blood cells and protein molecules are too large to get through the cellophane and so they remain in the bag. In this simple example, water would pass from the outside into the bag and would damage the blood cells, so in practice normal blood salts are dissolved in the water. Then only the waste products will pass out of the blood bag. Dialysis is the basis of artificial kidney treatment, of which there are two methods—peritoneal dialysis and hemodialysis.

In *peritoneal dialysis* the lining of the patient's own abdominal cavity, the peritoneum, is used instead of cellophane as a dialysing membrane. Dialysing fluid, containing salt, is run into the abdominal cavity through a plastic tube. Waste products pass out of the blood into the fluid, which is removed through the plastic tube after a few minutes. The process is repeated many times with many fresh 'washings' with dialysis fluid. Forty-eight hours of treatment twice a week can keep a patient with no kidneys in moderate health, but the procedure is uncomfortable. Another disadvantage is that infection may pass into the abdominal cavity and give rise to dangerous complications.

Hemodialysis. The kidney machine was devised by Kolff in Holland at the end of the Second World War. In the original apparatus a cellophane tube was coiled round a beer can. Blood from an artery was pumped through the tube and returned to a vein. The system was immersed in a bath of dialysing solution. This type of apparatus is still in use. An alternative is to pump blood over sheets of cellophane with the solution on the other side. Waste products in the blood move across the membrane into the dialysing fluid. A patient with no functioning

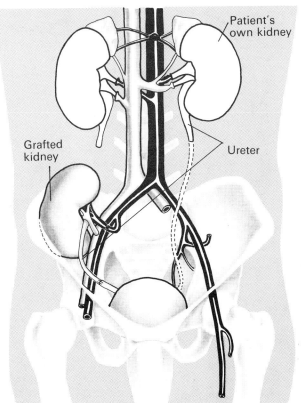

Patient's own kidney

Grafted kidney

Ureter

185

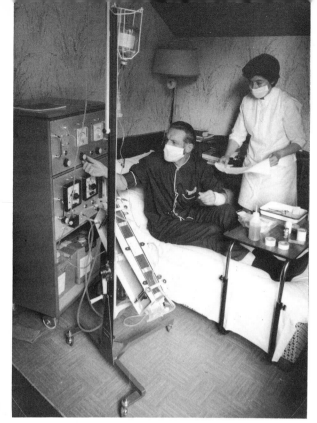

186

186 The development of a
home dialysing machine is a
recent innovation which has
greatly reduced the personal
inconvenience of regular dialysis. The patient and his wife
are seen here preparing to use
the home dialysis apparatus. In
the foreground may be seen the
dialysis cell, in this case of the
flat-bed type. Three overnight
periods of dialysis per week are
adequate to maintain the patient
in good health and enable him
to carry on working. He has
however to maintain certain
personal disciplines so far as the
nature of his food and the quantity of his drink are concerned.

kidneys can stay in good health if he uses this
'artificial kidney' for 12 to 15 hours, two or three
times a week, though he must also adhere to a
special diet and drink little fluid. It is a complicated
procedure, but people can be trained to dialyse
themselves in their own homes, provided they
have help from a devoted relative or friend.

The main difficulty in hemodialysis is getting
access to the patient's blood. One method used is
to insert two short plastic tubes into a limb, one
into an artery and the other into a vein. Blood
travels from the artery, down the tube and into a
longer tube which leads to the artificial kidney.
On leaving the machine, blood returns to the
body through the tube into the vein. When the
two tubes are not in use for dialysis, they are
joined together by a U connection to produce a
permanent 'shunt'. Plastic shunts are easy to use
but they can become blocked or infected, so their
life span is limited.

The alternative to a plastic shunt is an artificial
internal connection between an artery and a vein.
This is called a fistula and requires a minor
surgical operation. Blood flowing under high
pressure from the artery distends all the veins of
the arm or leg where it is connected to them by
the fistula. When dialysis is required, two large
needles are inserted into the dilated veins—
one to remove blood and the other to return it.
The obvious disadvantage of this method is two
needle pricks for each dialysis, but it is surprising
how readily patients are prepared to put up with
this discomfort, which can be minimized by a
little local anesthetic.

Kidney failure. Fatal kidney disease is not
uncommon, and it is particularly tragic when it
affects young adults in that most active time of

life, as it usually does. The three most common
fatal kidney diseases are glomerulonephritis,
pyelonephritis and polycystic disease.
Glomerulonephritis is a condition of unknown
cause in which the glomeruli of the nephrons are
destroyed. Pyelonephritis is a bacterial infection
of the kidneys. Polycystic disease is a condition
of maldevelopment of the kidneys in which cysts
develop and destroy the kidney substance.
All these diseases usually affect both kidneys and
by interfering with the function of the nephrons
they progressively impair the normal activity of
the kidneys. The result is kidney failure.

Fluid and waste products collect in the body.
There is edema (swelling or 'dropsy') especially
affecting the legs. The blood-forming cells are
depressed, resulting in anemia. The patient feels
ill and weak, with a pale complexion. The
accumulation of waste products may affect the
stomach causing vomiting, the bowel causing
diarrhea, and the heart causing inflammation of
its outer coverings and chest pain. The diseased
kidneys usually cause high blood pressure which
puts further strain on the heart and may produce
shortness of breath.

This distressing condition progresses to coma
and death. An unpalatable low-protein diet may
slow the process, but it cannot rebuild nephrons
that are destroyed. A patient in such a moribund
condition is not fit for an anesthetic, still less for a
major operation. Fortunately, regular dialysis will
transform his condition and this is the principal
reason kidney grafting has developed so much
more quickly than transplantation of other vital
organs. A dying patient can be made fit for
operation by dialysis. What is more, if the grafted
kidney is slow to resume function, dialysis will
keep the patient in reasonable health after
operation. Should the graft fail altogether, the
patient can be returned to dialysis and later
receive a second or third kidney transplant.

Logistics. From every million people in the
population, roughly 40 new cases of terminal
kidney disease occur each year. It is clear that the
nature and cost of the treatment could rapidly
become a serious drain on medical resources.
Regular dialysis is expensive in equipment and
very demanding on medical and ancillary staff.
Even if the patient is to undertake home dialysis,
he needs lengthy, highly skilled training,
and subsequent regular supervision is required.
For many patients or their relatives home dialysis
is a formidable undertaking and some flatly refuse
to consider it. The restrictions of diet and fluid
intake and, above all, the inexorable need to use
the machine every two or three days, make
regular dialysis far from ideal as a form of
treatment, even though with careful supervision
it is remarkably safe.

A good transplant is preferable. The patient is
independent of machines and his only

requirements are to take tablets daily and to attend clinics for regular follow-up. In fact, the life is similar to that of a diabetic. On the other hand, kidney transplantation is more dangerous than dialysis, and rejection of the graft is a serious blow to a patient who has pinned his hopes on its success. Nevertheless there can be no doubt that the best treatment for kidney failure is transplantation—both for the patient's return to relative normality and from the viewpoint of cost.

Kidney transplantation. The surgical technique of kidney grafting was developed in experimental animals at the beginning of this century. It was found that an animal could have a kidney transplanted back into itself—an autotransplant— and its other kidney removed, and live in good health with full life expectancy. It was this observation that led Dr Murray and his colleagues in Boston in the early 1950s to perform the first series of successful kidney grafts in man between identical twins. Since identical twins arise from the same egg, it was argued that they were biologically the same individual. A graft between such twins would, therefore, be the same as an autograft, with no possibility of rejection. The results of kidney transplantation between identical twins have been excellent and have justified these predictions.

Autografting has also been used successfully in diseases involving a single kidney. Surgeons can remove the kidney, cool it and then operate on it at leisure on a 'work bench'—perhaps to remove a tumor or repair a blood vessel—and then retransplant the kidney to its owner.

Transplantation between individuals who are not identical twins is less successful. After a few days urine production ceases, the kidney swells and becomes infiltrated with white blood cells called 'immunocytes', and the delicate blood vessels within the kidney become blocked or fragmented. In experimental animals, following this graft rejection, if the second kidney from the same donor is transplanted to the same recipient, it is destroyed more quickly than the first, indicating that the recipient has become sensitized or immunized by the first kidney. The process is similar to the protective immunity that follows an attack of an infectious disease such as measles. Subsequent exposure to the measles virus results in its rapid destruction so that more than one attack of measles is very rare. It seems that graft rejection is an unfortunate consequence of the extremely efficient immune protective apparatus that we all possess.

Unfortunately, the body cannot distinguish between harmful bacteria or viruses and potentially life-saving organ transplants. All are considered as 'foreign invaders' and the result is the production in the blood of antibodies and defensive immunocyte cells, which cause graft rejection (see illustration 81). Since the body defenses are so important and well developed it is hardly surprising that efforts to overcome them have often met with failure.

187

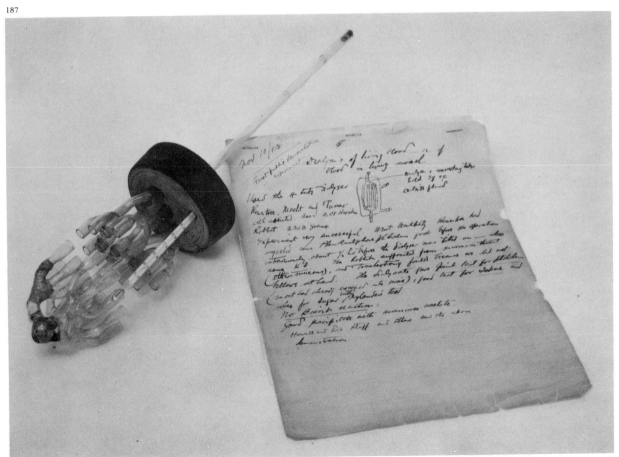

187 The principle of hemodialysis is the diffusion of unwanted substances from the blood across a semi-permeable membrane into a solution closely resembling the blood plasma. Diffusion occurs from the region of high concentration to the region of low concentration of the selected substance. The feasibility of this process in the living animal was first demonstrated by J. J. Abel (1857-1938) in 1912. The photograph shows his original dialysis apparatus with a note in his hand describing the successful experiment. Blood from the animal passed through the glass tubes, which were joined by tubes of a celloidin membrane, the whole apparatus being submerged in the dialysing solution contained in a bottle.

Powerful drugs can impair the body defenses but they may do so indiscriminately. They prevent the graft rejection reaction, but also render the individual easy prey to bacteria, viruses and fungi that he would otherwise have been able to resist. Throughout the world, those interested in organ graftings have tried to know more of the nature of the rejection process and learn how to overcome it in a specific manner, so as not to impair other immune processes. There are reasons to believe that this may be possible.

The objective is similar to that of desensitization in certain allergic conditions such as hay fever, where repeated small doses of the pollen responsible may cure the patient. In many experimental models, and probably also in patients with kidney grafts, a situation can arise where the graft desensitizes the recipient specifically so that the rest of the body defenses are left intact. More knowledge is required of the exact factors at work before this principle can be utilized in a predictable manner. In the meantime doctors are obliged to use non-specific and potentially dangerous 'immunosuppressive agents' to inhibit graft rejection. The three most used are the antileukemic drug azathioprine, corticosteroids and antilymphocyte serum, which all act by damaging or destroying the immunocyte white blood cells. The corticosteroids also counteract the inflammation that occurs in the graft during rejection.

Tissue typing. The chemical factors that differentiate individuals and are responsible for graft rejection are called 'transplantation antigens'. A simple example is the well-known red blood cell classification into groups, but there is another important system of inherited *white* blood cell groups, distinct from the red cell groups. These factors can be identified on the surface of white blood cells by methods similar to, but more complicated than, those used to define red blood cell groups. An individual's 'tissue type' can thus be defined and compared to those of potential donors. Since tissue types are inherited there is a one in four chance of two brothers or sisters having the same tissue type, each child inheriting two linked factors from each parent. Since every individual has four factors, a child will always have at least two in common with each parent. The relevance of tissue typing to kidney graft results has been clearly shown in intrafamilial transplants. Grafts between brothers and sisters with identical tissue types have fared almost as well as grafts between identical twins.

The survival of grafts between unrelated individuals is rather poorly correlated to tissue typing, suggesting that there are other important transplantation factors not demonstrable by current typing techniques. Recipient reactivity is also of great importance. People vary in their response to a bee sting, and in a similar way there are marked differences in the capability of individuals to mount an aggressive immune response against a graft.

Following rejection of a graft, or even after a blood transfusion or pregnancy, transplantation antibodies may be produced. If these are found in the blood the outlook for a renal graft is poor. On the other hand, a history of blood transfusions, pregnancy or graft rejection without developing antibodies indicates poor recipient reactivity and bodes well for a kidney graft.

Donors. Kidneys for transplantation in man may be taken from live human volunteers, live animals or dead humans. The results of grafts between different species even within the primates are poor and until grafts within a species can be predictably successful, it is unlikely that animal donors will be used. The results of grafts between unrelated live donors are little better than those for grafts from cadaver donors: therefore the only living donors used extensively are close blood relatives.

Live related donors. Removal of a kidney is a major operation involving pain and some risk. Although life with one kidney is normal, if that single kidney is damaged in an accident there is no reserve on the other side. Therefore, removal of a kidney from a volunteer donor cannot be undertaken lightly. It is obviously essential to determine that the donor is medically fit, and special care is taken to assess the function of both his kidneys. X-rays are taken to make sure that there are no structural abnormalities of the kidneys that might prejudice the operation. Tissue typing is then performed and if there is a high degree of compatibility between donor and recipient and all other investigations have proved satisfactory, then it is justifiable to proceed.

The advantages are that the operation can be scheduled at a given time. The kidney is unlikely to suffer damage from lack of blood supply since the operations on donor and recipient are synchronized. Also, as mentioned previously, the results of intrafamilial grafting are better than those between unrelated individuals.

Dead donors. To remove a kidney from a corpse with the object of saving a life can do no harm to the dead person and may be a gift of life to the graft recipient. This simple and surely obvious statement has, nevertheless, been beset with a web of ethical and legal circumlocution which has obscured the simple fact that should be intelligible and acceptable to all rational people. These are the doubts that have been raised.

Will the donor be really dead?
Death is not normally difficult to determine. In fact, nurses and many laymen can generally make a confident diagnosis that life has ceased when breathing and the heartbeat have stopped.

To be considered as a potential organ donor is an added safeguard against the fear of being buried alive that haunts some people, since they will be examined by a number of doctors of increasing experience, and in the extremely unlikely event of a mistake having been made, the first touch of the knife to remove the kidneys would result in bleeding and no harm would have been done. There are, however, situations where the diagnosis of death is not so clear and these are important in the context of organ grafting and require further consideration.

Most people dying in hospital are unsuitable as donors of kidneys, since they suffer from infection or cancer that could be transmitted to the recipient, or they have disease of their own kidneys. Suitable donors are patients dying from accidents, especially head injury, strokes and certain types of heart attacks, and tumors of the brain, which do not spread outside the skull. In each of these categories of disease it is often correct management to attempt resuscitation of the heart and lungs by artificial means, while the state of the brain is assessed. If there is no evidence of brain function after a variety of careful examinations and investigations have been made, artificial maintenance of the heart and lungs is usually discontinued, since to persevere can do no good to the patient who is maintained in a vegetable existence and will cause severe hardship and distress to his relatives, who visit not the person they loved but his inanimate shell. This has nothing to do with transplantation and the decision to stop resuscitation in these cases was being taken long before organ donation became a possibility.

When brain death has been diagnosed and the physicians have decided to stop artificial maintenance of the heart and lungs, *then* the transplantation team can be informed. Then the surgeon will be able to remove kidneys for transplantation before they have suffered severe damage from lack of blood supply.

Will the dying man be denied proper care because somebody wants his kidneys?

The categorical answer to this is 'no'. In every contact between patient and doctor there is a bond of mutual trust. When advised to have an operation for a stomach ulcer, the patient does not question the motives of the surgeon. The same trust exists in the case of patients who might become organ donors. If anything, more care will be given to them. There have been patients considered as possible donors in small peripheral hospitals who, following transferral to larger and better equipped institutions where transplantation is carried out, have been cared for more effectively and far from becoming organ donors, have been discharged from hospital cured.

Would the donor have objected or do his relatives object?

In all cases of sudden death an autopsy is carried out, in the course of which all the organs are removed from the body. The previous wishes of the deceased are overridden as are any objections of the relatives—yet there is no public outcry. It is accepted that the examination is a necessary part of the State's duty to investigate the circumstances of the death.

In organ donation the mass media have frequently taken a contrary view. Naturally the views of the patient in his lifetime should be respected and if the relatives are available, then they should be consulted and if they object then their objections also should be respected. In practice, however, the situation may be very difficult. In cases of sudden death, the views of the deceased may not be available and the relatives may not be traceable in the short period of under one hour that can elapse before the organs suffer irreparable damage. In these circumstances again, different countries have their own practice, but many people, both lay and medical, feel that it should be permissible to remove organs for transplantation unless the 'donor', or his parents in the case of a child, has registered a specific objection.

The law

There is no reason why organ removal should frustrate the processes of law. In fact, if there is a close liaison between the coroner's office, the pathologist and the transplantation team, the coroner may even be helped by the procedure. The surgeons removing organs can report in detail to the pathologist the internal findings in the abdomen. They can remove blood and urine specimens in a fresh condition so that determinations of alcohol and drug content can be made accurately. They have to discover whether organs are diseased or damaged, because that would make them unsuitable for transplantation, and information on any such damage can be made available to the officials concerned. In practice most coroners are helpful towards transplantation and are prepared to do their utmost not to prevent treatment of patients by organ grafts.

No matter what is the exact state of the law, the only way to ensure that sufficient kidneys are available for transplantation is through the attitude of the medical profession itself. Doctors are now aware of the valuable treatment that kidney transplantation has to offer and so is the public. Pressure by the public on the medical profession will probably eventually convince doctors that it is their duty in helping mankind not only to treat their own patients, but also to co-operate with the transplantation team when one of their patients is liable to be a

188 An effective program of kidney transplants requires the provision of suitable material for grafting. The view of the public and legislature on the provision of kidneys varies widely from country to country. In some, people are urged to carry with them a statement of willingness to provide organs for transplantation if by mischance they should be involved in some fatal accident. The card shown here is widely distributed by the government in the UK. Similar permission may be given for many other organs which, like the kidney, will not remain viable for long after death.

188

Kidney Donor Card

Your kidneys could help someone to live after your death

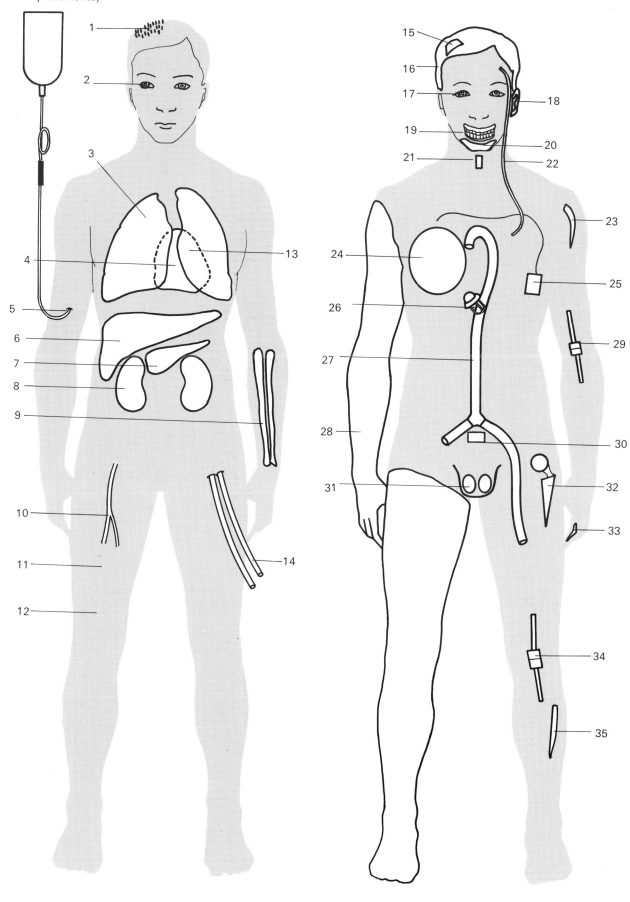

Homografts and heterografts (biological replacements)

Prostheses (man-made replacements)

Extra-corporeal machines

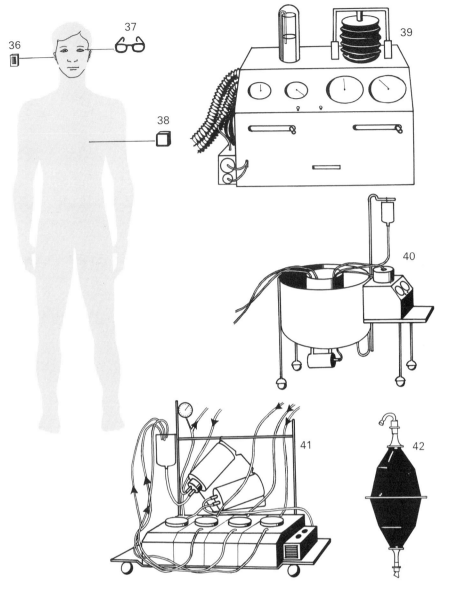

189 The ingenuity of the bio-engineer has combined with the dexterity of the surgeon to make possible a wide range of replacements, repairs and life-support systems for man. The left-hand figure shows the organs and tissues which can be usefully replaced, either, as in the case of skin or bone grafts, from the same individual, or from another donor, human or in some cases animal. The range stretches from cosmetic hair transplantation (1) to the familiar blood transfusion (5), which is in fact a graft of a fluid tissue. Of the organ grafts listed, kidney transplantation is by far the most successful at the present time. Most of the others are in a comparatively early, experimental stage. A major problem in maintaining function in a foreign graft is the host's immune response to it which tends to damage or destroy the transplanted organs (see chapter 5, illustration 81).

When replacements of metal or plastic are used, this immunological problem is greatly reduced. The second figure illustrates the manifold uses of these materials in the support or replacement of human organs. Into this category fall prostheses as diverse as false teeth (19) and a plastic cloth artery replacement (27). Metal and plastic replacements of the hip joint (32) have remobilized people otherwise incapacitated by arthritis (see illustrations 120 and 121).

On the right is shown a selection of the machinery which is available for improving or maintaining natural functions which have become defective.

1 Hair
2 Cornea
3 Lung
4 Heart or heart valve
5 Blood
6 Liver
7 Pancreas
8 Kidney
9 Bones in arm or leg
10 Blood vessel
11 Bone marrow
12 Skin
13 Supplementary animal heart or animal heart and lungs, or supplementary human heart or human heart and lungs
14 Links to baboon or other animal
15 Small plate in skull
16 Hair
17 Lens
18 Artificial ear
19 False teeth
20 False jaw
21 Artificial larynx
22 Drain for excess fluid round brain
23 Shoulder joint
24 Artificial breast (female)
25 Heart pacemaker (internal)
26 Heart valves
27 Main blood vessel
28 Artificial limb
29 Elbow joint
30 Bladder simulator
31 Artificial testicles
32 Hip joint
33 Knuckle joint
34 Knee joint
35 Metal plate
36 Hearing aid
37 Spectacles
38 Heart pacemaker (external)
39 Ventilator
40 Kidney machine
41 Heart-lung machine
42 Artificial liver (perfusion column)

suitable donor. It is surely an ethical obligation to inform the transplantation team and endeavor to help other patients in great need of treatment.

Results of kidney transplantation. More than 20,000 kidney grafts have now been performed throughout the world and the results have been collected by the Organ Transplant Registry. How long a kidney graft may last is not known, but present information is as follows:

1. If the donor is an identical twin, there can be no immunological rejection. The two-year functional survival of such grafts is nearly 90 per cent and the longest surviving graft is 18 years.

2. If the donor is a close blood relative but not an identical twin, the two-year functional graft survival is 75 per cent and the longest surviving graft is 15 years.

3. If the donor is an unrelated cadaver, the two-year functional survival is around 50 per cent and the longest surviving graft is twelve years.

These worldwide figures provide an idea of the average results, although some centers do better and others worse. The 'transplant survival' quoted here is less than the patient survival, because after a graft has failed it is usually removed. The patient goes back to artificial kidney treatment until he can be offered a new graft. The results of second transplants are little different from those of first grafts.

A graft that has functioned well for two years may still deteriorate subsequently. Five- and ten-year graft survival figures are not available in sufficient numbers for analysis but it would appear that late deterioration is more likely in grafts taken from cadavers than with live donors. It has always been assumed that this was due to late rejection, but progressive damage resulting from the initial lack of blood supply may be another important factor.

The quality of life of a patient with a graft that is functioning well can be excellent. Men may do heavy work; women may lead a normal life and even go through a normal pregnancy and deliver a healthy child. Usually, however, pregnancy is discouraged in women with kidney grafts because of the risk of high blood pressure and kidney infection, which are not uncommon in normal pregnant women. If anyone has any doubts of the value of kidney transplantation it is certainly not the patients.

The most serious complications after a graft are the side-effects of the corticosteroid drugs. They cause gain in weight and a bloated face—serious disadvantages in anyone, but particularly distressing for young girls—and predispose the patient to infection, duodenal ulcers and arthritis. The object of using immunosuppressive drugs is to reduce the corticosteroids to a minimum, and possibly stop them altogether.

Immunosuppressive drugs are given in high doses in the first few months after grafts. The patient is then in serious danger of picking up infections. Even a normally mild illness such as chickenpox can be lethal. After a few months, when the corticosteroid dosage is cut, the patients regain some of their ability to resist infections, without rejecting their graft. Some degree of specific desensitization would appear to have occurred.

In institutions which use antilymphocyte serum, treatment with the serum is stopped as soon as possible since it can cause alarming sensitivity reactions with swelling of the face and limbs, high temperature and joint pains. This serum is made from the blood of animals injected with human lymphocytes. It has proved difficult to obtain preparations of antilymphocyte serum with consistent and predictable properties, so many transplantation teams do not use it. Their results seem to be little different from those from institutions that give the serum.

Transplantation of other organs. Although artificial heart-lung machines are available—in fact their development has heralded a new era of heart surgery including heart transplantation—these machines can only be used for a few hours. They then tend to damage the blood and the altered blood can cause fatal lung disorders.

It has been said that the heart is 'just a pump', but it is a pump of such extraordinary qualities that no man-made substitute has ever approached it in performance. The heart beats on average 60 times a minute for 60 to 70 years. It regulates its action according to the body's needs and it has its own inbuilt 'power pack'.

The gas exchange function of the lung can be undertaken by machine for a few hours but contact of blood with the artificial gas exchange membrane eventually damages the blood with fatal consequences.

The functions of the liver are so manifold and complex that no machine could replace them all.

Thus, in the foreseeable future it is unlikely that there will be sufficient advances in biochemical engineering to produce reliable, compact, implantable artificial organs. The lack of artificial long-term organ substitution (with the

190 Blood is usually transferred from the patient to the artificial kidney from a vein in the arm, which has been specially prepared by a minor surgical operation which joins it to an adjacent artery, slightly distending it so that it can be readily entered with a needle, if necessary by the patient himself. In this photograph the distended vein is partly concealed by the tube leading to the kidney machine (below in picture). The blood returns to the patient through a needle into another vein.

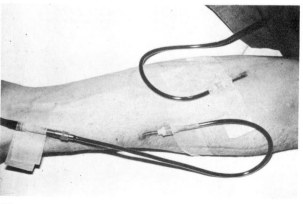
190

exception of the artificial kidney) is the main reason why grafts of other vital organs have lagged behind the kidney. Examples worthy of brief consideration are the heart, liver, lung and pancreas.

The heart. Severe coronary artery disease and certain rare conditions of the heart muscle can damage the heart muscle irreversibly. Patients with hearts so affected, who cannot leave their beds, are potential candidates for heart grafting. The operation, although complicated, is within the range of techniques available to any major heart surgery center—this explains the extraordinary number of heart transplants that were carried out a few years ago, when it seemed to some surgeons that not to follow the trend constituted professional failure. There was unwarranted adulation of heart grafting followed by its repudiation by the 'mass media'.

The American Dr Norman Shumway, who pioneered experimental heart grafting, has pursued an active program of heart grafting in man and has treated more than 90 patients. His results using 'heart beating cadaver' donors are very encouraging: some 40 per cent of his patients survive two years, a figure very similar to the pooled results of kidney grafts from cadaver donors. The longest surviving patient with a heart graft is now over six years since operation. Thus it is clear that worthwhile results can be obtained with this procedure using conventional immunosuppressive agents, provided the donor hearts are of excellent quality. (See chapter 4.)

The liver. Fatal liver disease is very common in Asia and Africa and moderately common in the U.S.A., but is relatively rare in the U.K. There are two categories of disease, namely primary malignant growths, which are much rarer than secondary growths that have spread to the liver from elsewhere, and non-cancerous diseases of the liver—the various forms of cirrhosis. The outlook in liver disease can be difficult to predict, so patients are only considered for liver grafting when it is obvious that they are dying. Frequently they are referred too late and die before a donor liver can be found.

The operation is a very major undertaking and would be extremely dangerous even in a healthy person. Moreover, there is no satisfactory method of helping the patient over the operation, since we do not have an artificial liver. Dr T. Starzl in Denver has recently obtained encouraging results using 'heart beating cadaver' donors, more than 20 per cent of his patients surviving a year. Two survived six years. In England, one patient lived more than five years after operation.

The lung. Fatal lung disease is tragically common but is frequently accompanied by lung infection and, as has already been explained, infection is a major hazard for a patient with any

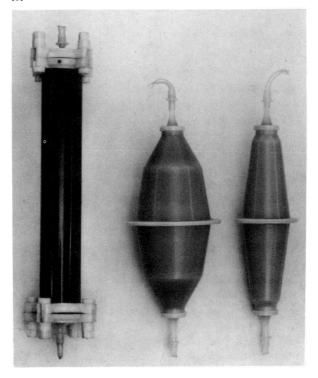

graft because he will invariably be given immunosuppressive agents. Following transplantation, the lung is extremely vulnerable to minor damage from rejection which other organs might survive. The delicate lining of the air sacs ceases to fulfil its function of gas exchange, with fatal consequences. These are probably the reasons why lung grafting has been extremely disappointing. Most grafts have failed soon after operation, although one patient in Belgium survived for nine months.

The pancreas. The pancreas is an important organ of digestion, but its most vital function is the production of the hormone insulin. Failure of insulin formation results in diabetes. Fortunately, insulin and insulin-mimicking drugs can control most of the features of diabetes, but in some patients, particularly children, serious damage to the eyes and kidneys occurs despite conventional treatment. Pancreatic grafting has been attempted in such patients, but results have not been encouraging. Most of the pancreatic grafts have controlled the main features of diabetes, but since the longest survivor is only two years, doctors do not yet know whether a pancreatic graft will prevent the eye and kidney changes. The pancreas is not particularly susceptible to rejection, and most patients have died from infection.

The future. Despite many years of intensive work by scientists all over the world, there has been little recent practical advance in kidney transplantation. The results obtained now scarcely differ from those of five years ago; a static situation which is unfortunate and contrary to the prediction of many. In fact, there have been important advances in knowledge of the

191 Charcoal, suitably prepared, has the property of extracting toxins and unwanted drugs from the circulation by adsorbing and binding them tightly to the surface of the charcoal granule. Blood from poisoned patients or those with liver failure may be fed through a column of tightly packed charcoal granules to make use of this property. The photograph shows three types of charcoal-filled columns which have been used at King's College Hospital Liver Unit in London. The liver may be the target of an attack by bacterial or viral infection and is susceptible to damage by many chemical poisons. Its susceptibility is largely due to its function as a detoxifying organ where many noxious substances are rendered harmless to the body. It also has other, greatly varied chemical activities, vital to the maintenance of life and health. These can only partially be supported by extra-corporeal devices, and the ability successfully to carry out liver transplantation will be of great benefit to many sick people. This operation is now feasible. Two patients have survived six years after operation in Denver, Colorado, and there has been one five-year survivor in the combined Cambridge University/King's College Hospital series. Immunological problems are less of an obstacle than in other transplants, and the main cause of failure has been technical difficulties related to drainage of the biliary tract.

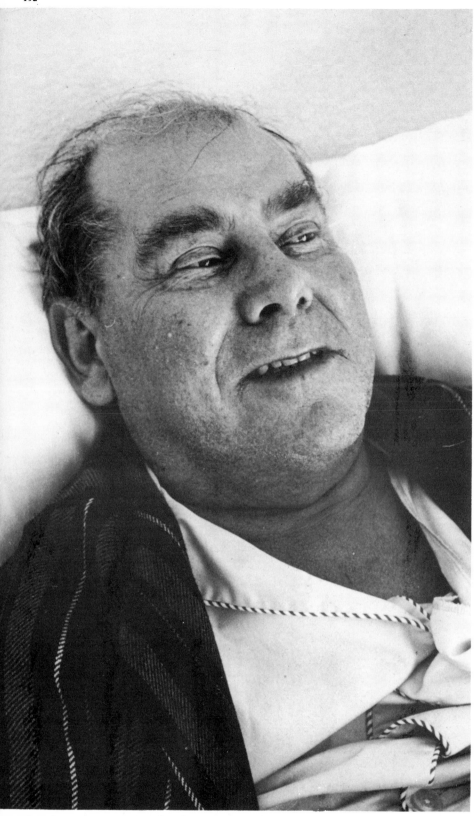

recipients within two years irrespective of tissue typing and conventional immunosuppression. The most important difference between patients who do well and those who do not seems to lie in their innate reactivity. Those who do badly are the ones who readily form antibodies when exposed to transplantation antigens, while those who do well tend not to form antibodies. It should not be too difficult to devise a laboratory test, using immunocytes of the potential recipient, to predict which of the two categories he belongs to. Those with a favourable test would be given a transplant with the expectation of an 80 per cent two-year graft survival, while the 'unfavorable' patients would be treated by regular home dialysis until more knowledge was available to facilitate their receipt of a kidney graft.

The results of kidney grafting would also be improved to an important extent if more donor kidneys were available and surgeons were not driven in desperation to use damaged kidneys. This is particularly true in Britain where probably 20 per cent of kidneys never function because of damage resulting from delay in their removal from the corpse. The result is an unnecessary and dangerous operation causing disappointment to the patient and his family. In the future the public and the medical profession everywhere may accept that unless there have been specific objections, organs may be removed from those who have died in hospital. In the normal course of events they would be used for grafting if they were suitable. A sufficient number of kidneys would then be available for transplantation and damaged organs would no longer be grafted.

Rejection is the central poorly understood barrier to success in organ transplantation. When it can be overcome predictably a new era of surgery will be born. No longer will grafting be a dangerous procedure reserved for desperate and dying patients. It will become a commonplace treatment for deficiency of any organ or tissue, and a desirable alternative to many unsatisfactory and prolonged current treatments by medicines.

192 A new frontier in transplant surgery was crossed when cardiac transplantation was achieved by Dr Christian Barnard and his team in South Africa in 1967. Dr Philip Blaiberg, shown here, was the second recipient of a heart graft. Although he was to die 19 months after the operation, he established beyond doubt the feasibility of operations of this kind. Two other patients have lived more than six years after this operation.

mechanism of rejection, but the new information only shows the system to be more complex than previously believed, and therefore makes any practical steps to rejection control seem more remote.

A spectacular improvement of kidney transplantation results might, however, be achieved without a scientific 'breakthrough'. It is known that approximately 50 per cent of cadaver kidneys will be rejected by their

12 Sex and Reproduction

Emotionally and psychologically sex is quite separate from reproduction. Anthropologists like Margaret Mead have shown that sex is mainly a form of social behavior. All young animals, including humans, display considerable sexual activity long before they are physically or emotionally capable of rearing young and this sexuality continues, particularly among the higher primates, long after reproduction has ceased to be physiologically possible. Few men or women enjoying sexual intercourse are motivated at that instant of time by a desire to reproduce.

The work of Freud founded the notion that sexual sublimation is an important psychological force. The current drive towards greater sexual freedom arises largely from his demonstration that sexual repression and enforced conformity can be a damaging factor both to the individual and to society. Freud and his followers have also been responsible for the fact that sex has now become a topic of polite conversation and is at last becoming even a subject for education and debate.

The introduction of effective and acceptable contraception has also had an effect upon sexual morals and behavior comparable in many ways to that made by the camera upon the artist. Whether or not we are at present witnessing a revolution in sexual morals and ethics is debatable, since evidence is hard to obtain, but there can be

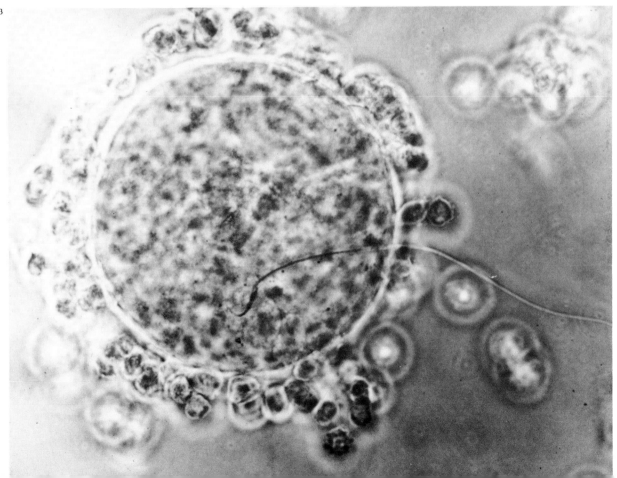

3

193 The moment of conception. The electronmicrograph shows a single sperm, the thread-like structure to the right, soon after entry into the ovum. The individual human sperm cell is only ·06 mm long: the photograph is of a rat sperm and ovum, virtually indistinguishable in appearance and structure from the human equivalent at this stage. The tail of the spermatozoon, which propels it to the ovum, is discarded after fertilization has been achieved. Changes in the wall of the ovum prevent a second sperm from entering. The nucleic acids which form the genetic material in the head of the sperm combine with those of the nucleus of the ovum, and from this mixture arises the genetic program for the new individual.

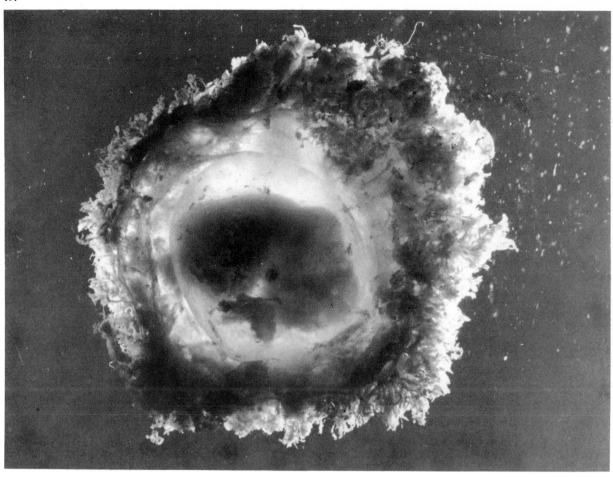

194-6 The extraordinary processes of fetal differentiation and development are well shown in this series of photographs of the human fetus at 8, 10 and 12 weeks of development respectively. At eight weeks little more can be seen than a lobed body with a limb bud protruding at top right. The eye spot identifies the head end of the fetus which is curled under the center of the structure. By twelve weeks (196), there has been striking differentiation of limbs and organs. Head, body, limbs and even digits of the fetus are now clearly differentiated, the whole enclosed in the fluid-filled amniotic sac within which the fetus floats freely, connected to the placenta by the umbilical cord which conducts blood to and from the developing individual. Another view, at ten weeks (195), as well as indicating the fetus within the amniotic sac, demonstrates the fine structure of the placenta which, by growing into the soft lining of the uterine cavity of the mother, effects an intimate communication between the maternal and fetal circulations (see illustration 201). At eight weeks the fetus is about 40 mm long; by the tenth week it is 250 mm long.

little doubt that the separation of sex from reproduction by the provision of adequate contraception must be the mainspring of any such revolution.

Meanwhile the role of the doctor in dealing with his patients' sexual problems is largely that of confidant and educator. Many patients gain enormous reassurance merely from learning that their sexual problems are common and are not regarded by their doctor as abnormal. The physician, with his knowledge of the wide variations of sexual behavior, is often able to give just that reassurance which permits his patient to accept and enjoy his or her own particular form of sexuality. Arising out of the work of Masters and Johnson, various mechanical aids to sexual gratification have been developed, but so far little reliable research into their efficacy has been carried out. Such aids have been widely and successfully marketed, but the medical profession as a whole has little scientific interest in their use.

Infertility. About one in ten of all couples find themselves to be infertile. The fault can, of course, lie with either partner, but statistically the woman is about ten times as commonly responsible as the man. Knowledge of the basic physiological processes of human reproduction is still patchy and incomplete but of recent times a great deal has been learned of the fundamental processes by which the ovum ripens, is prepared

for fertilization by a fully developed sperm, and then, when fertilized, implants itself in the lining of the uterus. The hormonal control of the processes is better understood, and this new knowledge has already resulted in the development of the powerful pro-fertility drugs which are used to induce the process of ovulation in women who have previously failed to produce ova.

Male infertility can follow as a result of incomplete descent of the testicles into the scrotum, which ought to be diagnosed in early childhood and corrected. In rare cases it can follow from injuries and it may also be caused by virus infections, in particular mumps, when these occur after adolescence. Only occasionally are surgical procedures of value in the treatment of male infertility. Severe hormone deprivation in the male is usually accompanied by infertility, but this is seldom diagnosed as the man rarely attempts sexual intercourse.

Pregnancy can be achieved by artificial insemination of the woman. In rare cases in which normal sperm production and ejaculation occurs, but coital difficulties inhibit successful insemination at intercourse, artificial insemination with the husband's semen (A.I.H.) is used. If the man is infertile, artificial insemination using semen from a donor (A.I.D.) is nowadays available.

Female infertility may be either primary, the

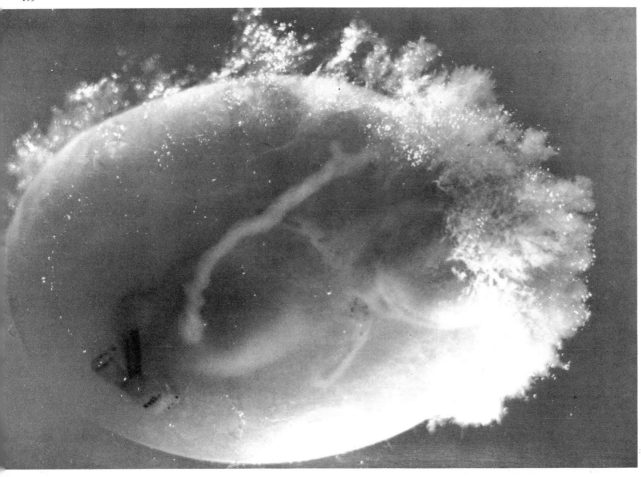

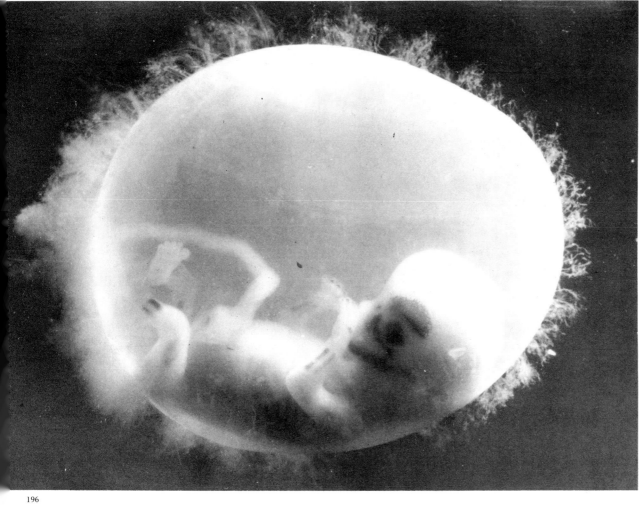

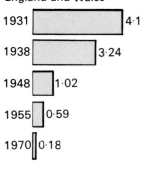

1931	4·11
1938	3·24
1948	1·02
1955	0·59
1970	0·18

197

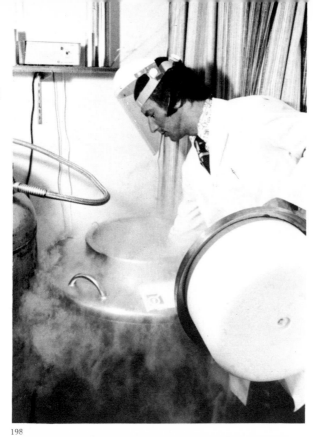

198

197 Over the past forty years maternal mortality has diminished very considerably in all developed countries. The diagram shows the decline in England and Wales. The reasons for this fall are many: they include a gradual change to a situation where the majority of deliveries are conducted in hospitals, better care of the expectant mother, and the availability of blood transfusions and antibiotics.

198 Human sperm may be stored at very low temperatures for long periods. After removal from its liquid nitrogen coolant, seen in the photograph above, and careful thawing, it will regain its mobility and fertilizing potential. This technique has long been used in stock breeding. The use of stored sperm has now made it possible for conception and pregnancy to be initiated in what would otherwise have been childless marriages, where spermatogenesis in the male is rendered defective by disease or where, sometimes for genetic reasons, the sperm, though apparently normal, is unable to fulfil its fertilizing function.

199 The laparoscope, a fine tube introduced into the abdomen, enables the contents of the lower abdomen to be visualized directly. This photograph of an ovary, the pale egg-like structure in the lower part of the illustration, was taken through a laparoscope. The fine, finger-like projection from the open end of the Fallopian tube, which guides the ovum on its path towards fertilization and implantation, can also be seen. Abnormalities can be diagnosed and even operations performed under laparoscopic control. For example, the Fallopian tube can be closed off by cautery (the local application of a heated filament), a form of sterilization which avoids the need for major surgery.

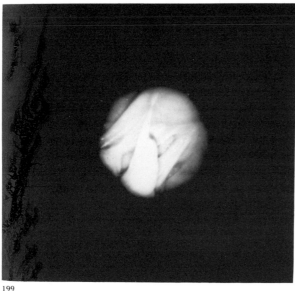

199

woman never having been pregnant at all, or secondary, that is following either an abortion or childbirth. Primary infertility may be congenital and such cases are often resistant to treatment. Some forms of primary infertility are due to moderately severe hormone imbalance and may be successfully treated with drugs. Otherwise the most common cause of female infertility is blockage of the fallopian tubes caused by infection. It is of interest to note that little more than two decades ago tuberculosis of the tubes was regarded as the most common cause of sterility in women; it is now rarely seen.

The investigation of female infertility usually involves the removal under an anesthetic of a sample of the uterus lining for analysis. Usually an attempt is made to test the fallopian tubes and

the recent introduction of the laparoscope has enabled the gynecologist actually to visualize the ovaries, taking a small biopsy if necessary. It is also possible to determine the exact site of any blockage by a special X-ray called a hysterosalpingogram, which photographs the tubes as they are shown up by a water-soluble dye, injected through the neck of the uterus.

With much improved diagnostic techniques have gone improved techniques of surgical repair of blocked fallopian tubes, but only a charlatan would *promise* his patients automatic success after such an operation.

The removal of a ripened ovum by use of the laparoscope, fertilizing it outside the body and implanting the fertilized egg into a uterus hormonally prepared to receive it, is in the experimental stage. Considerable expertise is needed to maintain this ovum alive outside the body even for the shortest time, to fertilize it, and then to insert the fertilized ovum via the cervix into the uterine cavity where it is hoped implantation will take place, exactly as if it has been fertilized during its passage down the fallopian tubes.

Such techniques open up numerous novel ethical dilemmas. There seems no problem where the ovum is taken from the woman and the sperm from her husband, but the removal of an ovum from one woman and implanting it once fertilized in the womb of another may be possible within the foreseeable future. Such a procedure may be useful in cases of congenitally inherited diseases passed down the maternal line. Perhaps we take these ethical problems too seriously for we have long accepted the transplantation of living infants—a technique which we call adoption.

Pregnancy and childbirth. Till early in the present century, death in labor was a serious possibility faced by every woman. Even in advanced countries reliable medical statistics are largely unobtainable for before the end of the First World War; it can be shown, however, that maternal mortality and morbidity has declined dramatically in the last 40 years.

Not only are women far less likely to die in childbirth today, but the experience is also far less likely to be unpleasant or painful and is unlikely to be followed by chronic ill-health. The physical process of pregnancy and childbirth is, by its nature, timeless and unchanging; so to explain the dramatic fall in the risks this process now carries we must examine medical and social factors which may influence it. In England in the 1920s only 10 to 15 per cent of women had their babies in hospital, whereas nowadays the corresponding figure would be 90 to 95 per cent. There is no question, therefore, that nowadays specialized obstetricians are much more likely to be involved. On the other hand, the concept of ante-natal care was already in existence by the 1920s and yet the first really dramatic fall in maternal mortality can easily be shown to be associated with the discovery of the sulfonamides. The subsequent discovery of the antibiotics which accelerated the decline in mortality and morbidity; the increasingly ready availability of stored blood for the treatment of severe maternal hemorrhage; greatly improved anesthetic facilities and higher standards of nutritional health—all have contributed.

Sir Dugald Baird, the well known Scottish obstetrician, says: 'The recipe for easy and efficient childbearing is simple, applies to all societies and is little more than commonsense, viz: first pregnancy soon after physical maturity, a high standard of health and physique, cessation of childbearing by the age of 30 and the restriction of the total number of children born to certainly not more than four.'

Over the last half-century, there has also been a very great improvement in the chance of a pregnancy ending with a live and surviving baby. In the 1920s, out of every 1,000 deliveries, about 80 babies would either be born dead or die within a week of delivery, and this figure has now fallen by about three-quarters. The improved prognosis for a living child arises out of a better knowledge of the physiological processes influencing the development of the fetus within the uterus. Once the fertilized egg implants itself in the lining of the uterus it develops a placenta through which it receives its essential nourishment. By the use of the placenta, the fetus is able to behave like any other tissue, taking what is needed from the mother's blood and disposing of waste. We now speak of the feto-placental unit as a separate entity within the uterus, and the study and protection of this feto-placental unit is really the main task of the obstetrician between conception and birth.

The obstetrician has, of course, a duty to manage the pregnancy and labor in such a way as to expose the mother to the minimum possible danger to life and subsequent health and well-being. This protection of the woman from possible ill-effects of pregnancy and labor may occasionally conflict with the interests of the fetus, but the high drama whereby the obstetrician is seen as adjudicating as to which shall live, mother or child, belongs more to emotive argument than to real life.

The detection and treatment of maternal disease is vital, as the feto-placental unit is very much under the influence of the mother's general health and of the good physiological function of the uterus. In its turn, the function of the feto-placental unit affects greatly the mother's maternal response and numerous 'feedback' systems have already been elucidated.

The interaction of the feto-placental unit with

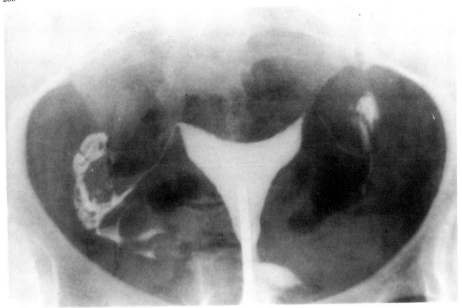

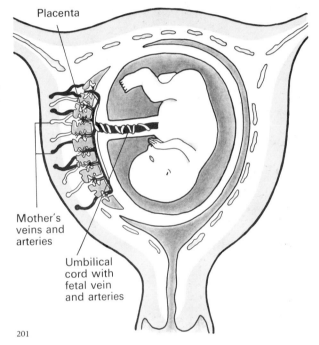

Placenta

Mother's veins and arteries

Umbilical cord with fetal vein and arteries

201

the maternal organism is so complex and as yet so little understood that the most important observations are those showing that the unit is functioning as a whole, rather than those which try to define the minutiae of malfunctions. Thus, indication of a steady and continued fetal growth keeping pace with the accepted norm indicates that the feto-placental unit is functioning correctly. Obstetricians have long attempted to do this clinically by assessing the growth of the fetus by palpation. X-rays were used, before their potential dangers were appreciated, to confirm that growth was progressing normally. This is no longer acceptable practice.

Since the Second World War, ultrasonic techniques have found wide applications in medicine. This involves the use of sound of high frequency, above that which can be detected by

200 An X-ray picture (hysterosalpingogram), in which a water-soluble radio-opaque liquid has been injected into the uterine cavity through a metal tube introduced from below, seen in the centre of the picture. The liquid has filled and outlined the Y-shaped uterine cavity, passed along the fine Fallopian tubes (extending from the arms of the Y) and then filled their lateral ends and spilled into the peritoneal cavity (visible as diffuse white patches). The picture was taken during the investigation of an infertile patient, but it showed that there was no obstruction in either Fallopian tube and that the uterine cavity was normal. The ovary releases its mature ovum into the potential space within the abdomen in which all of the organs lie. Known as the peritoneal space, it is this which becomes inflamed in peritonitis, and scarring can easily deny access of the ovum to the mouth of the Fallopian tube.

201 A diagrammatic representation of the feto-placental unit. The two circulations, maternal and fetal, can be seen entering the placenta from opposite sides. Within it they are closely apposed, but they remain separate. Although it used to be thought that the blood cells of the fetus never entered the maternal circulation, recent research has shown that in fact this not infrequently occurs. This sometimes leads to antibody formation in the mother against the fetal blood cells. If these antibodies cross the placental barrier, they attack the fetal cells, producing a severe anemia and release of blood pigments from ruptured red cells (bilirubin) into the fetal circulation. High levels of bilirubin can injure the brain. The recognition and therapy of rhesus incompatibility (see chapter 5) has provided a dramatic episode in the development of obstetrics and neonatal medicine.

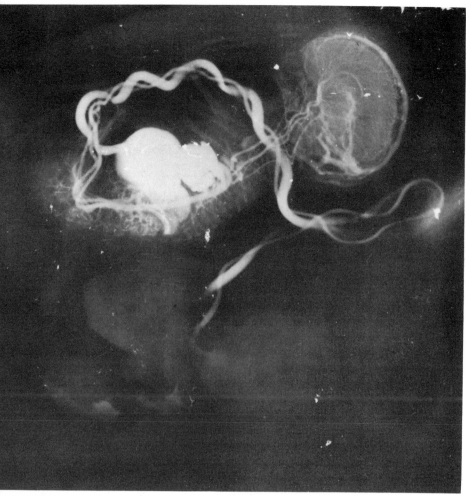

202 The fetal circulation demonstrated by high-speed angiocardiography (cine radiography of the passage of radio-opaque dye injected into the fetal circulation). This picture was taken half way through pregnancy when most of the blood leaving the fetal side of the placenta returns to the left side of the heart and from there passes to the rapidly growing fetal head. Very little blood passes to the fetal lungs which are of course not functional until after birth.

203, 204 Sound waves at ultra-high frequencies can be used to give a precise and detailed picture of the developing fetus within the womb, without any risk of damage. In a modified form of sonar scanning the varying capacity of the tissues and structures of the fetus and placenta for reflecting sound waves gives rise to an image on a television screen. Ultra sound is used to chart the growth and development of the fetus both as a means of detecting any deficiencies in its nourishment and as the most accurate method of assessing age and thus ensuring correct timing of delivery. It is used to detect a multiple pregnancy, though it does not enable sex to be determined; and it can reveal malformations such as spina bifida and hydrocephalus at an early stage. Its use to locate the position of the placenta enables the obstetrician to

the human ear. Ultra-sound is able to detect the outline of soft tissue tumors within other soft tissues of the body and, in this respect, is far superior to X-rays. Its use in obstetrics is widespread and important. It can be shown that the transverse diameter of the fetal skull, known as the bi-parietal diameter, increases uniformly with fetal age and maturity. Thus, serial estimation of the bi-parietal diameter of the developing fetus provides the most reliable estimate we have of fetal growth.

A further technique by which the functioning of the feto-placental unit can be assessed is to introduce a needle through the abdominal wall and into the amniotic cavity, withdrawing some of the amniotic fluid. This is then tested chemically and for enzymes, and the cells found within the fluid are cultured and then examined by special staining techniques. By these methods, a reasonably reliable estimate of the gestational age of the fetus can be made.

When an obstetrician has reason to feel that fetal growth is not progressing adequately it is now possible to assess fairly accurately the growth of the fetus using one or more of the techniques described. Accurate detection is a modern development and enables the obstetrician to assess the possible need for terminating the pregnancy by induction of labor or by Cesarian section. In such cases, the subsequent labor

would be particularly carefully monitored, since the fetus found to be at risk in pregnancy would certainly remain at risk during labor.

Apart from the minor disorders, such as nausea and vomiting, varicose veins and piles, the most common disease complicating pregnancy is 'toxemia' of pregnancy. This is essentially a disturbance of kidney function, often a mild illness with swelling of tissues with retained fluid and some leak of blood proteins into the urine. In a few cases it may be severe, with greatly raised blood pressure and fits, and may even threaten the mother's life. As we do not understand the cause and mechanism of this disease treatment is empirical. Full rest for the mother, with adequate sedation to ensure that she relaxes both physically and mentally, is often extremely beneficial and enables the pregnancy to be continued under close supervision until the fetus is sufficiently mature for the induction of labor to be performed. The early signs of this disease are unlikely to be appreciated by the patient herself; this is why it is so important that women attend for frequent ante-natal examinations in the later stages of pregnancy.

Childbirth. Once labor has started, the feto-placental unit is subjected to considerable strain. Every time the uterus contracts in its attempt to thrust the fetus through the genital tract into the outside world, the uterine wall also contracts, and because of this, maternal blood supply to the placenta is reduced.

If the placenta is already strained and working at its full capacity with no reserve, then this temporary, but repeated, reduction in efficiency will cause true deprivation of the feto-placental unit—a condition called fetal distress in labor. It has been estimated that the journey of about 4 inches through the mother's pelvis carries hazards as great as the infant will have to face from all causes in the next 40 years of life.

Early detection of malfunction of the feto-placental unit in labor has always been the aim of obstetricians and the methods employed have become increasingly sophisticated. Oxygen deprivation in the fetus causes a change in its heart rate. This can be revealed by careful monitoring throughout labor and particularly during delivery. Accurate monitoring can now be achieved either by the use of an abdominal device which picks up the fetal heartbeat and records it graphically, or by attaching a wire to the fetal scalp as soon as the cervix has dilated enough to allow such a procedure to be done. The wire then records the electro-cardiographic (E.C.G.) tracing of the fetal heart. Both methods, the fetal E.C.G. being the more accurate, have the great advantage of being operative even at the height of a uterine contraction—a time when listening with a stethoscope is extremely difficult and unreliable. The tracings, and particularly those of the fetal E.C.G., provide other technical data which gives clear and reliable indication of possible fetal distress.

The biochemist has also become involved in the modern management of labor. Once the cervix is dilated and the fetal head is beginning to descend, it is feasible to obtain a small drop of fetal blood which can be analyzed for its degree of acidity and for various important constituents which indicate the state of oxygenation of the fetus, etc. These form a reliable and scientific basis for diagnosing or excluding fetal distress. So far, the technique requires a fair degree of skill and the ready availability of expensive equipment for biochemical analysis of minute quantities of blood. A skilled technician is usually needed. It seems likely that improvement in the technique itself and in the analytical equipment will result in the technician no longer being needed on every occasion.

Spontaneous abortion. In every reproductive process there is some fetal loss. For those pregnancies which have established themselves and inhibited menstruation so that the woman knows herself to be pregnant, there is a spontaneous abortion rate of about 15 per cent. Recently it has been shown that there is very high embryonic wastage in the very early stages before pregnancy can actually be diagnosed, and that there are probably as many spontaneous abortions as there are pregnancies which lead to birth. It is believed that the vast majority of aborted embryos are abnormal and that the whole elaborate process of spontaneous abortion is really a protective mechanism whereby embryonic malformations are eliminated rather than being allowed to produce abnormal individuals.

Most abnormal embryonic and fetal development is congenital in origin. Such phenomena obey the Mendelian rules of inheritance and the chances of recurrence can be mathematically computed. Alternatively, abnormalities arise as 'chance' mutations in the particular ovum or sperm concerned. The whole question of the inheritance of congenital defects is rapidly being clarified and all parents who have produced an abnormal baby can nowadays be advised by a competent geneticist on their chances of doing so again in future pregnancies.

A second cause of congenital abnormality is when the pregnant woman develops a viral infection which crosses the placental barrier and affects the fetus. Rubella—German measles—has been definitely proven to cause severe abnormality in this way. If such an infection occurs in early pregnancy, the risk of bearing an abnormal child is high and, in most countries, abortion would be offered to the mother after a

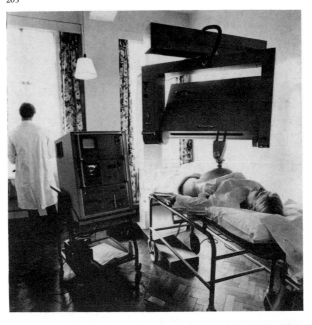

avoid the possibility of serious hemorrhage in the rare cases where the placenta lies across the mouth of the womb (placenta praevia), and makes it possible to prevent damage to the placenta in amniocentesis (where samples of the amniotic fluid are withdrawn through a needle in looking for chromosome and certain other abnormalities in the fetus). 203 shows the equipment in use, and below is an ultrasonic scan of the full length of a fetus seven weeks after conception, showing distinctly the head and limbs.

204

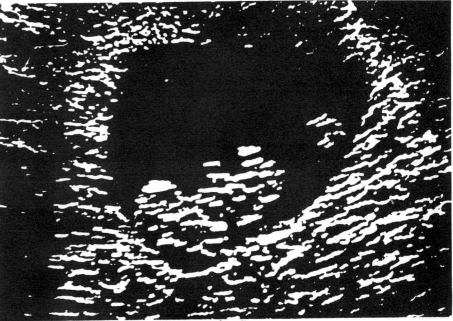

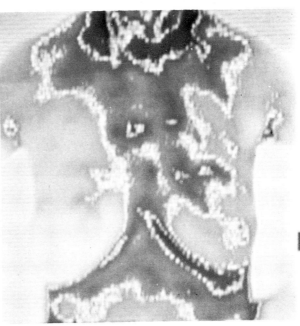

205 Thermography is a non-invasive diagnostic technique which measures variations in surface heat production. Locally increased blood supply and metabolic activity are associated with tumors, and these generate higher temperatures which can be observed in asymmetries of the surface heat production pattern. In this scan of a woman with an advanced cancer in the left breast the asymmetry is clearly evident. The equipment is adjusted to show up gradations in temperature in the range required, the higher temperatures being indicated by the darker tones. In this case the difference in surface temperature between the right and the left breast is about 3°C.

205

full explanation. The possibility that other viral diseases varying from the common cold to infective hepatitis may also cause fetal malformation is under active investigation, but statistical studies with adequate controls are exceedingly difficult to carry out.

The whole subject of fetal abnormality is currently of particular interest because we are at last beginning to develop reliable techniques for the diagnosis of congenital abnormalities *in utero*. A sample of the amniotic fluid can now be analyzed to show if there is fetal abnormality. If abnormality is diagnosed then abortion is likely to be recommended.

Induced abortion. Induced abortion is one of the most important factors in the voluntary control of human fertility. It has been used widely in all industrialized and urbanized societies, especially as the idea of family planning has gained acceptance. For the whole world, induced abortion, criminal and legal, is of far greater importance numerically in family planning than all forms of contraception and sterilization put together. By 1972, 58 per cent of the world's population lived in countries with liberal abortion laws permitting abortion on grounds other than purely medical. In practice, however, there remain vast differences in the way these laws are applied. In much of the U.S.A., abortion is freely available and there is no restriction in its usage except that of cost, and a similar situation applies in the U.K. In India, however, although there are estimated to be at least 3,500,000 criminal abortions annually, the existence of a liberal law has not so far affected medical practice substantially, and in 1973 only about 72,000 therapeutic abortions were reported. Clearly it remains of paramount importance to convince the medical establishment of a country that it is preferable to perform therapeutic abortions rather than to force those who seek abortion to use the illegal means.

The hazards of medically induced abortion have in the past been grossly exaggerated. No such procedures are without risk to the woman, but in countries where reliable statistics have been kept it can be shown that these risks are lower than those entailed by continuing with a pregnancy to term. Possibly the most significant risk of therapeutic abortion is when the operation is carried out rather late and the cervix of the uterus is over-dilated, resulting in its incompetence in future pregnancies and thus leading to unwanted spontaneous miscarriages. The true incidence of this complication is not known, but it is certainly small and fortunately the condition, when it does occur, is readily treatable. In early pregnancy, a relatively new technique of abortion using vacuum aspiration requires no, or only minimal, dilation of the cervix. The relative simplicity of the procedure means that it can

often be performed without an overnight stay in hospital and both short and long-term complications should be rare.

It has become clear that the vast majority of therapeutic abortions performed in western society are done on basically social grounds. To some extent the gynecologist performing such an abortion is undertaking a relatively new role and his actions are based on social as much as on medical reasoning. Medical historians may in the future see this development as the start of a fundamental change in the doctor's role in society.

Advances in gynecology. The gynecologist is nowadays better able to detect, assess and treat the wide variety of diseases which are peculiar to women; he has also become more deeply concerned with the social aspects of his speciality. These include contraceptive advice or female sterilization where desired and appropriate, aid with many sexual problems, and the alleviation of many minor discomforts which women in past generations have accepted as inevitable.

Gynecological operations are now infinitely safer and less uncomfortable than they used to be. As a result, women with a degree of disease or discomfort which their grandmothers would have accepted as normal, will now seek alleviation. This is particularly true in the diseases associated with uterine and vaginal prolapse, where the genital tract, usually having been dilated by childbirth, begins in middle age to sag or weaken, with consequent ill-effects upon the bladder and bowels. Whereas a generation or so ago many afflicted women wore internal pessaries to support the sagging vagina and uterus, such treatment would be recommended nowadays only in very elderly women or in the presence of other serious illness where operation would be too risky.

The complex hormonal control of menstruation is becoming better understood. Furthermore, highly effective synthetic estrogens and progesterones are now available and purified forms of the pituitary hormone responsible for their normal secretion are used to stimulate the ovaries, particularly in cases of infertility due to lack of ovulation. In addition, other synthetic drugs such as Clomiphene are available as stimulants to the ovaries.

With this relatively new hormonal armamentarium, disorders of menstruation, including painful periods, are far more readily treated on a medical basis and many women are now saved from a surgical operation which would previously have been inevitable.

The menopause or change of life is an extremely variable physiological phenomenon. The age at which it occurs is constantly becoming later and whereas 20 years ago menstruation after the age of 45 was unusual, nowadays it is common up to

206, 207 Minute scrapings from the cervix of the uterus can be used to exclude cervical cancer or to diagnose it at a very early stage, long before symptoms or signs are apparent. The diagnosis is based on the microscopic appearance of the cells in the scrapings, and these are illustrated in the photographs here. The malignant cells (207) have much larger, variably shaped nuclei, which have taken up more of the cell stain than the normal nuclei (206). The smear in 207 also shows evidence of cell division, a feature most carefully sought in making diagnoses. This approach to early diagnosis of disease is clearly highly desirable. Many cancers are curable if detected in their early stages. However, it must be remembered that we are still in the very early stages of evaluation of many of these methods, and that, though promising, many have not yet reached the stage of justifying widespread availability to the population. There is a price to be paid, economic, social and emotional, and all screening procedures have to be assessed as to whether benefits outweigh cost.

the age of 50. For many women, cessation of menstruation is an uneventful and virtually symptomless event, usually preceded by an irregular and possibly variable menstrual cycle. But the falling hormone levels may cause depressing emotional and physiological changes. Management of the menopause by the use of hormones has, until recently, been strongly deprecated because it may cause vaginal bleeding. In practice, however, there is no doubt that many women may be relieved from severe symptoms, in particular from serious depression, by such hormones. Recent work has also suggested that small doses of estrogens may prevent the loss of calcium from bones which is itself frequently responsible for severe backache in older women.

The use of estrogens in the alleviation of minor disorders associated with the menopause is now widely accepted. It is an example of the way in which doctors are accepting a role in improving the quality of life, rather than restricting their efforts to the detection and treatment of disease.

Gynecological cancer. Cancer occurs when a few cells cease to respond to the body's normal growth and regenerative control. This group of cells grows randomly, forming a tumor which displaces, invades and strangles surrounding tissues. Parts of such malignant tumors may be carried by the blood or lymphatic flow to other parts of the body where they lodge, gain access to the blood supply and grow anew as secondary deposits. It is often believed that cancer cells grow rapidly. In fact most body tissues, when regenerating after injury or disease, can and do grow faster than any malignant growth. However, regenerating tissues remain subject to a 'feedback' control, which inhibits further growth once they have attained an appropriate size.

Although the mechanisms of control of cell growth are not understood, it would seem that stimuli freeing cells from these controls can vary widely; chemicals, viruses and particular forms of chronic irritation have all been shown to induce special forms of cancer.

Diagnosis of cancer is made by examining a piece of the tumor tissue and/or a few cells scraped from the surface of the tumor. The latter technique, known as cytological (cellular) diagnosis, has been brought very much into prominence in the diagnosis of cancer of the cervix. G. Papanicolau in the U.S.A. first showed that cells in the vagina, suitably stained, could show up the existence of extremely early cancers of the cervix which could not have been diagnosed by clinical inspection. By this simple screening procedure, therefore, gynecologists are able to detect cancer of the cervix before it has produced any symptoms and before it has even developed clinical signs.

Cancer of the cervix is an emotive form of

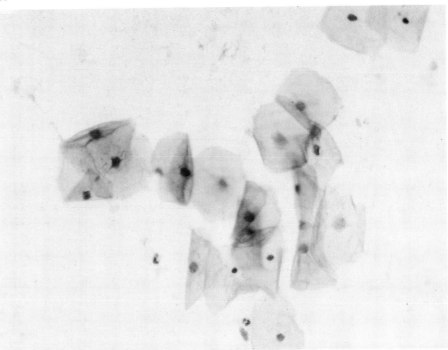

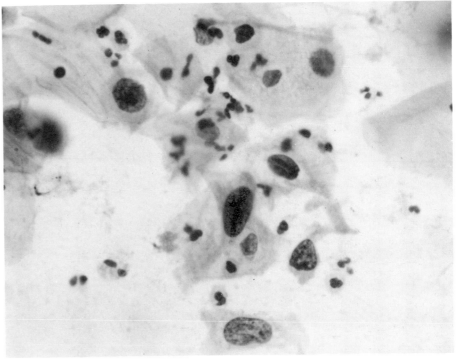

207

cancer since it tends to attack women in their late reproductive age while they are still likely to have dependent children. It is the form of cancer theoretically most readily 'eliminated' by mass screening and by treatment before it has become established. If all cases were in fact detected at the pre-clinical stage, usually known as *carcinoma in situ*, a cure rate of approximately 99 per cent could be anticipated. Even when established, this disease has a relatively good prognosis and about 75 per cent of women with early cancer of the cervix will be free from recurrence five years later.

Very rarely, following full-term delivery or

abortion, some of the placental tissue lying within the uterine cavity develops neoplastic change, and from this may come either the relatively benign form of hydatidiform mole, or the highly malignant *chorion carcinoma*. The chorion carcinoma was, until very recently, almost invariably fatal, and the disease was particularly distressing since the victims were invariably young women of reproductive age.

Around 1958 Dr Li, working in Hong Kong, started to use a drug called Methotrexate in the treatment of chorion carcinoma, which is common in that part of the world. The cure was dramatic and the treatment is now accepted world wide. In uncomplicated cases a genuine cure rate of more than 80 per cent can be anticipated, and even if the disease has already spread to other parts of the body when first diagnosed, combined treatment with Methotrexate, and irradiation of the secondary deposits, still yields a true cure rate of over 60 per cent. Uncomplicated cases can be genuinely cured, and many such women have subsequently borne normal children.

Cancer of the uterus proper, and strictly this is cancer of the endometrium or uterine lining, has a fairly definite symptom, namely vaginal bleeding after the menopause, and it is one of the most curable of cancers. If all women who experienced even the slightest vaginal bleeding after the menopause, or whose menstrual pattern at around the menopause becomes highly irregular, were submitted to a diagnostic cervical dilatation and uterine curettage (D. & C.), most cases would be detected early and could be successfully treated.

Cancer of the breast, by far the most common of the cancers associated with reproduction, remains a formidable killer and the cure rate has changed little in recent years. Recent advances in soft tissue X-rays—xerography—have added significantly to the early diagnosis of the disease and also, where the disease is treated entirely by irradiation therapy, have provided objective criteria for the assessment of treatment. Recently, the technique of thermography, whereby the breasts are photographed in terms of heat using an infra-red camera, has enabled early cancers to be detected in this way. It is possible that the breast responds cyclically, as do the ovaries, to hormones produced in the pituitary gland and that this cyclical stimulation may eventually overrun itself and result in cancers. If so, continued use of the contraceptive pill may help to prevent cancer of the breast.

It would seem logical that all women should learn the simple technique of monthly self-examination of their breasts. They should then seek advice at once if they detect a lump. If the doctor is uncertain, xerography and thermography are available for confirmation. All definite lumps should be surgically removed and pathologically examined. Early diagnosis and treatment of breast cancers certainly can save lives.

Hysterectomy. Hysterectomy is part of the usual treatment for cancer of the cervix or uterus, but such cases account for less than 5 per cent of all hysterectomies performed. The main reasons for the operation—which some doctors think is over-used—are heavy and irregular periods at around the time of the menopause, often associated with the existence of completely non-malignant fibroid tumors of the uterus. Essentially this means that the uterus is removed because there is no effective means of controlling its malfunction. In the past, the ovaries were also removed to ensure that further surgery would not be necessary to remove an ovarian cyst, malignant or not. This abrupt castration was frequently followed by severe menopausal symptoms which, a few years ago, were largely untreated except by reassurance and tranquilizers. Nowadays, the tendency is to leave the ovaries, so that in fact the woman does not go through a menopause until later. One great advantage of performing hysterectomy is that, should the woman later develop menopausal symptoms, they can be effectively and safely treated by estrogens without the possibility of uterine bleeding.

Contraception. Even in technologically advanced countries, unplanned and also unwanted pregnancies remain distressingly common occurrences. It is estimated that of all legitimate births in the U.K. and the U.S.A., at least one quarter are unplanned, though they may of course be not unwelcome by the time the child is born.

The prevention of an unwanted pregnancy begins with sex education and in the past doctors have been little concerned in this area. No educated person could now be unaware of the world population explosion, or of the relatively enormous demands upon limited natural resources made by individuals in the developed countries as opposed to those as yet undeveloped. The medical profession (as well as sociologists and educationalists) is inevitably concerned in this problem and certainly the ordinary doctor is being forced to take an active part in sexual and contraceptive education.

Until the development during the past 20 years of the oral contraceptive and of the plastic intra-uterine device, only the male sheath or condom was widely available and used for contraceptive purposes. Even today the condom remains the most common single method of contraception in both the U.S.A. and the U.K. The advent of the pill, however, has provided an esthetically acceptable and highly efficient contraceptive for the first time.

Intra-uterine devices, initially promoted as safer than the oral contraceptive, have proved to carry with them risks of infection and of menstrual irregularity which have considerably impeded their acceptance. Furthermore, they do not provide anything like the same security against an unwanted pregnancy. Most gynecologists would tend to recommend them only where the pill was contra-indicated or had proved unacceptable in use.

It is always extremely difficult to estimate the effects of contraceptive practice upon population trends. Now that virtually two-thirds of the world's population live under liberal abortion laws there can be little doubt that therapeutic abortion is an important factor in fertility control. Nevertheless, in those countries where large numbers of abortions are suddenly being performed and notified following changes in the law, birth rates have fallen only very marginally, confirming the belief that previously criminal abortion must have been widely used.

In both the U.S.A. and the U.K., gynecologists finding themselves suddenly called upon to perform many more therapeutic abortions have developed an increasing interest in female sterilization. The modern operation is performed through a tiny opening in the abdomen with the aid of a laparoscope, allowing women to be sterilized with a very short stay in hospital or even as out-patients. It should be noted that once a woman has been sterilized, the operation is for all practical purposes completely irreversible.

The technique of vasectomy, or male sterilization, has been known for many years but its use as a form of deliberate sterilization was extremely limited until about 1954, when it was taken up as part of the family planning program in India. Well over 12 million vasectomies have been carried out in India and it can now be confidently stated that it has no physical effect upon sexual performance or enjoyment. Currently it is being widely used in the U.K. and, to a lesser extent, in the U.S.A. Reversal of vasectomy with restoration of reproductive potency has been fairly widely practised in India and, less commonly, in the U.K. It would probably be fair to say that in the ordinary case the chance of success is slightly better than 50 per cent.

Population control—future prospects. It has only recently become possible to plan the birth of each individual child by the use of highly effective methods of family planning appropriate to different religious persuasions. In those countries where the position has been studied, it has been shown that if all unwanted pregnancies were prevented, the resultant birth rate would be highly acceptable demographically. It would follow, therefore, that the community does have a responsibility to make the means of family planning available to all parents so that they can obtain the family size they desire. By retaining the principle that the decision on family size remains firmly with the parents, the politically unacceptable idea of population planning is avoided and the desired results are still likely to occur.

The most hopeful sign for the future lies in the fact that in western countries where contraception, sterilization and abortion are all freely available, they are now being used effectively on a voluntary basis and the birth rates in these countries are rapidly falling to replacement levels. In the less developed countries, it can already be shown that the idea of restricting fertility is much more acceptable than had been believed and that, ironically, governments and the medical professions of such countries often lag far behind the climate of opinion among ordinary citizens.

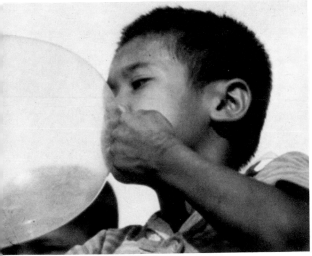

208

208 The condom in its various forms has been used both as a protection against venereal disease and as a contraceptive. It remains one of the most widely used methods of contraception and, being relatively uncomplicated and inexpensive, is suitable for widespread use in the countries of the third world with their problems of rapidly increasing population. The child in the picture, though perhaps not yet ready to employ such devices, is putting a rubber sheath to an alternative use. It is by game play like this that familiarization and education can be achieved at the same time.

13 Childhood and Infancy

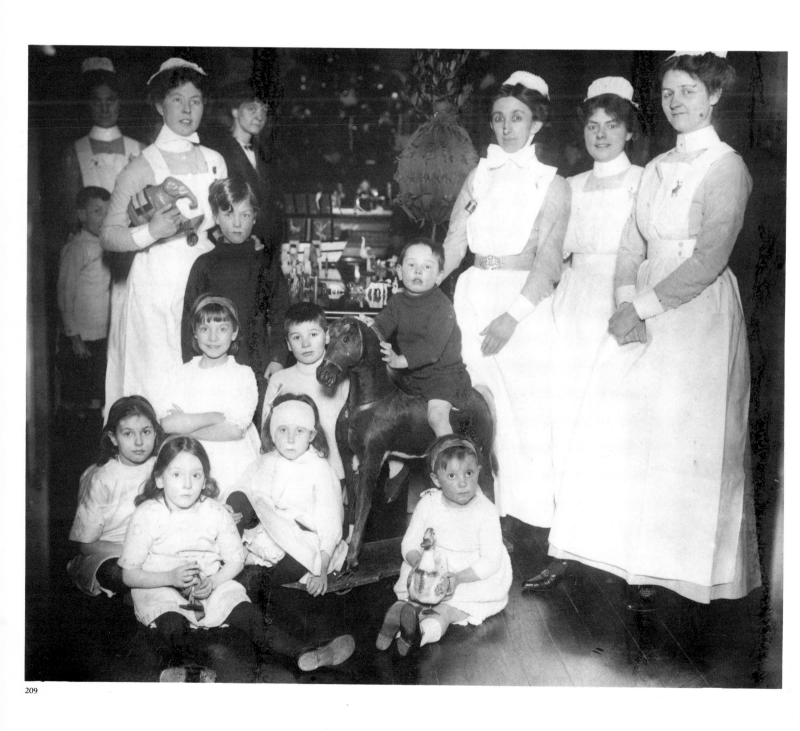

209

Hippocrates, the father of medicine, was aware that children presented special problems to the doctor: a 'textbook' of pediatrics was published by Thomas Phaire in 1553; and we can read reports from the 17th and 18th centuries which demonstrate concern over the terrible death rates among children. At some points in time the number of babies dying in the city of London, for example, outstripped the number who were born. Not only did all the babies who were born die, but several who had been brought into the city from outside also perished. Yet it is paradoxically true that pediatrics only began to emerge as a major speciality in medicine when these very high mortality and morbidity rates in children began to fall substantially. Most of the deaths were due to infections and although the child, particularly the baby, is more prone than the adult to infections and suffers more from their effects—for instance, the baby with gastroenteritis can rapidly become dehydrated and die—nevertheless the nature of common infectious diseases is not markedly different in children from their nature in adults. Therefore it was only when the infectious diseases were overcome that doctors became aware of the many special medical problems of children. Many children's hospitals were founded during the 19th century, but it was not until as late as 1929 that the British Pediatric Association was formed. The American was started in 1932. Since the Second World War the speciality of pediatrics has boomed and the number of doctors specializing only in diseases of children has increased tremendously.

Most medical specialities deal with a part of the body: the pediatrician, however, specializes in a whole group of people—namely children— and his initial emphasis is on how diseases affect the child. His approach is therefore more *patient*-oriented than *disease*-oriented. He has to be aware of the interrelations between a disease and its effects; to think of asthma, for instance, not simply in terms of respiratory function, but of its effects on what the child can do, how it will alter his school life and what influence it will have on him socially and within his home.

It is true that the last decade has seen the development of a number of pediatric subspecialities. There are now pediatric cardiologists, pediatric neurologists, pediatric nephrologists, and several others, but the emphasis of all these doctors is first on the children and only secondly on the part of the body they have decided to specialize in.

Child development. To understand the effect of disease on a developing body, the doctor must have a thorough understanding of the course of normal child development. An enormous amount of information has now been gathered about the process of growth and development. Physical

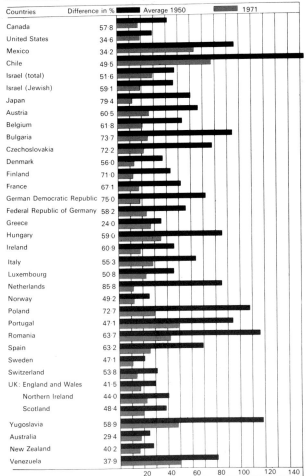

210

Infant deaths per 1,000 live born, and per cent decrease

Countries	Difference in %	Average 1950	1971
Canada	57·8		
United States	34·6		
Mexico	34·2		
Chile	49·5		
Israel (total)	51·6		
Israel (Jewish)	59·1		
Japan	79·4		
Austria	60·5		
Belgium	61·8		
Bulgaria	73·7		
Czechoslovakia	72·2		
Denmark	56·0		
Finland	71·0		
France	67·1		
German Democratic Republic	75·0		
Federal Republic of Germany	58·2		
Greece	24·0		
Hungary	59·0		
Ireland	60·9		
Italy	55·3		
Luxembourg	50·8		
Netherlands	85·8		
Norway	49·2		
Poland	72·7		
Portugal	47·1		
Romania	63·7		
Spain	63·2		
Sweden	47·1		
Switzerland	53·8		
UK: England and Wales	41·5		
Northern Ireland	44·0		
Scotland	48·4		
Yugoslavia	58·9		
Australia	29·4		
New Zealand	40·2		
Venezuela	37·9		

20 40 60 80 100 120 140

growth has been charted and measured; biochemical changes which underlie other changes, such as the onset of puberty, are beginning to be understood; and all the processes of change within the baby around the time of birth have also been intensely investigated.

The functional development of the child and its understanding by the doctor was given a tremendous boost in the 1940s and 1950s by the work of Arnold Gesell and his colleagues in America, and more recently by Ronald Illingworth in the U.K. and many others all over the world. And nowadays the pediatrician has to be concerned about his patients not just from the time of birth, but from the time of conception.

The field of genetics has continually expanded throughout the century. Certain diseases were known to be inherited and the patterns of dominant and recessive inheritance had been discovered by Mendel in the 1860s. Clearly this new knowledge had applications in medicine, but the mechanisms of genetic disorders were not known in any detail until after the Second World War.

In 1949, M. Barr in Canada made a remarkable observation. He was studying the effects of fatigue in the brain of a cat when by chance he noticed that certain nuclei in its cells contained

209 It was only towards the end of the 19th century that pediatrics became a specialized branch of medicine. A famous early children's hospital was the Hospital for Sick Children in Great Ormond Street, London, where the Christmas group shown here posed in 1913. The children's ward of today is quite different. Infections and their consequences used to be the major cause for the admission of children to hospital, but now inborn and congenital abnormalities represent the greater proportion of cases. There has also been a growing awareness of the emotional damage which may be occasioned to the child by early separation from the mother, and in many hospitals, when admission is vital, both mother and child are accommodated.

210 This diagram comparing infant death rates per thousand live births in thirty-five different countries shows very great variations in infant mortality, particularly between the developed and developing worlds. The rate of decline in infant mortality rates between 1950 and 1971 has also varied widely from country to country, but it is nevertheless the case that every country has seen a dramatic improvement in this twenty-year period. There are many factors responsible for this success. They include a general improvement in education, nutrition, hygiene and housing, immunization and the development of antibiotics which have countered the infective causes of death. Of course the population effects of lower infant mortality rates are far-reaching, and the pursuit of voluntary measures of population control seeks to match the humane achievements of alleviating the ravages of 'natural' population control.

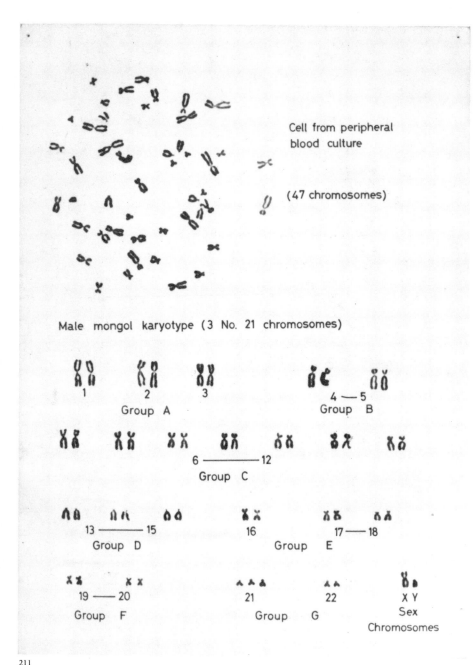

Cell from peripheral blood culture

(47 chromosomes)

Male mongol karyotype (3 No. 21 chromosomes)

1	2	3	4 — 5
	Group A		Group B

6 ————— 12

Group C

13 ——— 15	16	17 — 18
Group D		Group E

19 —— 20	21	22	X Y
Group F	Group G		Sex Chromosomes

211

small black dots. At first he attempted to relate them to fatigue, and it was his lab assistant who pointed out to him that the nuclei with the black dots belonged to the *female* animals. It was rapidly shown that females could be distinguished from males by means of these 'nuclear sex spots', which were in fact the large female sex chromosomes.

The implications of this discovery for medicine were important because it led to the microscopic study of human chromosomes and eventually to the identification of a whole group of abnormalities known as the sex chromosome anomalies. In certain syndromes, the individual has not one nuclear sex spot, as the normal female has, but two or three or more, and these can be seen in the cells of affected individuals right from birth. Soon it became possible to produce cell cultures in which actual human chromosomes could be clearly seen and counted. In this way another fundamental and important discovery was made by Lejeune in 1959 when he demonstrated that children with mongolism—or, as it is now called, Down's syndrome—had 47 chromosomes instead of the normal 46.

Quite a number of other chromosome anomalies have now been described, and these genetic developments have led to a huge expansion in the possibilities for genetic counselling. Today, cells from the unborn child can be examined and some genetic diseases confirmed or ruled out. The same technique, amniocentesis, also shows the sex of the child in the womb, but it would not be used. solely for that purpose. Even without the aid of such tests, the pediatrician may have the task of advising parents about the risks of having a handicapped child, based on their family history. When the risk is very high, parents may want to stop the pregnancy and an abortion may be carried out. There are now literally hundreds of conditions ranging from quite common ones such as achondroplasia (a familiar form of dwarfism

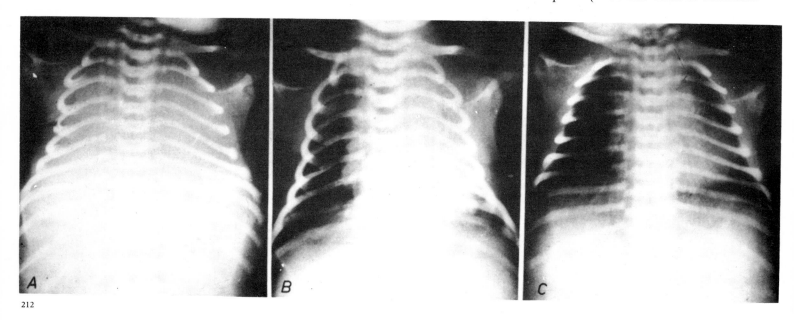

212

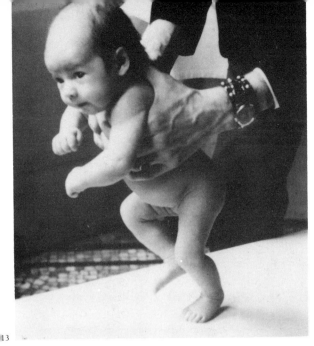

13

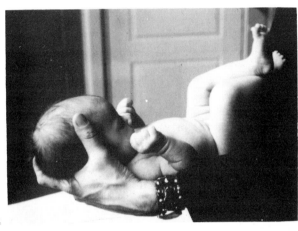

14

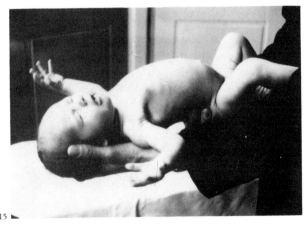

215 ►

hours and should otherwise be left alone. Nowadays, however, the birth of so many babies in hospital has led to an expansion in the study of the newborn baby and its abilities.

The newborn baby has a disproportionately large head, but his overall body shape is like that of an adult. The development of his central nervous system is very much further advanced than was once thought. Complicated responses can readily be demonstrated in the newborn period. Some of the best known of these are primary walking, the Moro response and the placing response. These responses underlie the later development of normal adult function. The child's visual and auditory systems have also been extensively studied: for example, from birth the child responds selectively to sounds in the human speech range in preference to pure tones and mechanical noises. Because of this basic understanding of the normal pattern of neurological action within the child, doctors know what to look for and when to be suspicious of a baby's function from birth if it seems to indicate some condition such as cerebral palsy (the brain damage of the spastic child). In advanced centers today all children with cerebral palsy are detected before the age of one, whereas in other parts of the world this condition may not be diagnosed until the child is two, three or four, by which time secondary deformities may have developed.

Not all functions of the baby can be studied at birth. One cannot see how a child's concept of shape and space is developing until such time as he demonstrates these abilities. One cannot see how he copies until he is three or four and beginning to use a pencil. One can suspect at five that a child may one day have difficulty in learning to read, but one cannot say that he has this difficulty until he has been exposed to school and has failed at reading. Working, however, in collaboration with psychologists, doctors now have a good idea of the process of normal development and can use this in early identification of handicapping conditions.

As the infant mortality from infectious diseases decreased, it became clear that certain groups of babies were particularly at risk of dying in the newborn period. Initially these were grouped as 'premature babies', defined as all babies with a birth weight of under five pounds. More recently it was realized that two types of baby were particularly susceptible: there was the short gestation baby, who was normal in weight and development for his age but was born early at perhaps 32 weeks and therefore weighed less than five pounds; and there was the baby of normal gestation who had spent 40 weeks in the womb but weighed less than five pounds because of intra-uterine malnutrition.

Both groups of babies may have difficulties

211 The chromosomes, which carry the genetic material in every one of the many billions of cells in the body, are situated in the nucleus of each cell. The normal human being has 22 pairs of chromosomes (autosomes) and one pair of sex-chromosomes, XX in the female, and XY in the male. A number of disorders are due to abnormalities of the chromosomes, and it is possible to culture white blood cells outside the body and by special techniques to photograph the chromosomes under great magnification. The images of the individual chromosomes are then cut out and arranged in pairs. In the condition known as mongolism, now usually referred to as Down's syndrome, there is an extra chromosome, and this is revealed in this karyotype where there are three instead of two no. 21 chromosomes.

212 At birth the infant lung is airless and unexpanded. An X-ray may be used to diagnose the state of inflation of the fetal lung. The X-ray A shows a not yet inflated, and therefore radio-opaque, chest. The succeeding radiographs (B and C) show the effect of the first few breaths, C demonstrating the fully expanded and radiolucent lungs. Failure of the newborn lung to expand may occur in the premature birth, where the lung has not yet developed the detergent-like surfactant material which holds the delicate air-filled cavities open after inflation. The blue baby which used to die in asphyxia soon after birth can now be saved by the use of special ventilating apparatus which gently and rhythmically pumps air into the lungs under pressure. It is also now becoming possible to prevent this situation for, by treating the mother appropriately if there is time, surfactant production by the fetal lung can be stimulated early.

213-15 The baby is born with a number of inbuilt instinctual reflex responses, of which sucking is the most familiar. Close observation of these primitive reflex activities is of great value in diagnosing abnormalities in the development of the brain. Two such reflexes are shown here. 213 shows primary walking. During the first three months of life, if the baby is supported and moved forward, regular 'stepping' takes place. This response becomes harder to elicit from about 12 weeks onwards. The baby illustrated is 4 weeks old. Illustrations 214 and 215 show the Moro response. If the newborn baby's head is rapidly lowered, a complex response is observed. The arms initially come together, then they are extended, and the hands and fingers open. Subsequently the hands and arms come together across the midline. This response disappears at about 3 months, except in some forms of brain damage such as cerebral palsy.

where the limb-bones are abnormally shortened but the skull, chest and pelvis—and intelligence—are normal) to excessively rare ones with strange names, like the Marisesco-Sjögren syndrome, where detailed knowledge based on genetic and cytogenetic studies is available. Here the pediatrician is able to give the parents detailed advice about what effect the particular abnormality is going to have on the baby, following a diagnosis made shortly after birth.

The newborn baby. Some people used to think that the newborn baby was a relatively inert vegetable which simply required milk every four

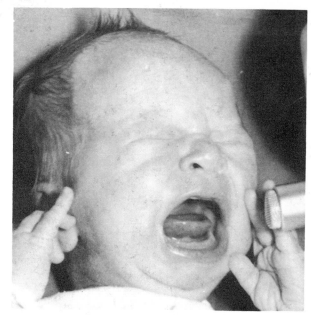

216

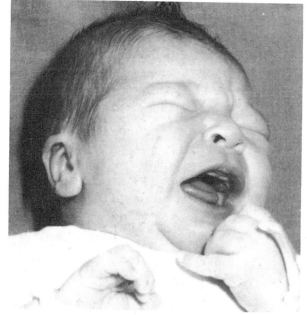

217

216-18 Another approach to the early diagnosis of abnormalities in brain development is the systematic analysis of the baby's cry. In the studies carried out by a group of Scandinavian researchers from which these illustrations were taken, the pain cry (216), produced by a small stimulus such as the prick of a vaccination or a gentle pinch, is studied as distinct from the less energetic cry of hunger (217). 218 shows the form in which the cry is recorded graphically. A represents the word 'now' spoken by the person carrying out the examination at the moment the stimulus is delivered. The baby responds after a moment with the first expiratory cry (C). After a second moment of latency there is a short sound on the intake of breath before the following expiratory cries. The time sequences were studied and the first long cry, C, subjected to close analysis of its sound characteristics. This information was related to familiar auditory observations such as the high-pitched cry of a child with cerebral damage or the so-called Cri du Chat, and to other means of diagnosing abnormalities such as the analysis of chromosomes in Down's syndrome shown in illustration 211.

219 The incubator has radically improved the outlook for the premature baby. It acts as a partial substitute for the womb, providing a relatively constant environment in which temperature and oxygen supply can be controlled and which can be kept relatively sterile. The picture shows a premature baby being nursed in an incubator. The baby is being fed intravenously via a scalp vein and a catheter is being introduced via the umbilical vein so that arterial blood can be sampled for its oxygen content.

during the newborn period but they are rather different. For example, the respiratory distress syndrome (hyaline membrane disease) is more common in the baby of short gestation. His lungs are not adequately developed and he can become hypoxic (short of oxygen). On the other hand the baby of low birth weight ('small-for-dates') is much more likely to have suffered in the uterus and may be brain-damaged and have periods of oxygen insufficiency in the newborn period.

Some of the difficulties of intervening in

such situations are illustrated by the complications which arose once these small babies began to be treated energetically. It seemed reasonable, as the babies were often anoxic, to place them in the controlled environment of an incubator and to give them oxygen. However, babies who were placed in pure oxygen were found to be liable to develop retrolental fibroplasia, a condition which causes blindness, and it was recognized that high concentrations of oxygen were toxic to the baby. This discovery in the early 1950s forced pediatricians to reduce the concentration of oxygen they administered to babies. Careful studies later showed that this in turn increased the incidence of spastic diplegia (leg paralysis) and possibily other conditions.

What was happening was that some babies were getting retrolental fibroplasia as a result of too much oxygen, while other babies were suffering brain damage because of too little. Some babies in the course of three or four weeks suffered both conditions, ending up blind and with cerebral palsy. The solution to this dilemma came with the development of a means to measure the amount of oxygen in arterial blood, a sample being withdrawn through a catheter inserted via the baby's umbilicus into an artery. The actual concentration of the oxygen in the baby's blood is measured and the concentration that he is breathing is varied accordingly. In modern pediatric units where such aids exist the outlook for the baby who is small at birth has become extremely good.

Treatable diseases. Though the emphasis in pediatrics is on prevention, there are many conditions where prevention is not possible. Advances in the study of diseases in adults have been applied to children, who may present special problems. Thus the development of cardiac surgery in the adult was quickly followed by similar surgery for the child, where there are the added technical problems of the small size of the patient. Another example where treatments have been developed for adults and children is in leukemia. The new drugs which affect this condition have been so successful that in some instances it is now possible to speak of a cure. Again, children have their own varieties of kidney disease, and the artificial kidney machine has saved the lives of many. But although there are important aspects of managing children with these conditions, the medical principles are not too far from those for the adult patient.

There remain a host of problems, however, that are unique to childhood and which have attracted the attention of pediatricians over the last twenty years. A huge proportion of children suffering from them come under the blanket term of 'handicapped children'.

As the pediatrician was released from acute

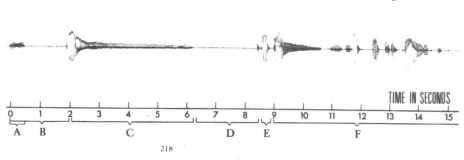

TIME IN SECONDS

0 1 2 3 4 5 6 7 8 9 10 11 12 13 14 15

A B   C   D   E   F

218

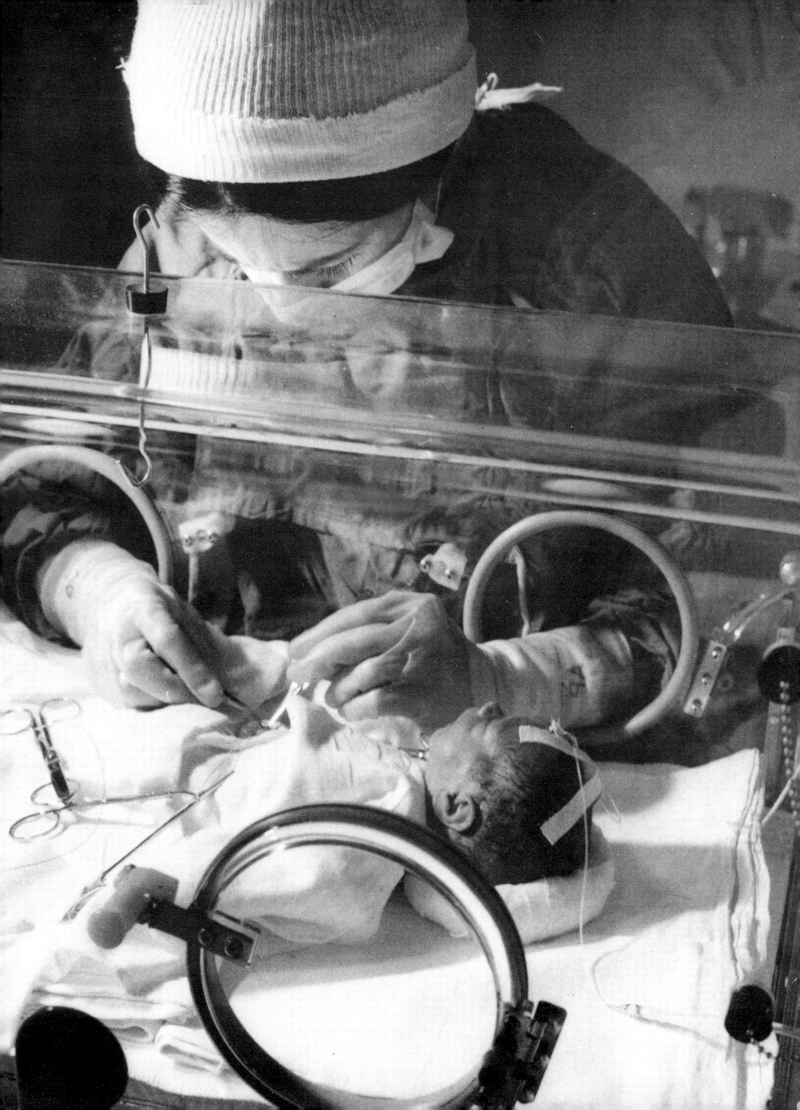

life-saving work on children with pneumonia, he began to find time to look at the many children who had been shut away in hospitals for the mentally handicapped or in homes for crippled children, and to try and sort out what was wrong with them and what had happened to them. From the late 1940s onwards children with cerebral palsy received a great deal of attention. The different varieties were identified: for example the child with shaky movements and a lot of instability is now said to have athetoid cerebral palsy, while the child with stiff limbs and contractures has spastic cerebral palsy. In some instances it became possible to see the cause of the condition and to prevent it, and while there are still about two cerebral palsy children for every 1,000 births, the severity of their condition has been much ameliorated by early identification, early management of the condition and early help for the family into which the child has been born.

Less successful, but by no means insignificant, are the efforts which have been made to treat spina bifida. In this condition the child is born with a gap in the mid-line of his back, through which the coverings of the spinal cord and part of the spinal cord itself protrude. The children are often born with complete or partial paralysis of the lower limbs, and the nerve supply to the bladder is often involved. Because of abnormalities of the nervous system they are very likely to develop hydrocephalus (water on the brain). During the 1950s a treatment for hydrocephalus was developed which involved the insertion of a one-way valve to allow excess fluid to flow from the head to a vein. This technical development resulted from collaboration between a neurosurgeon, Spitz, and an engineer, Holter (whose child had hydrocephalus), and led to an energetic attack on the problem of spina bifida.

Spina bifida occurs in some parts of the world at a rate as high as four per 1,000 children, although elsewhere the incidence is much less. With the knowledge that they could handle the hydrocephalus which was going to develop, surgeons made dramatic plans to treat the spina bifida in the back itself. A study carried out in 1959 showed that if the wound was closed early— within the first 24 hours of life—far more of these babies survived. Many of them had previously died from infections during the early weeks or months of life. Now babies were brought into centers immediately, the protrusion was removed or replaced in the spinal column as far as possible, and skin grafts were made to cover the open area. The initial results of this activity were extraordinarily promising and the percentage of babies surviving the first year of life went up to about 60 per cent. As time went on, however, it was realized that the quality of life for these survivors was not good. Despite the effectiveness of the valve, its presence did not lead to a permanent cure for the hydrocephalus and in consequence, as the child grew, the valve had to be replaced. There was always the risk that during replacement or at other times an infection would develop in the system because of the presence of the foreign body, and meningitis would occur.

Even those children who escaped such complications were often left with paralyzed or partially paralyzed lower limbs and incontinent bladders. Urinary infections might develop, followed by renal failure. Complex urino-genital surgery was necessary to relieve some of these symptoms. In more severe cases where the original lesion had been high in the back the child was very likely to develop a bent back (scoliosis) which proved very difficult to treat.

The problems raised by the treatment of this condition were not purely medical, but ethical as well. Was it reasonable to use immense resources and finance to extend the lives of these babies from a few weeks to six or seven years, when during that time the children would suffer so much—and when the families would suffer equally in caring for them? Today most pediatricians feel that the approach to spina bifida and other such conditions should be selective, and that not only life but the quality of life must be considered in planning to help such babies when they are born. The policy of most developed countries is now one of selective operation on those children whose prospects are best.

In addition to this work on children with physical handicaps, attention has focused in the last 20 years on children who were diagnosed as having a mental handicap. More and more people became aware that this simple label was not adequate to describe the wide variety of different types of problems which had previously been thus grouped together. While the child with Down's syndrome (mongolism) might suffer from simple mental retardation, other children had far more complex dysfunctions.

One group which has attracted a great deal of attention is that of children with autism. It has been possible to demonstrate that some of these children have basically normal intellectual potential, but they have extreme difficulty in communication—a difficulty which interferes with their emotional development as well as with their development of communication skills. Autistic children seem unable to look anyone straight in the eye; they often develop odd repetitive movements called stereotopies while failing to develop normal speech and language. Possibly the basic damage is a failure to integrate different subsystems of the brain, so that these can never really sort out the messages that are coming into them. Even within this relatively small group of children, as pediatricians today look at them more closely, there are found to be subgroups of the main group and children with different varieties of autism.

The first step, therefore, is adequate diagnosis and assessment of the child's particular difficulties, and then it is sometimes possible to plan a treatment or management program which may help the child to develop more normally.

Emotional development. With the work on normal child development which was mentioned earlier, there have been studies of the way the child develops within the family. From the late 1940s people began reporting that children in orphanages or homes suffered from slow, and indeed stunted, mental and emotional development. Investigations were started on the effects of removing a young child from his family and placing him in a hospital. Two-year-old children who were not visited by their families typically started off by crying continuously but then seemed to withdraw, and after a further period of time might appear happier but would not subsequently respond to their parents at all. Although the long-term effects of such deprivation of maternal care were probably overstated at first, doctors began to think more carefully about the influence of the hospital or institutional environment on a child. The importance of the parents for normal emotional development was recognized, and in most children's hospitals parents are actively encouraged to be present with their children as much as possible. Where a child does experience separation, child psychiatrists tackle the problem of how to help him, and a new understanding of the background to emotional development has led to a more rational basis for child psychotherapy.

Particularly in America during the last decade problems both of behavior and of learning in ordinary children have attracted a tremendous amount of pediatric attention. New diseases have been described such as dyslexia—an inability to read despite average intelligence; dysgraphia—difficulty with drawing; and dyscalculia—difficulty with numbers. Much attention has been given to hyperactivity in school children, and in some states as many as 20 per cent of ordinary schoolchildren have been given drugs to 'treat' this overactivity. Not all the enthusiastic activities of doctors with schoolchildren have been beneficial, however, and slowly a balanced attitude to the role of the doctor vis-a-vis the educational system is being evolved.

It is true that certain children are more likely to have difficulties in school. For example children who learn to talk late, after three, are especially likely to have difficulties in learning to read. The relationship between the findings the

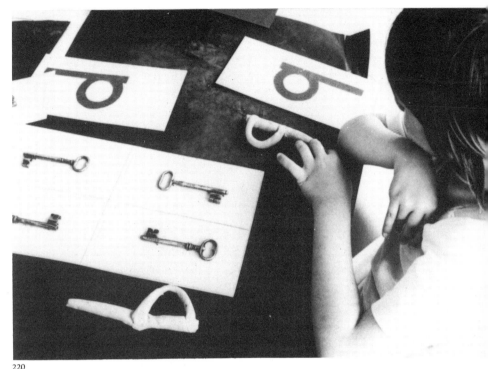

220

doctor makes and the child's performance in the school are not simple, and in order for the doctor to understand what is happening he has not only to study the child in his clinic, but also to watch his behavior and his activities in the schoolroom situation. More and more this is being done, and perhaps the most exciting prospect for the future is of collaboration between doctors, psychologists and teachers leading to far less failure in school, and the development of the full potential of many children who in the past have missed out because of lack of proper understanding of the difficulties that they are facing.

220 Children with learning disorders may have perceptual problems which make it difficult for them to distinguish between similar-shaped letters. This may be associated with some difficulty in distinguishing between left- and right-handed shapes, as here with the letters d, b, p and q. In this picture the child is being given help to overcome this learning difficulty.

14 In the Operating Theater: Surgery and Anesthesia

221 This picture records a historic operation, the first ovariotomy, carried out by the surgeon Ephraim McDowell in Danville, Kentucky, in 1809. The operation was successful, but the scene, with the patient laid out on a common table in the surgeon's house, does illustrate strikingly the terrors and hazards of surgery before the advent of anesthesia and asepsis. Perhaps the freshness of the country air partly contributed to the patient's escape from infection by the myriad germs which lingered in the doctor's 18th century clothes and about his living room with its comfortably glowing fire, but good fortune must have played a larger part.

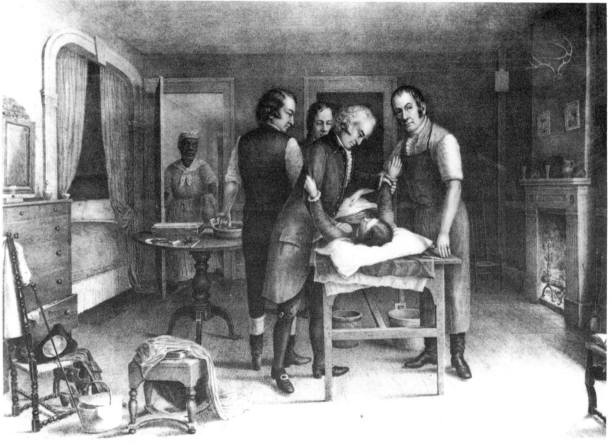

221

Attempts at surgical correction of physical illness have been well documented for thousands of years. However, it was not until the latter half of the 19th century that the techniques of surgery which today enable us to enter safely into any of the cavities of the human body to remove, repair or even replace damaged organs became basically different from that practised by our surgical forefathers.

The gleaming operating theater of today filled with complex scientific hardware and inhabited by a team of gowned, capped and masked professionals evolved from the fortunate juxtaposition of three events. Two of these, revolutionary in concept, and the third the result of a somewhat longer process, ushered surgery into its most productive and exciting era.

First was the discovery and use of anesthesia. Second, and of equal importance, was the acceptance of the germ theory of disease and shortly thereafter, the discovery of an acceptable method markedly to decrease bacteria

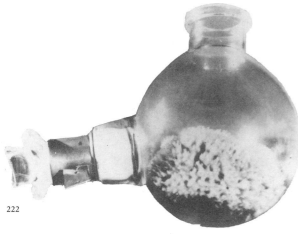

222

in the surgical environment. The last was initially accomplished by antisepsis, that is, the killing of microbes already present, while in more recent times asepsis, which prevents the entrance of pathogenic bacteria into the operating area itself, has been practised. Third, although possibly not so dramatically apparent, was the

mantle of a surgeon. There was a steady progression in emphasis from his role as expert anatomist to that of physiologist, and often to research scientist as well. He is now one important member of a team who is very dependent upon the co-operation of colleagues in ancillary fields for the success of his surgery.

Since time immemorial man has been seeking ways to relieve pain. The ancient Greeks recommended the ingestion of mandragora roots for lessening this dread symptom. A thousand years later Arabian physicians could only offer a soporific sponge to produce a modest analgesia. Through the centuries, however, only alcoholic beverages or opiates were available in any practical sense, and these fell far short of the mark in offering either a safe or a reliable anesthetic. As late as 1839 a distinguished French surgeon wrote: 'To escape pain in surgical operations is a chimera which we cannot expect

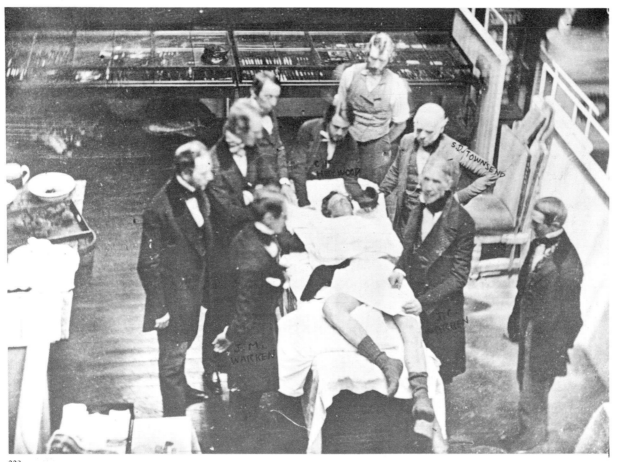

223

change in the surgeon himself. No longer was he a man of little education learning his trade by apprenticeship, looked upon as a social inferior and as a member of a trade associated with pain and the aura of death. By the late 1800s he had developed his skills through a program of more formal training, although the classic residency programs which we know today did not evolve until the 1920s and 30s. He was eventually forced to pass rigorous examinations of both theory and practice before being allowed to assume the

in our time'. Yet only seven years later, on 16 October 1846, the physicians and students present in the surgical amphitheater of the Massachusetts General Hospital in Boston saw the first operation performed under ether anesthesia. While there is some claim of an earlier use of this anesthetic agent, most authorities would accept this demonstration as a reasonable first date. John Collins Warren, the distinguished Harvard surgery professor who performed the operation, was alleged to have exclaimed:

224 The extraordinary sophistication of the modern equipment for inducing and maintaining anesthesia is evidenced in this photograph. When considerable muscular relaxation is required, it may be necessary to paralyze all muscle activity. In this case the anesthesiologist becomes responsible for maintaining the patient's respiration by means of an automatic pumping device (seen at the front of the machine, on the left). The thermometer-like gauges are used to monitor the flow of up to four anesthetic agents at once, either gases, stored in the cylinders on the right, or vaporized liquids from the bottles suspended next to the gauges.

225, 226 Joseph Lister (1827-1912) struck the first blow against the second major hazard of surgery, sepsis. The discoveries of Louis Pasteur (see chapter 1) convinced him that the infection and putrefaction which so often followed operations that were technically masterly were due to microorganisms coming from the air, the surgeon's hands, the very instruments which reached into the patient's body. In a radical attack on the ubiquitous germs, Lister insisted upon high standards of cleanliness, reinforced by the use of carbolic solutions, even including a fine spray to sterilize the air. The detail from an engraving shows his carbolic spray in use around 1880. The photograph shows Lister at the age of 64 (seated in center), twenty-five years after he performed his first 'antiseptic' operation, in a ward of King's College Hospital. In the same year as this photograph was taken, he said in an address to the surgical section of the British Medical Association in Dublin: 'Since the antiseptic treatment has been brought into full operation and wounds and abscesses no longer poison the atmosphere with putrid exhalations, my wards, though in other respects under precisely the same circumstances as before, have completely changed their character, so that during the last nine months not a single case of pyaemia, hospital gangrene or erysipelas has occurred in there.'

227 The evolution of modern surgical technique may be traced through this photograph and the succeeding three photographs overleaf. This picture taken at the turn of the century shows an operating theater scene at University College Hospital Medical School in London. The anesthesiologist can be seen at the patient's head. The origin of the term 'theater' is evidenced by the audience of students seated in rows and observing the spectacle. It is clear that there are many potential sources of infection from them and elsewhere which threaten the patient. Observation of surgery today is often by way of a television link (see 229).

'Gentlemen, this is no humbug'. Indeed, it proved not to be. Within one year there was hardly a single major operation performed in the civilized world without ether anesthesia. Other agents shortly came into use. Chloroform, which was rather more pleasant than ether, was popularized, particularly for obstetrics, by Sir James Young Simpson of Edinburgh. The use of anesthesia for obstetrics met some opposition on theological grounds since fundamentalists adhered to the biblical injunction that children should be 'brought forth in pain'. All opposition was swept away, however, when Queen Victoria elected to have a chloroform anesthetic for one of her parturitions.

The anesthesia utilized at the turn of the century is to modern anesthesia rather what an early commercial aircraft is to the jet liners which criss-cross our skies today. Basically they both get you where you wish to go, but when one considers the safety, reliability and comfort provided, the trips are barely comparable!

Progress in anesthesia proceeded along two separate but mutually dependent channels. The first concern was to develop safer and better anesthetic agents; the second, to be able to deliver these agents in a controlled manner. Modern inhalation anesthetics, in contrast to ether and chloroform, are minimally irritating to the breathing passages and lungs. They are practically odorless and, when given in proper dosages by trained anesthesiologists, have few unwanted side effects on vital organs such as the heart, liver and kidneys. The anesthetic machines which are now available can deliver up to three separate types of anesthetic agents singly or in combination, with constant monitoring of the amount of each agent being given at any particular point of time. These agents are for the most part non-explosive and non-inflammable.

Conduction anesthesia, in which sensory nerves to the desired area are blocked by injection of an anesthetic agent, was introduced in 1885 by a surgeon, William Halsted. It is of some interest that the first agent used was cocaine. As a result of the experiments on himself, Dr Halsted became an addict; he eventually overcame the addiction, but only with the greatest difficulty. At the present time, however, non-addicting drugs are used. The most common type of conduction anesthesia is spinal anesthesia. In this technique a needle is inserted into the fluid-filled sac which surrounds the spinal cord, and an anesthetic agent is injected into this sac, producing anesthesia of all the nerves below the area of injection. No medication is actually injected into the spinal cord itself. The employment of spinal anesthesia is usually limited to surgery involving the lower half of the body, including the lower abdomen. If the level of anesthetic is carried any higher than this,

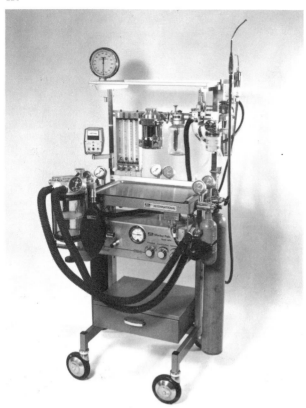

224

there is some risk of interfering with the muscles of respiration. Whether a spinal, local or general anesthetic is used is generally dependent upon the type of surgery to be performed. For some operations, a combination of nerve block plus local anesthesia is desirable. In some cases the choice is dependent upon the wishes of the patient. Some people prefer to remain awake although drowsy during the surgery; others wish to be completely asleep.

Prior to surgery drugs are administered to dry up the secretions of the respiratory tract. This reduces the irritant effects of some volatile anesthetics and helps pulmonary function during the operation. The dry mouth which the patient may experience is a small price to pay for this protection.

If a general anesthetic has been decided upon, the actual beginning of unconsciousness, the induction, is usually initiated by the intravenous injection of a rapidly acting barbituate, thiopental. This technique allays the apprehension and fear that many people would feel if a mask were placed over their face for induction by means of inhalation. However, the depth of anesthesia, which varies for different operations, is usually maintained by the use of anesthetic gases rather than by continued injections of the intravenous medication.

A remarkable recent advance has been the introduction of muscle-relaxing drugs as an adjunct to the anesthesia. There are two types: a long-acting one called curare which was first derived from arrow poisons used by South American Indians; and a shorter-acting one, succinyl choline, an analog of a body chemical necessary for proper muscular action. These enable the surgeon to obtain easy access to body cavities, particularly the abdomen, without having the patient brought to the very deep and possibly dangerous levels of anesthesia required for total relaxation of the powerful body wall musculature.

These drugs may, as part of their effect, paralyze the muscles of respiration. Control of the patient's breathing is then taken over by the anesthesiologist. The lungs are inflated by compression of the anesthetic bag, either manually by the anesthesiologist or mechanically by a machine which can take over this function but which is supervised by the anesthesiologist.

Barring any special technical problems encountered during surgery, the period during anesthesia when the patient's vital functions are carefully followed and he is well oxygenated is probably the least hazardous. Much as in flying, the take-off and landing is much more dangerous than the usually routine middle of the flight. The patient's vital signs such as his pulse,

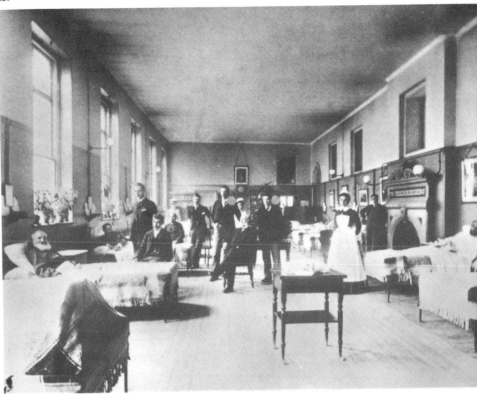

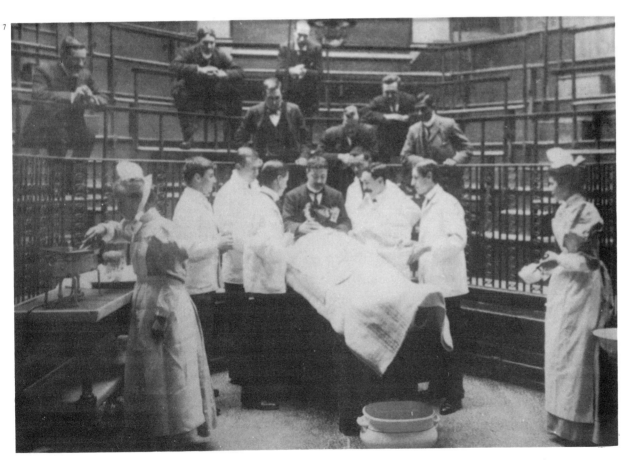

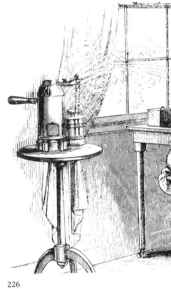

respiration and blood pressure are monitored constantly. If the operation is of great magnitude, these vital signs are followed by electronic gadgetry and visually displayed. This is usually done by means of an oscilloscope screen built into the monitoring equipment. However, permanent records can be obtained of any portion of the data should it be desired. The patient's temperature is also constantly monitored. This is very important in patients who are brought to the operating room with fevers or when patients are cooled for certain operations to lower their metabolic rate. With some very complicated procedures such as open heart surgery, more

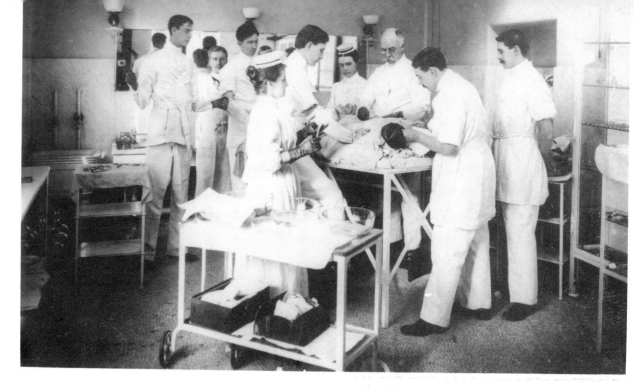

228

228 Transatlantic differences in style and the pioneering enterprise of the New World are manifest in this photograph taken at the Roosevelt Hospital, New York City, just two years after the scene at University College Hospital on the preceding page. Doctor McBurney, well known for his contribution to abdominal surgery, is operating, gowned and gloved but not capped or masked. Here the onlookers are themselves in theater garb.

sophisticated data such as cardiac output, blood oxygen content and blood acidity can be followed as well.

It was apocryphally stated by some surgeons as they rejoiced in their technical expertise that only two problems remained to be solved before they could scale further heights of excellence: anesthesia and lighting. Just as the former discipline has been able to keep pace with modern surgical advances, so has the engineering genius applied to the problem of lighting the operating room. Modern lighting, although often taken for granted, has enabled the surgeon to see clearly into every recess of the human body without excessive heat and without disturbing shadows. This has been a noteworthy adjunct to the modern surgical equipment.

All modern operating rooms are air-conditioned, but in a special fashion. A complete air change can be accomplished every two to three minutes, and with the use of special filters, over 99 per cent of all solid particles only one twentieth the size of a red blood cell can be eliminated. Thus, the system not only provides comfort for the patient and the operating room personnel, but eliminates all contaminates in the air which could carry bacteria with it.

Anesthesia is so timed that the patient awakens at approximately the time the surgery is over. This can be very precisely controlled, and there is no danger of the patient waking up during surgery. After surgery the patient is taken to a special area called the recovery room where especially trained personnel watch over his postsurgical state until he is awake and alert enough to be returned to his room.

Today we all accept the germ theory of disease as self-evident, a truism, an unassailable scientific fact. Such has not always been the case.

Bacteria or animalcula were in fact described by the Dutch physician van Leeuwenhoek in 1683. However, the demonstration that these minute living things could cause specific diseases was many hundreds of years in coming. Building on the work of others, but with the insight of his own genius, Louis Pasteur provided the irrefutable scientific experiments which laid to rest the theory of spontaneous generation of microbes (see chapter 1). The work of Pasteur laid the foundation for another fundamental revolution in surgery, the introduction of the antiseptic method.

It was the British surgeon, Joseph Lister, later to become Lord Lister, who recognized that wound infections, the overwhelming scourge which made what would be considered a minor surgical procedure today hazardous in the extreme, were due to germs gaining entrance to the operative area. He used carbolic acid as an antiseptic for local wound dressings and as a spray in the operating room. He chose this particular compound apparently because it had been used to keep down the odor in sewage which was at that time a great problem throughout the major cities of Britain. Within one year he was able to reduce by 300 per cent the mortality rate of his patients requiring amputation. However, because of the cumbersome nature of the carbolic acid method, antisepsis gradually gave away to asepsis. The earliest rational approach to this problem was championed in the first half of the 19th century by an Austrian obstetrician, Ignaz Semmelweiss. Although he was able to lower the death rate from puerperal fever (infection of the newly-emptied uterine cavity) by simply having the attending physicians soak their hands in chloride of lime before examining their patients, he was

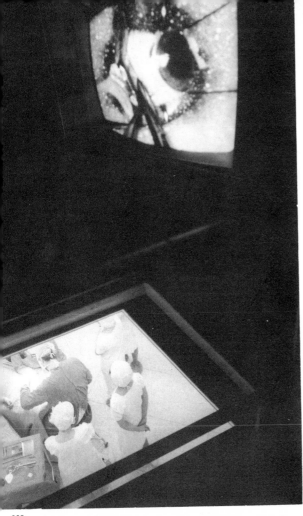

scorned and mocked for his efforts. It was an idea whose time had not yet come and which was revived only when the germ theory of disease and its transmission by passive carriers was finally understood. Important contributions came in rapid succession from many centers of medicine throughout the western world. From Germany in 1875 came the concept of scrubbing the patient's skin and the surgeon's hands prior to the operation. This was shortly followed by steam sterilization of surgical instruments and drapes. William Halsted of the United States popularized the use of rubber gloves as well as caps to cover the hair. Gauze face masks were first worn by the French surgeon Paul Berger. The operating gown in its present form seems to have come from Italy.

Our present-day environment encompasses all these barriers to pathogenic bacteria in a much more sophisticated fashion. Entrance to the surgical suite and the operating room itself is barred to all except those who have an obvious need to be present: the physicians in attendance, surgical nurses and students or house officers directly involved in the care of the patients. Glassed, enclosed observation booths in many large medical centers have taken the place of the tiered rows of benches for students and other physicians present at the turn of the century. In

229 Closed-circuit television is now widely used to give medical students an optimal close-up view of the surgeon's working field while preventing the possibility of their being a source of infection. This picture shows an eye operation in progress which is being viewed on a television monitor.

230 A modern operating theater prepared for an orthopedic operation. Positioning of bone and fixation devices is monitored by X-ray apparatus within the theater. At the patient's head is the anesthetic machine and, in the foreground, the portable X-ray control console. The covering of the occupants of the operating theater with gowns, caps, masks, towels and overshoes is now almost complete. Illustration 6 on page 15 shows the completion of the trend towards total asepsis.

229

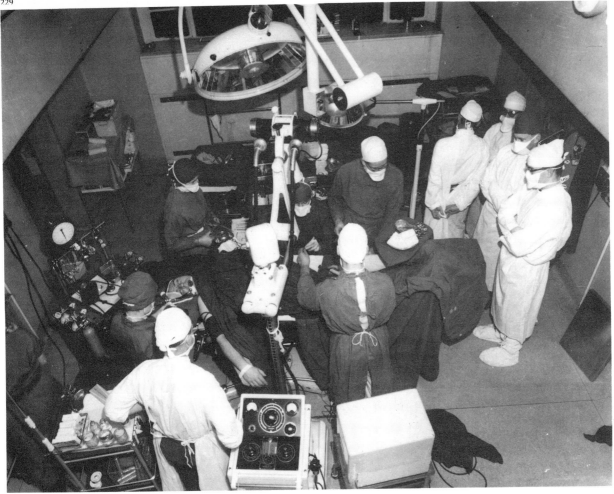

230

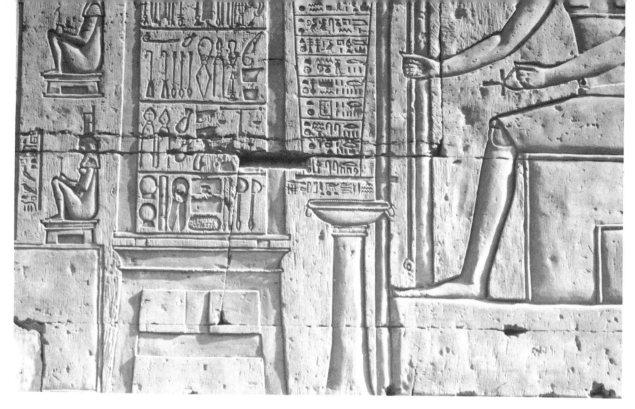

231, 232 Many similarities can be observed between the surgical instruments depicted on a wall surface in the Temple of Komombo on the east bank of the Nile, built by the Ptolemies about 69 AD, and those contained in the modern set of orthopedic instruments laid out for a spinal operation, in which, among others, scalpels, forceps, hammer and chisel may easily be recognized. In other fields very specialized surgical instruments have been developed to meet specialized requirements. Miniaturization is required for the microsurgery of eye and ear (see illustration 178), the heated cautery wire is used for the rapid arrest of hemorrhage from the small blood vessels, and a super-cooled probe is used in some eye operations (see illustration 163) and for the therapeutic destruction of tissue in certain areas such as the pituitary gland.

more recent years closed circuit television cameras have relayed the operation to an audience seated comfortably in an auditorium.

The surgical team changes all its street clothes outside the operating suite and dresses in pyjama-like tops and bottoms made of cotton or other non-static producing material. Shoes are covered with disposable paper booties which have built-in grounding strips.

Although modern anesthesia rarely calls for the use of an explosive inhalation agent, all floors are constructed so as to preclude any building up of static electricity. While the patient is being put to sleep, the surgeon, now masked and capped, scrubs his arms and hands for five to ten minutes with a suitable germicidal agent and on entering the operating room he is handed a sterile gown made of cloth or moisture-proof special paper material. Now properly gowned and having donned very thin flexible sterile rubber gloves, he and his assistants, who have also scrubbed and are sterilely attired, approach the anesthetized patient. As the patient's skin has bacteria on its surface, the operative site as well as the surrounding area was shaved before surgery and scrubbed in much the same manner as the surgeon scrubbed his hands. Then large sterile drapes are spread over the patient exposing only the area where the incision is to be made.

Basically speaking, two objectives must be met to make any surgery possible. First, there must be a way to control and avoid hemorrhage (hemostasis). Secondly, there must be a reliable method of reclosing any opening made in the patient's skin and musculoskeleton to gain access to the underlying organs. Control of hemorrhage is possible because of the surgeon's knowledge of anatomy. This enables him to avoid cutting or

injuring major vessels during the course of his dissection. Those vessels which must be cut are first clamped with special instruments called hemostats and then tied or sutured shut.

The purpose of a suture is to hold severed tissue together mechanically until enough natural healing has taken place to maintain the integrity of the divided structures. Until recently the surgeon has had a choice of two main types of suture material; one that the body absorbed over a period of time and one that remains in place for the life of the host. The former type, commonly called catgut but actually obtained from the lining of sheep intestine, is reabsorbed by the body in about two or three weeks. It is thus ideal for use in subcutaneous tissue where prolonged holding power is not necessary or in areas where the potential for infection is high, since in that situation it would be disadvantageous to have a permanent foreign body in the wound. It is now possible to synthesize this type of absorbable suture and thus eliminate the variability of strength that occurs with any natural product.

Until very recently the non-absorbable sutures have been manufactured from naturally-occuring fibers, either cotton or silk. In recent years however more and more synthetic non-absorbable sutures made from plastic have been utilized for their unique advantage. Just as increasingly sophisticated instrumentation has enabled surgeons to achieve greater technical proficiency, so stronger and more inert suture material in sizes finer than the finest hair has extended technical possibilities to their outer limits.

Having reviewed the aseptic precautions, the anesthetic safeguards and the numerous

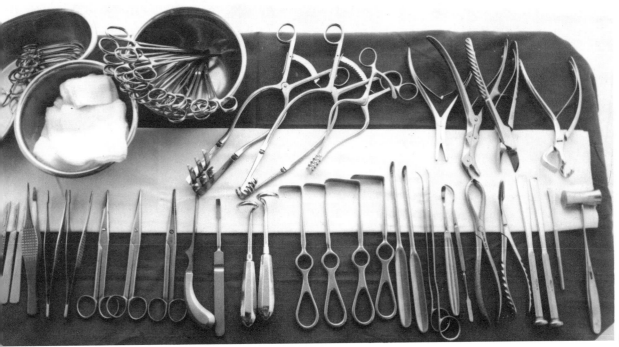

technical advances as part of the complex milieu into which the surgical patient entrusts himself, what remains to be discussed is that very human and therefore somewhat indefinable factor, the surgeon himself. Perhaps if one accepts the latest fanciful novel, the offerings of television and the occasional stereotype which our medical colleagues are apt to promulgate, a surgeon appears as a somewhat stubborn extrovert who is given to action, even if it be intemperate, rather than to introspective and contemplative reflection. This may well be a survival from the days when all surgery, because of its danger, was dramatic and the surgeon was the absolute master of the operating room, a somewhat regal figure, the cynosure of all eyes, before whom nurses trembled and house officers worshipped. The surgeon of today can be considered a physician who, by virtue of his specialized training and skills, is also able to operate. He is, ideally, a physiologist who not only has the ability to remove a gall bladder but also to understand the disease process which eventually brought the patient to surgery.

The formal training of a surgeon is long and arduous. Following graduation from medical school he has to go through five to seven years of special training. During this time under close supervision he will have done hundreds of operations of gradually increasing complexity, and will in addition have spent many hours in learning the methods of pre and postoperative care. It is of vital importance that the surgeon comes to accept the fact that doing operations, i.e. achieving greater technical expertise, must be balanced against the experience that comes with the understanding of disease processes, and against learning what is called, for lack of a better term, good judgment. Learning when to operate as well as how to operate is a slow process at best and probably one that never ceases.

By the end of this century the development might be seen of some form of ultrasonic jet, which would divide the tissues at the same time as it sealed the small blood vessels, as a replacement for the scalpel. New techniques of theater sterilization will almost very probably have removed the scenario of gowns, gloves and masks. The careful electronic monitoring of the patient and the automatic replacement of blood and fluid and balancing of various salts and hormones will prevent surgical shock during operations. One thing is certain, and that is that a hundred years from now surgeon and patient alike will feel about our own present operating rooms much as we, smug in our own 'modern' surgical environments, look back upon the operating rooms of 1881 as merely a crude beginning.

15 Drugs in Modern Medicine

233 An early 17th century print showing the mixing of medicinal balms and ointments. Ancient folk medicine, which used plant remedies arrived at by chance or chosen on the grounds of some superficially apparent association with the ailment they were to treat, was the ancestor of today's scientific pharmaceutical industry. Some of these remedies continue in use alongside the drugs derived from fungi, the products of the synthetic chemical industry, human and animal hormones, and the refined variants produced by the molecular chemist. Among them are digitalis, a derivative of the common foxglove, important in the treatment of rhythm disturbances of the heart, and vincristine, an extract of the garden periwinkle plant, still among the range of drugs which doctors use in combination against leukemia (see illustrations 67 and 93).

234 Sir Alexander Fleming (1881-1955) whose discovery of the antibiotic properties of the mold *Penicillium notatum* gave the world penicillin in what may truly be called one of man's greatest triumphs in the treatment of infectious disease. He shared his Nobel Prize with Sir Howard Florey and Sir Ernest Chain who realized the potential of Fleming's discovery and translated it into a therapeutic reality. In this photograph Fleming can be seen holding in his hands the culture plate shown in the next illustration.

235 A historic photograph with caption in the hand of Alexander Fleming reading 'Print of the culture plate which started the work on Penicillin (25 years old and rather dried up) AF'. The lethal effect of material diffusing from the mold (large white colonies on left) on the much smaller colonies of staphylococci (right of plate) is clearly visible. The discovery occurred as a result of the

The history of therapeutics is fascinating and exciting. Since prehistoric times man has used drugs to alleviate the pain, anxiety and discomfort of disease. The most primitive approach is represented by folk remedies. These concoctions were based on trial and error, good luck or a philosophical or magical concept. Ancient Egyptian physicians developed many such remedies, some of which are still used today. In the famous Ebers Papyrus there are directions for compounding over 800 prescriptions which include some effective cathartics. For each folk remedy that was beneficial, there were hundreds whose efficacy relied upon the suggestibility of the patient (and his doctor).

Remedies were designated according to the physical appearance of the drug, the characteristics of the plant from which it was derived or the place where the plant grew. Paracelsus believed that a breast-shaped plant would help diseases of the breast and that yellow substances were beneficial in jaundice. The willow tree—a source of salicylate (the active constituent of aspirin)—was originally suspected to be effective for arthritis because willows thrive in damp, marshy land. Dampness was—and sometimes still is—thought to cause rheumatism. It was much later that the true reason for the efficacy of salicylate was realized. Many important discoveries were made fortuitously: for example opium, which is still harvested from oriental poppy pods in the manner originally described by the Greek physician Dioscorides, was discovered many centuries ago to be an effective analgesic and tranquilizer.

Individual doctors improved on this approach by wedding the idea of a folk remedy to their own research and analysis. Thus William Withering, an 18th-century English physician,

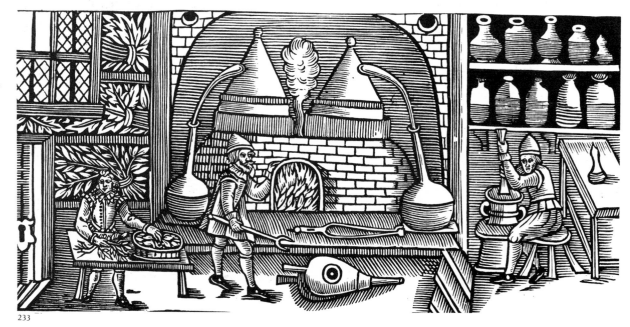

233

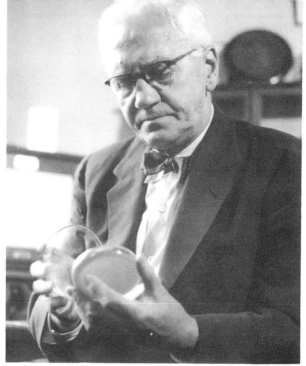

234

Rubrum, the first sulfonamide, was one of the many aniline dyes being tested in 1932. This chemical contains the sulfonamide nucleus which is effective against streptococcal infections, bacillary dysentery, meningitis, puerperal fever and some types of blood poisoning.

The sulfonamide molecule is also the basis of three other chemically related groups of drugs—the sulfones, which are used to treat leprosy, the sulfonylureas, a group of drugs that has enabled many diabetics to avoid insulin, and the thiazide diuretics—the first diuretics to be administered as tablets, rather than by injection.

The next chapter in the story of chemotherapy was another fortuitous discovery. Penicillin was discovered by Alexander Fleming in 1929 as a result of the accidental contamination of a culture plate with the mold penicillium. In 1940 Chain and Florey isolated penicillin as the active

chance contamination of this culture plate by the penicillin mold. The lid had accidentally slipped off during a course of experiments on the staphylococcus germ which Fleming was conducting at St Mary's Hospital in London in September 1928. Fleming later wrote: 'There are thousands of different molds and there are thousands of different bacteria and that chance put that mold in the right place at the right time was like winning the Irish Sweep'. It needed Fleming's alertness and observation to be added to this chance for him to notice the effect the fungus was having on the germs instead of just throwing the plate away as a spoiled experiment.

pursued with great skill and imagination an old wives' remedy from Shropshire. As a competent botanist he realized that not all the many ingredients of this remedy for dropsy were active and that the source of the cure was the foxglove plant. Withering laid the basis for the modern treatment of heart failure with digitalis. His classic monograph on the foxglove cannot be improved on today for its wise advice to the physician using digitalis.

There are many important therapeutic developments that could be mentioned but in a limited space it is impossible to discuss them all. This chapter confines itself to some of the more striking, fortuitous and interesting major advances that have been made. The examples illustrate general principles which apply to many other drugs.

The first effective chemotherapeutic agent was discovered in 1630 when the cinchona bark from Peru was used by the Jesuits in the treatment of malaria. The active ingredient, quinine, was later isolated by two French organic chemists, Canestou and Pelletier. Quinine is still useful today for malignant cerebral malaria. This discovery was followed by the synthesis of a whole series of antimalarials. These proved very valuable to armies fighting in the East in World War II.

It was 300 years before the next discovery came about, at the hands of Paul Ehrlich, the father of modern medicinal chemistry, who synthesized the first organic arsenical, arsphenamine. This is an effective treatment for syphilis. Prior to this all drugs were extracted from plants.

The next major discovery, which placed another important series of drugs in the hands of the doctor, also arose purely by chance as a spin-off of the synthetic dye industry. Prontosil

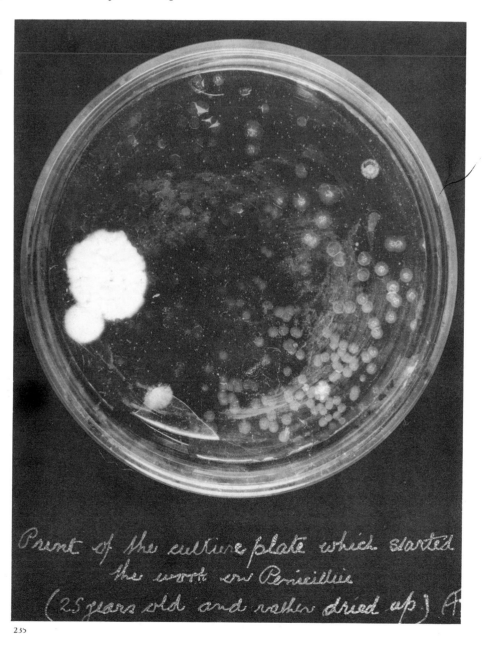

Print of the culture plate which started the work on Penicillin (25 years old and rather dried up) A

235

constituent of the mold penicillium. This led to the award of the Nobel Prize to all three men in 1945. This antibiotic was soon followed by others. In 1943, the antibiotic streptomycin was isolated from a strain of a soil fungus, *Streptomyces griseus*. Streptomycin is still used in the treatment of tuberculosis. This was the first of a number of antibiotics which followed the joint efforts of research workers and pharmaceutical companies. Chloramphenicol, **an** antibiotic that is active against many more infections than penicillin or streptomycin, was the first of the broad spectrum' antibiotics. It was followed in 1952 by the tetracyclines, so named because their chemical structure is based on four attached cyclic benzene rings.

The first, chlortetracycline, appeared in 1948 and was followed by oxytetracycline and tetracycline. Later members of the family were demethylchlortetracycline, which has a longer duration of action and is given twice daily, and doxycycline (released in 1966). This tetracycline, unlike the others, can be used in patients with kidney failure.

The tetracyclines and chloramphenicol were the first of many broad spectrum antibiotics. For some time many felt that the panacea for every

infection had been found. It was several years before the disadvantages and problems associated with the 'blind' prescribing of antibiotics became apparent. The first such discovery was in 1962, when it was found that chloramphenicol caused permanent damage to the bone marrow. Although this complication is uncommon (one case in 40,000) it is always serious. Nowadays, chloramphenicol is only recommended for serious infections such as septicemia and meningitis.

Meanwhile, the synthetic chemists were developing new broad spectrum penicillins. The first of these was ampicillin, which was followed by amoxycillin. In the last few years several orally active broad spectrum penicillins, effective against resistant organisms, have been synthesized.

Another group of broad spectrum antibiotics, the cephalosporins, were originally isolated from a sewage outlet on the coast of Sardinia. New members are being synthesized each year.

In all these examples the pharmaceutical chemist has isolated chemicals either from plant sources or fungi or as a by-product of the chemical industry. Another source of drugs is the body itself. The story of the discovery of the corticosteroid hormones produced by the adrenal glands is related in chapter 3. The

236

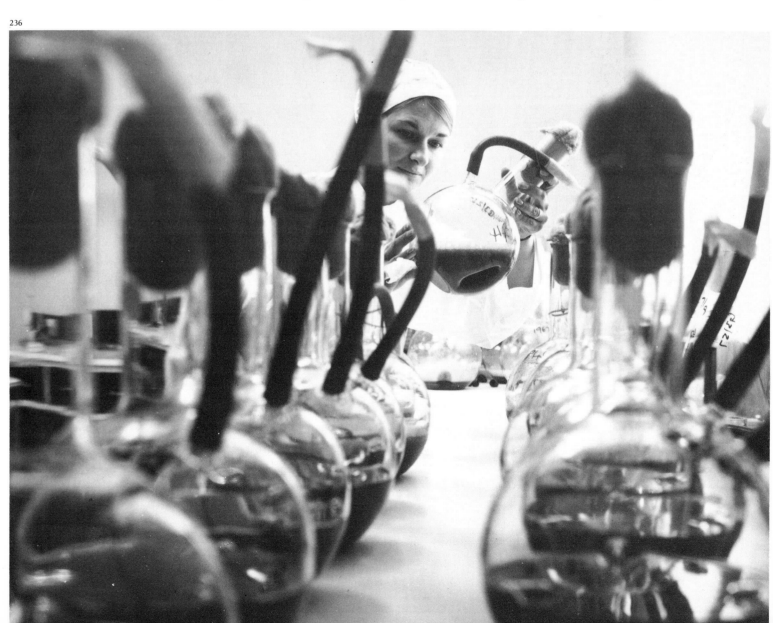

organic chemist has manipulated the steroid molecule to synthesize many potent new steroids. These have fewer side-effects than the natural hormone (hydrocortisone) and have much more anti-inflammatory effect. The contraceptive pill is another synthetic hormone with which most people are familiar.

The story of the discovery of general and local anesthesia, already described in chapter 14, is another important part of the history of therapeutics.

Vaccines have abolished diseases like diphtheria and small pox. Their origin and development has been considered in chapter 1.

Any discussion of the advancing history of therapeutics would be incomplete without a reference to the placebo phenomenon. The word placebo implies to many people a make-believe medicine, one devoid of effect other than that achieved by suggestion. In ancient times, most of the popular medicaments were probably placebos, capable of little that was either good or bad. Such remedies as unicorn's horn, moss from the skull of a hanged criminal, eunuch fat and dried mummy, despite their popularity, almost certainly capitalized solely on the desire of most patients to be well. Patients who ingested such ancient medications were lucky if they were not harmed by them.

Even in the 18th and 19th centuries much of what the medical profession did in the way of therapy depended on the credulity of both doctor and patient, and on the healing powers of time. There was little reason for rejoicing, for example, around the turn of the 19th century, over the attempts of European physicians to improve on the old advice of Pliny that a mouse be eaten once a month to prevent toothache. A Dr Gerbi in Pisa advised crushing a worm between the thumb and forefinger of the right hand before touching the aching tooth. A Weimar court physician varied the treatment by substituting the more esthetic ladybird for the worm, and an official commission confirmed the immediate relief of toothache by this method in two-thirds of patients. An English paper pointed the way to even greater success: 'Fill your mouth with milk and shake it until it becomes butter.'

It is only since the advent of modern medicine's many powerful drugs that physicians have begun to study systematically the symbolic power for good and harm that resides in the act of prescribing pills or injections. Before 1945 the word 'placebo' had never appeared in the title of a medical article, and was not even listed in the main indexing services for medical literature. In the decades since, however, scores of articles have been published in all parts of the world, either testifying to the power of the placebo or attempting to explain it.

As one might expect from the psychological

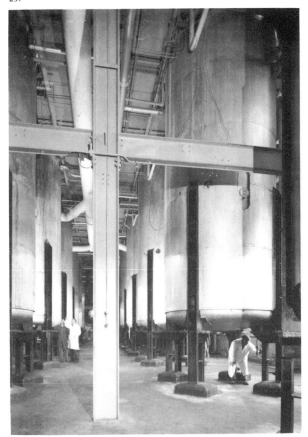

component of the placebo effect, the field of mental illness is well represented in the literature on the placebo. Anxiety, tension, psychoneurosis, melancholia, psychosomatic illness, behavior disorders in children, schizophrenia—all have been reported to respond to inert medication. Some of the 'responses' have been in the direction of worsening, but more often improvement has occurred. Indeed, some psychiatrists have questioned how much of 'specific' psychotherapy—even when it is of a highly formalized and theoretically grounded type—is not just an elaborate way of capitalizing on the placebo phenomenon.

One of the most dramatic examples of the indestructibility of the placebo effect was a study performed at Johns Hopkins a few years ago. Fifteen neurotic outpatients were asked to take sugar pills, with the instructions: 'Do you know what a sugar pill is? A sugar pill is a pill with no medicine in it at all. I think this pill will help you as it has so many others. Are you willing to try this pill?'

All but one took the placebos, and of these everyone reported improvement, a change concurred in by their doctors. Eight of the patients said they accepted the fact that the pills were sugar, while six thought the tablets really contained active drug (three of these reported 'side reactions' from the pills). Four patients said the pills were the most effective ever prescribed for them, and five wanted the placebos to be continued; attribution of improvement was

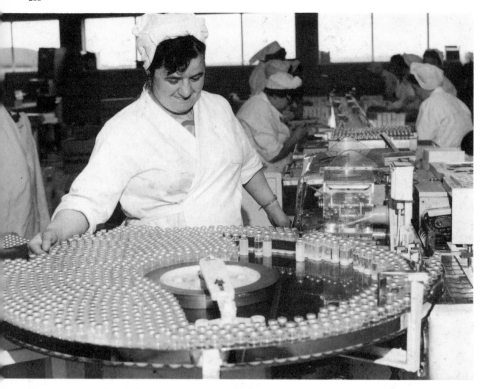

secretion of gastric juice. The same investigators were able to prevent vomiting from ipecac in a pregnant woman by assuring her that this nauseating drug would *relieve* the excessive vomiting from which she suffered.

The placebo also has the capacity for producing harm. While most 'side-effects' after placebo are subjective—nausea, thirst, headache, dizziness, sleepiness, insomnia, fatigue, depression, numbness, difficulty in concentrating, hallucinations, feelings of cold or warmth, itching and the like—some side-effects are of the kind verifiable by the observer. These include vomiting, tremor, fast heart beat, diarrhea, changes in blood pressure, pallor, skin rashes (sometimes of alarming severity), hives, unsteadiness of gait, and swelling. In one study, a patient who had travelled to Miami on holiday called his physician to complain that his medicine had so weakened him as to cause a near-drowning in the surf; a hasty check of the records showed the patient to be on placebos.

One of the questions bedevilling students of the placebo since the early 1950s is the relation between personality and response. Are there people who will predictably reap benefit from an inert pill, and others who tend to react negatively to all maneuvers with therapeutic intent?

In the first study of this question, Professor Lasagna and his colleagues analyzed the characteristics of patients whose post-operative pain responded consistently to placebos, and of patients whose pain never responded. Most fell

238, 239 From apparently crude beginnings emerges a pure, sterile, life-saving substance, insulin. The isolation of pure insulin by Sir Frederick Banting and Charles H. Best in 1921, which completely transformed the outlook for diabetics, previously doomed to an early death, is described in chapter 3. Today animal pancreases are collected from slaughterhouses to provide the raw material (239) for the production process, the other end of which is seen in 238, where machinery is being used for the counting and packing of insulin ampoules ready for use by diabetic patients.

unrelated to whether the patients thought the pills to be placebos or not. (In Czechoslovakia a few years ago, a patient was reported to be 'addicted' to placebos, and suffered dreadfully when the placebos were withheld!)

Psychiatric illness is not, however, the only medical field in which the placebo has been shown to have an impact. Almost any type of pain may respond—pain after surgery, pain during or after childbirth, angina pectoris, dental pain, and the distress of cancer. In the treatment of 150 patients with headaches due to tension, the common cold, sinusitis, premenstrual tension or eyestrain, one investigator found that placebos relieved pain completely in 43 per cent of cases, and partially in another 31 per cent; others have come to similar conclusions.

Cough, insomnia, seasickness, chronic bronchitis and the common cold may all yield to the placebo. Patients with osteoarthritis and rheumatoid arthritis have shown both subjective and objective improvement. Peptic ulcer, gastritis, and dyspepsia have in some studies shown amelioration after placebo in 92 per cent of patients, a showing so impressive that certain gastroenterologists have speculated on whether most of the hundreds of 'treatments' for ulcer are not merely placebo remedies.

Nor is it only subjective complaints that respond to placebo; variables that are extremely 'objective'—such as blood pressure and sputum production—have also displayed change. In the classic series of Cornell studies on the subject Tom, who had a large gastric fistula, placebos and manipulation of the emotional situation produced impressive changes in the appearance and movement of the stomach, and in the

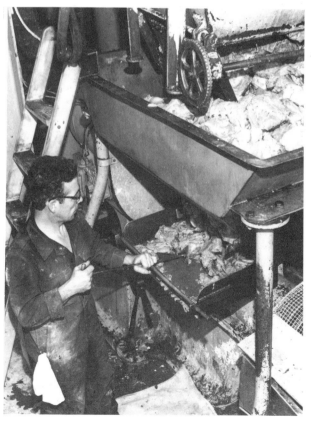

between the extremes, sometimes obtaining relief, sometimes not. Neither age nor sex seemed important determinants of placebo reactivity. Women were no more likely to respond than men, and the 'reactors' ranged in age from 35 to 64 (although placebo reactors tended to be older). I.Q. scores of reactors and non-reactors were similar. Where differences did appear was in the psychological test results; reactors tended to be more anxious and less hostile, voluble and weepy on interview. They also had a more positive attitude toward hospitals and medical personnel and were considered more co-operative by the nurses.

Since that time a number of other investigators have analyzed the same problem, with contradictory results. In one camp fall the researchers who claim that the whole thing is a matter of chance—that there is no predisposition to respond to placebos. (This seems as reasonable as saying that one person is just as easy to hypnotize, or sell insurance to, as the next one.) In another camp are those inclined to find some common characteristics running through all placebo reactors, and whose studies have to some degree substantiated the earliest experiments. Most reasonable, probably, is the premise that there is no constellation of traits that will enable one neatly to pigeonhole people as 'reactors' or 'non-reactors'. Most of us are suggestible to some degree, and the likelihood of responding to placebos, and the nature of the response, will be determined to a great extent by the setting, the symptom being treated, and the specific medical figures involved, as well as by the personalities, past experiences, anticipations and fears of the subjects.

Part of the difficulty in teasing out psychological contributions to the placebo phenomenon lies in the dual nature of the effect. Only part of placebo 'success' or 'toxicity' is due to suggestibility—the rest is attributable to spontaneous improvement or deterioration, or unrelated phenomena that are temporally but not causally related to placebo-taking.

Years ago, for example, hospitalized patients awaiting elective surgery at the Massachusetts General Hospital were given a placebo solution to prevent insomnia. Over two-thirds of them fell asleep in less than an hour, but the same 'success rate' was observed in another group of patients who received nothing of any kind! In other words, the supposedly stressful situation was not especially bothersome for the majority of subjects—at least in regard to falling asleep. A psychological study of the 'reactors' in this study could hardly have shed light on personality-placebo relationships.

This second component also accounts for some of the other effects attributed to placebos in therapeutic situations. Hospitalization per se

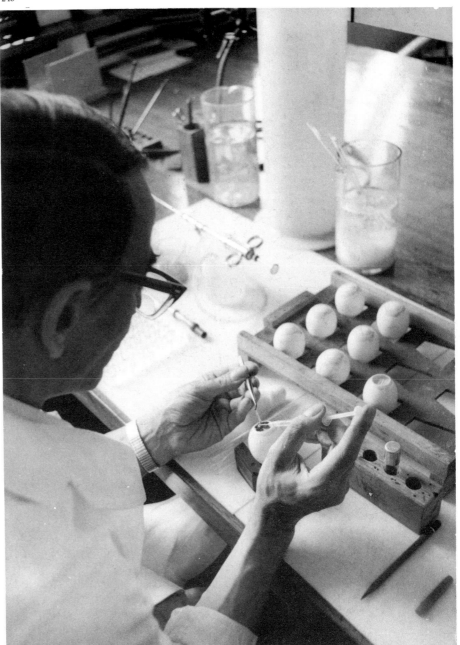

can cause a drop in blood pressure. Certain diseases, like serious depression, are intrinsically cyclic phenomena; many ailments will run their course whether treatment is provided or not.

Spontaneous change is probably the likeliest explanation for such reported placebo cure rates as 83 per cent in scalp ringworm, or the 50 to 75 per cent clearing of pathogenic organisms from the throats of children given placebos. Similarly, while certain 'toxic' reactions to placebos may be psychogenic, others may represent simply the rash or headache that was coming on anyway at the time the placebo was taken. (Conceivably, however, an occasional patient may also be sensitive to some trace substance or coloring matter in the placebo pill.)

In therapy, placebos as such are not extensively used, although a good many remedies prescribed by physicians over the years have been in essence placebos. The indications for placebos are few

240 The production of antiviral vaccines involves the culture of attenuated forms of the virus in living tissues. In this photograph chicken embryos are being inoculated with an influenza virus at the World Influenza Centre in London. Thanks to the extreme mutability of the influenza viruses, large-scale immunization is not practical or economic, and periodic epidemics of varying intensity continue to take their toll of deaths. Inoculation programs on a limited scale continue for research purposes.

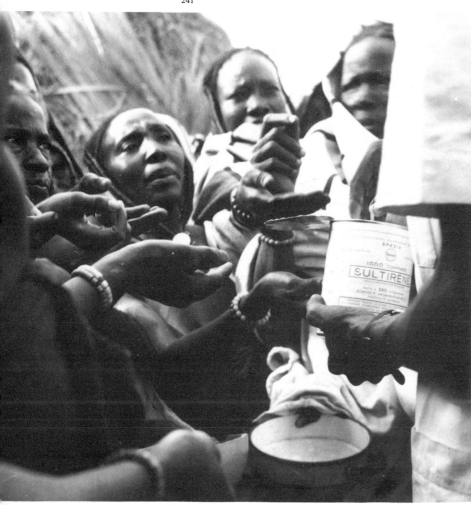

After discharge, he finds that he cannot get a good night's sleep without barbiturates. It is often difficult to wean these individuals off what they regard as an essential prerequisite for a proper night's rest.

Control over medicaments started in Europe long before food and drug legislation in the United States. The British Food and Drug Act of 1872 was followed in 1906 by the first bill in the U.S.A. The world was painfully reminded of the hazards of drugs by the sulfanilamide disaster, when 107 people, many of them children, were fatally poisoned by the solvent in which the miraculous new sulfonamide was dissolved. Although it had been checked for appearance, flavor and fragrance, its safety had not been tested. Twenty-five years later, the disaster recurred with the sedative thalidomide, which produced pathetically deformed babies in women who had taken it during early pregnancy. These events increased the demand for evidence of safety and efficacy.

Although initial discoveries are often made in small laboratories or university departments, further development of drugs is taken on primarily by the pharmaceutical industry. This reflects the enormous complexity of technical development and the numbers of personnel and the large amounts of money required to exploit and market a new drug. Potential new drugs are synthesized by organic chemists, either on the basis of chemical theory, or in an attempt to modify a molecule found empirically to be useful in treating human disease. These new chemicals are then subjected to evaluation in animals, attempting to assess the potential for desirable pharmacological activity as well as the potential for harm. In this evaluation we are limited by the availability and validity of animal models of human disease. Antibacterial drugs can be tested against the bugs we wish to kill. But how does one mimic schizophrenia in an animal? Animal tumors exist, but reliance in the laboratory is on transplanted tumors whose relationship to human cancer is questionable. If the laboratory investigations in regard to activity and toxicity are promising, and it appears that trial in man is justified, the drug is administered cautiously either to healthy volunteers or to volunteer patients suffering from the disease or symptom in question.

These early studies are really for the purpose of assessing what dosage range may be tried in later clinical trials, and what sorts of side-effects are likely to be seen in patients who receive the drug in such trials. These initial studies are often combined with chemical analysis of blood, urine, or other tissue fluids to study the absorption, distribution, biotransformation and excretion of the chemical.

The next step is to give the drug to patients.

241 The chemical attack on the microorganism, the beginning of the anti-microbial era, was heralded by the development of the sulfonamide series of drugs, originally a by-product of the aniline dye industry. The first of these, the dye Prontosil Rubrum, was used by Gerhard Domagk in 1932. Although largely superseded by the antibiotics, sulfonamides are still very valuable in the treatment of certain infections. Meningitis is one of these. When used on a wide scale, the drug may arrest the spread of an epidemic through a population. Niger is one of five countries between latitudes 8 and 16 North (the others are Sudan, Northern Nigeria, Chad and Upper Volta) that form the 'meningitis belt'. In the period since 1960 there have been approximately 40,000 cases and 3,000 deaths per annum in this region alone. The picture shows the distribution of sulfonamides to mothers in a village in Niger.

and consist primarily of situations where a physician needs to tide over a patient who expects medication while awaiting the results of diagnostic tests or where a doctor needs to 'pacify' a patient who demands drugs but doesn't need them.

Newspapers, radio and television have highlighted the tragic results of addiction to 'hard drugs' such as heroin and cocaine. In the U.K. this problem has not reached the proportions it has attained in the U.S.A. The introduction of addiction clinics run by trained psychiatrists was a major advance. Only doctors who have received special training in the addiction field can now prescribe narcotics to addicts in the U.K. Addicts sometimes resort to 'mainlining'—the injection into a vein of a solution of a variety of crushed drugs including barbiturate tablets. The provision of disposable syringes by addiction clinics has reduced the mortality from septicemia—a cause of death in addicts using an unsterile syringe for self-administration.

A more common type of addiction in general practice concerns the patient who has required barbiturate sleeping tablets for 20 to 30 years. These may have been prescribed originally as a short term measure for insomnia, perhaps during a stay for treatment in a noisy hospital ward.

Clinical trials compare a new compound either with an established drug or with a dummy tablet. To avoid any bias in the assessment of drug effects, patients must be treated under 'double-blind' conditions: the active and the dummy tablets or capsules, identical in appearance, are prepared by the pharmacy so that the results of the trial are not biased either by the patient's preference or by the doctor's preconceived ideas. Neither the patient nor the doctor supervising the trial knows which medicament is the drug and which is the dummy. At the completion of the trial the 'code' held by the pharmacy is broken and the results assessed.

Eventually, the available information on the drug, ranging from chemistry, method of manufacture, and criteria for purity down to clinical trials and reports of toxicity, are scrutinized by a national regulatory body, and a decision made as to whether the data allow marketing, or whether further studies are required to help decide about the drug's future. Ultimately, the true worth of the drug has to be measured after marketing by its use under naturalistic conditions by physicians of varying competence in different patient populations suffering from a variety of ailments often treated simultaneously with a number of other drugs. Because of this fact, it is only possible in the roughest way to anticipate the actual utility and safety of a drug on the basis of pre-marketing studies. Drugs are often recognized to have new uses only years after their introduction for their original purpose. A recent example has been the unexpected finding that amantadine, a drug originally developed as an anti-viral agent against influenzal infection, was of value in the treatment of Parkinsonism. Serious drug toxicity may be recognized several years after a drug has been introduced. Recent examples include the ocular and cutaneous side-effects of the beta blocking drug practolol, and the serious and sometimes fatal pseudomembranous colitis that is associated with the antibiotics lincomycin and clindamycin.

Regulations controlling the manufacture and evaluation of drugs have reduced the likelihood of another thalidomide disaster but legislation has produced its own problems. Many compounds that are rejected in animal tests might not produce the same toxic effects in man. For example, had penicillin been subjected to animal studies, it might never have reached man, since it causes death in guinea pigs. The inevitable result of legislation controlling drug development from early synthesis to introduction is an increased cost and duration of drug development, and hence a slowing down of investigation of new preparations.

A recent financial catastrophe followed the

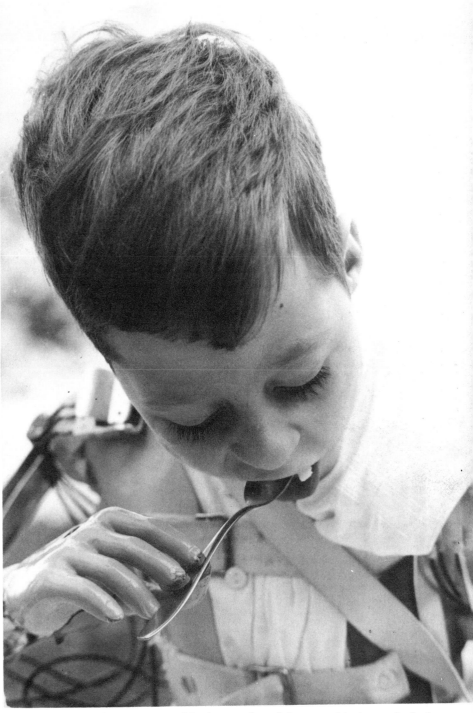

testing of a new beta receptor blocker, Tolamolol. After several million pounds had been spent by the manufacturer, this drug was given to animals at many times the normal human dose at the request of the American Food and Drug Administration (the F.D.A.) After many months of administration the animals developed breast tumors. When the results of these toxicity tests were known the manufacturer decided not to market the drug.

Another important problem is the cost of manufacturing small quantities of drugs used for rare conditions. The expenditure involved in marketing such compounds far outweighs the possible economic return. Most multinational companies provide these drugs as part of their

242 This photograph of a 5-year-old German boy learning to eat with a pneumatically-operated prosthetic arm is a poignant reminder of the thalidomide tragedy. Large numbers of otherwise normal children were born with pathetic limb deformities as a result of the tranquilizing drug thalidomide having been prescribed for their mothers during pregnancy between 1958 and 1961. This was an extreme example of the kind of disaster which procedures for scrutinizing and testing new drugs are designed to prevent. Disasters of this sort are extremely rare. They have to be seen against the considerable benefits of drugs and the enormous investment required to bring a new drug to the patient.

243 The ingenuity of the chemist and the drive of the pharmaceutical industry have created a vast profusion of drugs and medications, many valuable and some life-saving. However, there is considerable reduplication of these preparations. There are many variants of the same basic preparation with minor differences in formulation and action. An indication of the perils of polypharmacy is given by the mound of drugs shown in this photograph, all of which were taken by one patient at one time or another for dyspepsia. Even more worrying is the multitude of potent and active preparations prescribed for and hoarded by elderly people over years of chronic ill-health. The 20th century benefits introduced by the pharmaceutical industry have placed new responsibilities on the prescribing doctor. He must know a great deal to make his way through the unnecessary and confusing plethora of alternative products. This is necessary to reduce prescribing costs, to avoid the hazards of drug interaction, and to reduce the danger of mistakes by the patient.

service to medicine. This fact should be remembered when pharmaceutical companies are criticized for making vast profits. Much of the so-called 'excess profit' is spent on research for new drugs.

The effects of the drug may also be complicated by other medication, prescribed or self-administered, and by disease other than that for which the drug in question is given. Patients receiving drugs that sensitize the skin may develop rashes when exposed to sunlight. This sometimes happens with chlorpromazine, a drug used in the treatment of schizophrenia. Patients treated with long-term corticosteroids are more susceptible to infections. Drugs interact with one another in strange and unpredictable ways. They may potentiate or antagonize each other's good or undesirable effects. Some of these interactions are put to therapeutic use, for example, probenecid is given to delay the urinary excretion of penicillin. An example of drug interaction is the deleterious effect of certain cough linctuses and nasal decongestants on the blood pressure of patients with hypertension. Patients being treated for high blood pressure have to be warned about the effect of proprietary nasal

decongestants purchased from the chemist to counteract nasal stuffiness. This is a common side-effect of many blood pressure lowering drugs, for example guanethidine and bethanidine. Most nasal decongestants contain adrenaline-like amines, such as ephedrine, which clear the nose by constricting the blood vessels but in so doing cause a rise in general blood pressure.

Some blood pressure lowering drugs (such as methyldopa and clonidine) can cause depression. Sometimes, the depression is treated with tricyclic antidepressants (e.g. imipramine, amitriptyline, nortriptyline) which actually reverse the blood pressure lowering effects of the original drugs. The sensible physician stops the drug causing depression and chooses a suitable alternative, of which there are many.

There is an enormous proliferation of drugs. Thousands of single and combined preparations are available to treat any and all complaints. Debate rages between the medical and pharmaceutical professions about the need for many of these products. One wonders how much harm is done by the confusion generated by this abundance of medication and the similarity of

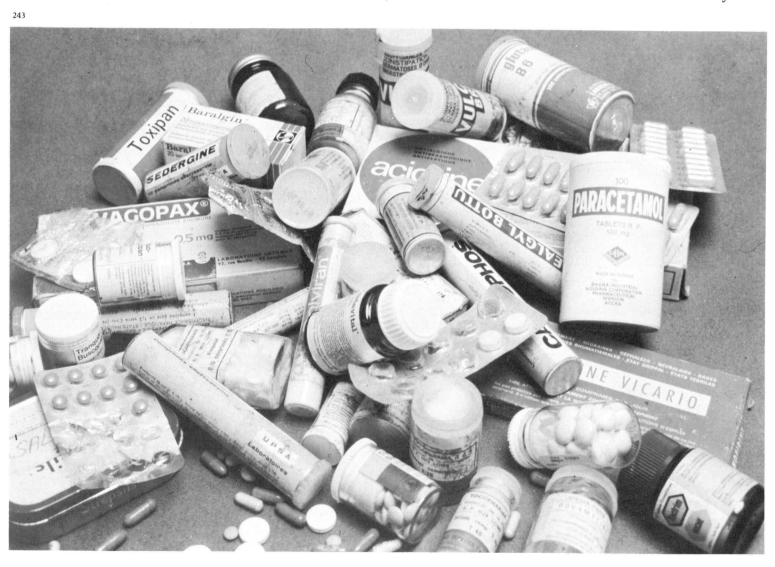

drug names. This causes confusion and may be dangerous, since drugs with similar names may have very different effects. The diseases caused by doctors and their therapy even have their own name. They are called iatrogenic diseases. The ready availability of potent therapy has increased the need for the prescriber to know and use his drugs only when indicated, in the smallest effective dose and for the shortest necessary time.

Errors can occur during manufacture, pharmacists can make mistakes, nurses can by accident administer the wrong drug or give an incorrect dose. We are increasingly aware of the difficulty patients have in carefully following directions. For this reason, drug regimes should be kept as simple as possible and adequate instruction of patients is vital. Patients receiving steroids, anticoagulants and other long term therapy are often supplied with a card, giving the name of the drug, the dose and frequency, and the reason why it is taken. This idea has been adopted by many general practitioners who provide written instructions to the patient in order to reduce the likelihood of errors when the preparation is taken or the prescription is renewed. Mistakes over medication are very common in elderly patients and some drugs can themselves aggravate this confusion. The good doctor appreciates the need for repeated explanation about disease and its treatment. The actions of each drug must be explained in lay terms that can easily be understood. Changes in drugs or their dosage are best made gradually, one drug being altered at each visit. Several visits permit the instructions to be repeated and remembered. Changes should be made gently to reduce the risk of side-effects, for example the excessive fall in blood pressure or blood sugar that may follow sudden increases in the dosage of potent antihypertensive or antidiabetic agents.

Some patients take their drugs less often than prescribed; others take more than the recommended dose, which may lead to drug toxicity. We have gone a long way towards the goal of an adequately informed population, but much remains to be done in the area of education of the patient before the full potential of many remedies can be realized.

Drugs have important economic aspects. The burden to society from disease and disability is great, and effective medicaments can, by saving lives or preventing loss of time from work, more than repay society for the costs of development and of purchase by the consumer. The cost of drugs is important also to the creative manufacturer, since his research and development expenditures depend on the income from his marketed products. Patent protection allows an innovative manufacturer a certain number of years from which to profit from his

ingenuity, but there is increasing resistance on the part of private third party payment groups and of national health schemes to pay what are deemed excessively high prices.

Another problem arises when patents expire, and physicians can prescribe drugs in so-called generic form, i.e. where the identical chemical is made by several different manufacturers. Traditionally, medical students have been taught that these different versions are interchangeable, but recent experience shows clearly that chemical identity may not be the same as 'bioavailability', a term used to indicate the actual availability of the drug for performing its task in the body. Some preparations, for example, while adequate in terms of ingredient content, are not absorbed properly from the gastro-intestinal tract and are therefore unavailable for achieving the desired results. For some ailments, failure of performance of this kind may be trivial, but for other diseases the result of sub-par performance may be catastrophic. The recent outbreak of phenytoin toxicity (phenytoin is an anti-convulsant) in Australia was caused by a change in the excipient contained in the medication. The former excipient, supposedly the inactive vehicle for the drug, had actually interfered with its absorption. This change was not publicized and it took some time before the altered bioavailability was recognized as being reponsible for the problem. Other drugs which can differ in their bioavailability are digoxin, ampicillin and the tetracyclines. New tests are now being developed to ensure minimum guaranteed bioavailability.

Most of the above has dealt with so-called ethical drugs, i.e. those requiring a prescription from a doctor. But a good many drugs are bought by the consumer 'over the counter', i.e. as part of the process of self-diagnosis and self-treatment. Since much of the population is afflicted with transient and trivial complaints, it is desirable for the public to engage in such self-diagnosis and self-treatment if it is done properly. There is little evidence that most of the headache remedies, cough suppressants, etc. consumed by the public produce harm, and many consumers are satisfied with their performance. On the other hand, certain serious situations do arise from abuse of over-the-counter remedies. One example is the so-called syndrome of analgesic nephropathy, wherein some individuals who have consumed large quantities of analgesic tablets or powders over a period of years end up with serious and sometimes fatal kidney disease. Another example of abuse is the chronic taking of medication that masks a disease that is not trivial or self-limited, but rather a serious ailment urgently requiring medical attention. The challenge to the medical profession and to the public is to devise ways for self-diagnosis and

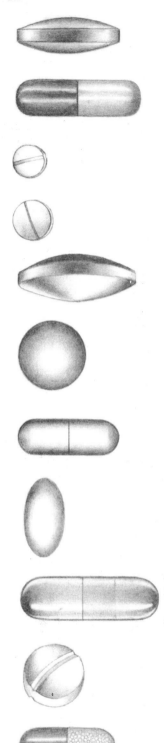

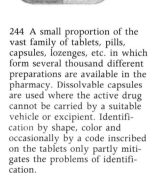

244 A small proportion of the vast family of tablets, pills, capsules, lozenges, etc. in which form several thousand different preparations are available in the pharmacy. Dissolvable capsules are used where the active drug cannot be carried by a suitable vehicle or excipient. Identification by shape, color and occasionally by a code inscribed on the tablets only partly mitigates the problems of identification.

self-medication to be exhibited so that public welfare is maximized.

For many types of disease, the available therapy is established and reasonably well documented as to its benefits, even though few *cures* are available through drugs. In the field of infectious disease serious bacterial infections, as well as infections by many fungi, can be dramatically modified or even eliminated by the use of drugs. Other infectious diseases can be prevented by the timely administration of vaccines. On the other hand, our ability to modify virus infections is still primitive. Digitalis, diuretics, and antihypertensive drugs are useful in the management of various forms of cardiovascular disease, but it is unclear whether any medicine that we have available at the moment definitely affects fundamentally the course of coronary artery disease or a stroke once it has occurred. In the field of cancer, we can now modify dramatically or even cure certain leukemias and lymphomas (such as Hodgkin's disease), but the physician is therapeutically impoverished when it comes to treating 'solid' tumors (such as cancer of the lung) which constitute the bulk of malignant cancers.

Useful drugs are available for treating pain, insomnia, schizophrenia and certain depressions, yet our ability really to normalize most patients with serious mental ailments is limited. The drugs available for treating arthritis, while useful, all have serious limitations in terms of both efficacy and safety.

In conclusion, drugs not only have a past and a present, but a future as well. We have learned much over the centuries in regard to evaluating remedies and to making them available for mankind. We are still a long way, however, from solving most of the problems of serious disease. Indeed, even for such minor ailments as the common cold, our ability to modify the course of disease is limited. While it would seem attractive to attack disease at its source and diminish our reliance on drugs, it seems more realistic for the moment to continue to search for new and better medicaments. Simultaneously, we must continue to do research on the causes of disease and on the mechanisms involved in the production of disorders of mind and body. Eventually, if our wisdom becomes great enough, we will be able to use drugs to modify disease in a way that is much more predictable and efficient than the methods presently available.

Glossary

Amines These simple but important nitrogen-containing compounds occupy a central role in human biology. They play an integral part in nervous transmission, both inside and outside the brain. Disturbance of amine metabolism may be responsible for functions as widely varying as disorders of mood and changes in blood pressure.

Amino acid The nitrogen-containing 'unit' chemical compounds which link to form proteins. The 'essential' ten amino acids cannot be synthesized in the body and have to be supplied in the diet. Deficiency of these leads to impairment of development and growth.

Amnesia Loss of memory which characterizes many neuro-psychiatric disorders. It also occurs after accidents involving the brain, in certain vitamin B deficiency states, and in the ageing of the central nervous system.

Amniotic The developing fetus within the maternal womb is supported and protected by a collection of clear fluid, the amniotic fluid, which is contained within the amniotic sac. Cells shed by the fetus, its secretions and excretions accumulate within the amniotic fluid. This may be drawn off by careful tapping (amniocentesis) and examined for chemical and microscopic clues indicating disease or disturbance of development of the fetus.

Anabolic Relating to anabolism, the process of building up of body structures which is promoted by the influence of certain hormones (e.g. insulin, testosterone, growth hormone) on nutrient intake. Catabolism is the reverse process of tissue or body breakdown which occurs in many infective diseases, in thyroid overactivity or in insulin lack (diabetes mellitus).

Anemia The commonest of blood diseases from which the human being suffers, anemia, occurs when the hemoglobin of the blood is inadequate. It may have many causes, such as dietary deficiency of iron, continued slow blood loss, and failure of the bone marrow to manufacture red cells.

Aneurism A localized 'ballooning' of a blood vessel, usually an artery, the diseased wall of which has slowly stretched in response to the pressure within. Modern surgery can excise and replace these weakened segments.

Angiography It is often valuable to pick out the blood supply to an organ to detect a major blockage or other signs of disease. This is normally achieved by radiological means (*see* Arteriography) but may also be carried out by passing specific, harmless dyestuffs through vessels and photographing them in passage. The regional circulation having been defined in this way, diagnosis may be improved or repair operations planned.

Anoxic Deprivation of tissues or organs of oxygen is known as anoxia. This may be due to abnormally low concentrations of oxygen in an artificial atmosphere, to lung disease which obstructs the pick up of oxygen by hemoglobin (q.v.), or to circulatory hindrance which prevents the access of oxygen-containing blood to the tissues.

Antibiotic Antibiotics are substances secreted by molds, fungi and even some bacteria, and inhibit the growth or multiplication of other species of microorganism, while being largely inoffensive to human cells. Penicillin, produced by the mold *Penicillium notatum*, is the classic example.

Antibody External substances introduced into the body (microorganisms, pollens, transplanted tissue, etc.) are 'recognized' as foreign by the host lymphatic defense mechanisms which respond by producing neutralizing proteins called 'antibodies', fashioned to 'fit' the foreign stimulus. In many cases the antibody inactivates an infective agent or prepares it for destruction elsewhere in the body.

Anticonvulsant The increased irritability of affected parts of the brain which results in epilepsy may be controlled by certain drugs, known as anticonvulsants. Phenobarbitone is a widely used anticonvulsant.

Antigen The (usually) foreign material, often a protein, which excites the body's immune response system and calls forth the antibody response (*see* Antibody).

Antihistamine Histamine is one of the body's potent amines (q.v.) released from cells damaged by physical, chemical or allergic attack. It may lead to considerable, sometimes dangerous, localized swelling of the skin and internal tissues, running eyes and nose in hay fever, and some forms of asthma. Antihistamine drugs block these unwanted effects.

Aorta The main channel which conducts arterial blood under pressure from the muscular left ventricle of the heart and from which large branches distribute the supply to the head, upper limbs, trunk and legs. It is a resilient tube approximately 2 centimeters in diameter with large quantities of elastic tissue in its walls. Its internal surface may become the site of atherosclerosis (q.v.).

Arteriography The process in which a radio-opaque dye is injected into a major blood vessel (e.g. the aorta, q.v.), outlining all of the branches of the vessel so that X-ray photographs may be taken. Obstruction, for instance to a coronary artery, can be identified and located in this way.

Arteriosclerosis Literally a thickening or hardening of the arterial wall, this term encompasses many changes affecting large and moderately large arteries in the body. The clinical effects of arteriosclerosis depend on the degree of obstruction to blood flow which ensues and which particular territory of supply is involved. Gangrene of the foot, coronary thrombosis and stroke are often due to arteriosclerosis of the limb, coronary and cerebral arteries respectively. Delicate arterial surgery may relieve arterial obstructions, but preventive measures aimed at delaying and preventing the degenerative changes in the arterial wall are now being actively researched.

Arthritis Disease of the articulating joint surfaces or the structures closely associated anywhere in the body is included in this rather general term. The least common variety is due to infection. The degenerative changes of age, osteoarthritis, are almost inevitable with the passing years, and are hastened by injuries or if the joint is congenitally abnormal. Rheumatoid arthritis is a chronic deforming and disabling disease thought to be due to immunological attack upon an altered joint lining (*see* Autoimmunity).

Arthroscopy Inspection of the interior of a joint with a specially fashioned telescope, now often employing optical fibers.

Arthrosis This term distinguishes a non-inflammatory change in a joint, e.g. degenerative change due to ageing, from the inflammatory changes of arthritis. The terms are however often used interchangeably.

Atherosclerosis Literally 'hardening of the gruel'. This is the term

185

now widely applied to the fatty, cholesterol-containing plaques which form on the internal surface of arteries an overlying clot, leading sometimes to complete obstruction. Its profile can be demonstrated by arteriography.

Autoimmunity When the body's immune responses are stimulated, not against 'foreign' materials but against 'self', the autoimmune state so caused may lead to severe damage to normal body tissues.

Bacillus Rod-shaped microorganism, of which there are many subtypes. Though many strains of bacilli may be responsible for infection in man (e.g. urinary tract, bowel or bloodstream infections), others may live within the human bowel without causing disease unless resistance to infection is lowered. The familiar colon bacillus, *Escherichia coli*, has been extensively studied in the laboratory and its metabolism and genetic characteristics have provided much new information of value to the understanding of disease in man.

Bacterium The name of the whole family of microorganisms, including bacilli, cocci, spirochetes, etc., but excluding fungi and the ultra-microscopic viruses. They inhabit the planet in unimaginable numbers and variety, and fortunately only a few cause disease in man. The great majority occupy an important and, in human terms, valuable place in our ecosystem.

Barbiturates A class of drugs widely used in the past for their sedative and narcotic properties. Because of the frequent development of drug dependence, and the commonness of abuse and suicidal use, there are powerful moves to restrict the general use of barbiturates, though several well defined and important indications for their use (e.g. epilepsy) remain.

Biopsy The removal of a small fragment of tissue from an affected organ, usually as a 'core' cut by a fine needle inserted into the tissue under local anesthesia, for microscopic or chemical diagnostic examination.

Cancellous The structure of bone is very dependent on its function. The tubular, ivory-like cortex (q.v.) of the long bones of the limbs, for example, gives great strength and rigidity to the structure. A much less dense, spongy bone occupies part of the interior. This cancellous bone gives strength along lines of special stress and strain.

Capillary The finest division of the vascular system, supplying blood to the tissues through hair-fine, tubular structures, the wall of which is essentially one cell-layer thick and so permeable that oxygen and nutrients readily pass out to the tissues and waste products diffuse in from them.

Carcinogenic Certain chemical substances or physical factors which provoke cancerous change in skin or other body tissues are described as carcinogenic. Many carcinogens have now been identified, some derived from tar and its products. Repeated application of radiation (even very strong sunlight over many years) may cause cancerous change in the skin.

Carcinoma This is a general term for malignant growths or cancers arising from epithelial or surface cells lining the various tubes, glands and cavities—even the skin—of the body. Cancers of deep, non-surface connective tissues (e.g. bone and muscle) are known as sarcomas.

Cartilage The gristly material which gives structural support to the nose, the ears, the respiratory tubes, etc. Most bones arise from ossification of cartilaginous forerunners in the infant.

Catheter A catheter is a fine tube which is introduced into one or other of the cavities or conduits of the body. Initially catheters were used for drawing urine from the bladder. Special catheters have now been devised which can be threaded, through venous or arterial channels, into and beyond the heart. Blood samples and local pressure measurements can thus be obtained from otherwise inaccessible sites.

Cerebral palsy Failure of development of part of the forebrain, often due to injury to it during childbirth, resulting in abnormality of the neurological functions involved. When the motor areas of the brain are affected the limbs concerned are weak, stiff and uncontrollable, i.e. spastic. Though speech and movement may be grossly disordered, potential intelligence is often intact. Intensive retraining, drugs and surgery, can now do much to make life tolerable for people so affected.

Cervical Literally means 'apertaining to the neck', but usually requires further qualification. Cervical vertebrae, for example, are the bony segments of the spine in the neck region. A cervical smear is taken from the neck of the womb.

Chemotherapy Strictly, the use of chemical substances to attack in a specific way the agents (microorganisms, fungi, cancer cells, etc.) which are responsible for disease. The sulfonamides were an early example, still used in the treatment of meningococcal meningitis. In some senses, the antibiotics like penicillin should be included under this head, particularly as many antibiotics are now chemically synthesized.

Cholera An infective disease spread in contaminated water supplies responsible for great waves of death and disease until quite recent times. The cholera vibrio attacked the intestinal wall, which shed great volumes of fluid into its lumen (q.v.). The ensuing dehydration and vascular collapse quickly had lethal effects.

Cholesterol A waxy fat which is an important constituent of every cell in the body, playing a role in the structure of the cell membrane, and of the tiny organelles within the cell. Transported in the blood as part of the lipoprotein complex, when present in excess it is thought to play a key role in causing atherosclerosis (q.v.).

Chromosome The unit of inheritance is the gene, composed of deoxyribonucleic acid (DNA). Many genes strung together in functional sequences form a chromosome, usually a double structure with a contribution from each parent. Each species has its own characteristic number and shape of chromosomes. Abnormality of a single gene may cause inherited disease but this structure is so small that it causes no observable change in the structure of the chromosome. However, large chromosomal abnormalities (additional parts or whole chromosomes, loss of a chromosome) have now been detected microscopically as the cause of certain disease states. Most major chromosomal aberrations are incompatible with fetal development.

Cirrhosis Usually applied to liver disease in man, this is a condition of fibrous replacement of normal liver tissue with shrinkage and distortion of the organ and loss of function. Infections, drugs and alcohol are the main causes.

Coeliac Coeliac disease is essentially a disorder of the absorptive mucosal surface of the small intestine. In a very high proportion of cases, it is due to an abnormal reaction of the gut mucosa to a constituent of wheat, gluten. Withdrawal of gluten from the diet usually leads to recovery of normal function.

Coronary arteries Literally, the ring of arteries that 'crowns' the heart and supplies it with its own circulation. Arrest of flow in a coronary artery or a main branch by blockage will result in death or disordered function of the heart muscle in its area of supply—coronary thrombosis and myocardial infarction.

Cortex When an organ or tissue of the body is functionally separated into an outer 'shell' and an inner pulp, these are known as the cortex and medulla respectively (e.g. adrenal gland; bone; brain).

Cyanosis The blue color of lips, fingers, and sometimes cheeks and mucous membranes resulting from an increase in the deoxygenated (reduced) form of hemoglobin (q.v.). This may result from slowed blood flow with increased local oxygen extraction, or from disease of the heart and lung which impairs oxygen pick-up (*see* Anoxia).

Cytotoxic Certain drugs have a direct poisonous or toxic action on living cells. They may disrupt the metabolic processes of the cell or hinder its multiplication. Although clearly harmful, these effects may be used therapeutically in the treatment of cancer or leukemia, when the tumor cells may be selectively damaged and their unruly proliferation brought to a stop.

Diabetes One of the earliest diseases of man to be recognized and described, diabetes is, in its most severe form, made obvious by the tremendous thirst and urination caused by the uncontrolled loss of glucose from the body. It was a fatal disease until the isolation of insulin in 1921 made it possible to replace, by injection, the key hormone the absence of which causes this lethal condition.

Diuretic The accumulation of fluid in the body in some diseases of the heart, kidneys or liver may be reversed by the use of diuretic drugs which promote increased urinary excretion of salt and water by selectively inhibiting reabsorption in the kidney tubules.

Diverticular Diverticular disease is a condition where small 'outpouchings' form along the length of the intestine, most often in the colon. Infection occurring in one or more of these causes much pain and fever, sometimes with local abscess formation.

Dropsy The ancient term for fluid accumulation in the body. Though most familiar as swollen ankles or legs, fluid accumulation may also affect the lungs and make breathing difficult. Diuretics (q.v.) are used for treatment.

Eczema A condition where the chronically irritated skin reacts with thickening, increased cellular activity, and oozing, crusting, scaling and itching. It is often the result of sensitization of the skin to some external substance met with in the home or at work.

Electrocardiogram (ECG) Each beat of the heart is accompanied by the generation of tiny electrical currents which can be detected, amplified and recorded in an electrocardiogram. This gives important information about the health of the heart muscle and shows up any disturbances of rhythm.

Electroencephalogram (EEG) As with the heart, brain action also generates micro-currents which can be picked up at several points over the brain and recorded in an electroencephalogram. The normal pattern of wave activity is disturbed by tumors, infection or epilepsy. The self-observation and willed control of certain dominant cortical electrical rhythms form the basis of so-called biofeedback, being actively explored as a method for the self-treatment of disorders regarded by some as psychosomatic.

Electrolyte The salts which go into solution in the body fluids and then ionize—sodium, potassium, magnesium, calcium chloride, bicarbonate, etc. Electrolytes have vital functions in the maintenance of normal cellular activity.

Embolus If the circulation is impeded by some body which blocks the vessel and which has been swept there by the blood flow, the body is described as an embolus. Though usually a blood clot, it may also be an air bubble which has entered the blood stream. Rarely, fat globules released from the marrow after bony injury may be responsible.

Endemic Endemic diseases lie dormant within a population, just a few cases appearing from time to time to point to some undetected cause. If the disease is infectious it may flare up to epidemic proportions, particularly if the level of immunity (natural or induced by inoculation) in the population falls to a low level.

Endocrine Endocrine glands (e.g. pituitary, thyroid, adrenal) secrete their product (a hormone) directly into the bloodstream, unlike exocrine glands such as the salivary or gastric glands, which secrete to the 'exterior'. (*See* Pancreas.)

Endoscope Most of the cavities, hollow organs and even blood vessels can be viewed directly through an appropriately constructed endoscope, in principle a long, flexible tube containing a multiple fiber light guide, the tip of which can be directed to its destination. As well as giving a direct view, the endoscope enables photographic records to be made.

Enzyme A term coined by Louis Pasteur to describe the fermenting powers of extracts made from yeast. 'Enzyme' (literally, 'in yeast') has now come to be applied to a vast array of organic catalytic molecules which spatially arrange reactive molecules to optimize reaction rates.

Epidemiology There is much to be learnt from the study of disease in defined population groups as well as in individual patients. Though first applied to the study of infection in human populations, epidemiology now extends to include all disorders—cancer, heart disease, psychiatric disorders, etc.

Epilepsy Sudden, unpredictable convulsions in apparently healthy, normal humans have been described since the earliest records were made. In some cultures people so affected have been worshipped as possessed of a holy spirit. In modern society, the condition is understood as a sudden discharge of nerve impulses from the brain, often the cerebral cortex, resulting in convulsive and uncoordinated motor activity and disorders of consciousness.

Epithelial Refers to the cells coating the 'outer' surface of gland, organ or tissue. The surface concerned may be deep within the body: for instance the renal tubules, which process the urine, lie deep within the kidney, yet are lined by epithelial cells. An epithelium is an external limiting layer of cells, often with highly specialized functions (e.g. excretory, absorptive, protective).

Erythrocyte (Erythro = red, cyte = cell.) The mature red blood corpuscle (there are 5 million of them in one microliter of blood) which transports oxygen in combination with the hemoglobin it contains to the tissues of the body.

Femur The thigh bone which, at its upper end, makes the important ball and socket joint with the pelvis. It is the neck of this bone, taking great stresses, which is liable to fracture in older people with thinning bones.

Fiber-optic A light path composed of many fine flexible fibers of glass which has been incorporated in most modern endoscopes (q.v.). As well as illuminating the area under inspection, the fibers will carry reflected light back to the observer's eye and are able to transmit images around an arc of curvature.

Fibrillation The uncoordinated flickering or fluttering of muscle, in contradistinction to powerful, well organized voluntary contraction. When it occurs in heart muscle, the pumping function of the chamber involved is greatly compromised.

Fistula A fistula is an abnormal communication between adjacent organs or tissues, or with the surface of the body. Thus, a fistulous connection between bladder and bowel may lead to recurrent infection of the urinary pathway by organisms from the gastrointestinal tract. A chronic fistula may discharge pus from an abscess deep within the body out onto the skin surface.

Gastro-enteritis Irritation, inflammation or infection of the stomach and intestine, leading to microorganisms or toxic substances, leading to vomiting, diarrhea and, frequently, abdominal pain. The loss of fluid from the bowel may be very considerable, and in small children or babies may even lead to lethal dehydration.

Gastroscope A specially adapted endoscope (q.v.) which is able to pass through the esophagus into the stomach and to provide a view to the observer's eye or to the camera of the internal surface of the stomach. Ulcers and cancers can be diagnosed at a very early stage in this way. Small samples of tissue (biopsies) may also be snipped through the gastroscope for microscopic examination and diagnosis.

Genes *See* Chromosome.

Geriatric Geriatrics is a branch of medicine and medical science devoted to the problems of the elderly. It is important to remember that this is in many ways an artificial division—many disorders of the old have their origins in youth and may differ little clinically from those of younger people. There are of course disease states which are seen much more commonly in the elderly, and social factors come to play a very large part in their management.

Germ The term widely used in popular parlance to describe the transmissible agents of disease. Not very precisely defined, it is used to refer to bacteria, viruses, fungi, and in fact all microorganisms.

Glycoside A complex chemical substance with glucose as part of its structure, usually derived from plant sources. Glycosides have great value in the treatment of heart disease. Digitalis and its derivatives (the cardiac glycosides) are probably the best known examples. They act by slowing and strengthening the contraction of the heart.

Goiter Swelling of the thyroid gland usually occurring because of its increased stimulation by thyroid-stimulating hormone from the pituitary. In iodine-deficient areas, goiters may grow to enormous size and may even threaten life by obstructing the airways.

Half-life Certain substances disappear from the body in such a way that their concentration halves every so many minutes or hours. Clearly, it would be very difficult to pick the precise time that the substance disappeared finally from the body, since its absolute removal grows slower and slower. However, the time in which its concentration halves remains constant across a wide range and can therefore be used to express its 'rate of decay'.

Hematology The study of disorders of blood and bone marrow. It is an important branch of medicine with many specialized techniques.

Hemodialysis *See* Renal dialysis.

Hemoglobin The chemical substance responsible for the redness of the blood. This iron-containing protein serves the vital function of carrying oxygen from the lungs, where it picks it up, to the tissues of the body, where it releases it. Some form of oxygen-carrying protein of this sort is an essential prerequisite of all higher forms of life.

Hemolysis Lysis is the breakdown of cells, and so hemolysis refers to blood cell (usually red cell) breakdown. Old cells are lysed continuously but increased rates of red cell lysis cause anemia and jaundice (from the yellow products of hemoglobin breakdown). Hemolysis may be the result of a fault in the red cell, the presence of toxic substances or infection which injure red cells, or overactivity of normal removal mechanisms.

Hemoperfusion The removal of circulating poisons from the blood by passing it through a column of adsorbent material (charcoal specially purified is most frequently used) which selectively binds the toxic material and allows the normal constituents to pass on.

Hemorrhage Loss of blood following injury is the most familiar form of hemorrhage but blood may be lost in the gastro-intestinal tract or into one of the body cavities and so be concealed. Clotting mechanisms usually stop hemorrhage unless they are defective.

Hemostasis A term applied to the mechanisms by which bleeding is arrested. It includes contraction of injured vessels, plugging of leaks with blood platelets, and the complex series of events by which the fibrin clot forms and closes off the injured vessels.

Heterotransplantation (*See* Homotransplantation.) The grafting of organs and tissues from one species to another.

Histology The study of cells and tissues under the microscope. Histology will often identify the nature of a disease process and sometimes point to its cause. The development of specific stains which pick out and identify certain cell constituents has greatly aided diagnosis and research. This approach may be even further refined by attaching a dye, often fluorescent, to an antibody which reacts only with a single antigen in the cell.

Homeopathy A system of medicine, differing from conventional medicine or 'allopathy', and working on the principles that 'like cures like' and that drugs become active in a highly diluted state.

Homotransplantation (*See* Heterotransplantation.) Exchange of organs and tissues within members of the same species.

Hormone The product of special cells or glands, which passes into the bloodstream and produces a specific effect upon other, usually distant, cells or tissues. Thus thyroxin from the thyroid gland governs the metabolic activity of all the tissues of the body.

Hypo- Below, beneath, under, or deficient.

Hypothalamus Part of the brain which forms the floor and part of the lateral wall of the third cerebral ventricle (q.v.). It has controlling functions over the pituitary gland as well as over sleep, body temperature control, appetite, etc.

Hyper- Above, increased, excessive.

Insulin Hormone produced by the beta cells, a constituent of the islets of Langerhans, tiny glands scattered through the pancreas and making up about one-hundredth part of its bulk. Principally concerned with blood glucose control, insulin also has important actions upon protein and fat metabolism. It was extracted, purified and used in the treatment of diabetes just over 50 years ago.

Isotope The function of various tissues and organs of the body may be monitored by the use of isotopes, usually the radioactive ones. An isotope is the form of an element (e.g. iron, hydrogen, iodine, etc.) which differs from the naturally occurring form in the structure of its atomic nucleus. This may confer special properties (e.g. radioactivity) upon it so that its progress through the body may be followed and deductions drawn about the normality or otherwise of the processes concerned.

Laparoscope An endoscope (q.v.) used to visualize the interior of the abdomen.

Lesion A general term indicating an alteration in a tissue due to disease or injury.

Leucocyte A white blood cell. It has the capacity to engulf foreign material, including bacteria, and forms part of the body's defense mechanisms.

Leukemia Disease of the blood, caused by uncontrolled proliferation of the cells producing leucocytes or lymphocytes.

Ligation Tying; the application of a ligature.

Lumen The cavity or channel of a tube, for example the space within the blood vessel or within the intestine.

Lymphatic Almost all organs and tissues of the body are supplied with a system of fine channels which drain the tissue fluid which accumulates outside the blood vessels. These fine lymphatic channels pass through small lymph nodes which filter off microorganisms, foreign particles and even toxic molecules and prevent them from passing back into the general circulation of the body. It represents an important first and second line of defense of the body against invasion.

Lymphocyte These white cells are formed in the lymphoid tissue throughout the body and in the thymus gland. They have an important function in the defense against infection, both in the production of circulating antibodies and by actual physical adhesion to invading agents.

Medulla *See* Cortex.

Megakaryocyte This is a giant multinucleate cell in the bone marrow, from which platelets are released to circulate in the blood. These platelets are involved in blood clotting and also physically aggregate to plug small holes in blood vessels.

Metabolism Essentially a shorthand word used to describe the totality of physical and chemical processes occurring in a living organism. Strictly describes the changes wrought in food between the points of ingestion and excretion. It includes the processes of anabolism (building up) and catabolism (breaking down).

Microbe Another term for microorganism, bacterium (q.v.) or, more popularly, germ (q.v.).

Mitral valve The valve between the left atrium and left ventricle, said to resemble a bishop's *mitre*. It is particularly susceptible to damage in rheumatic fever and its disease leads to imperfect function of the pumping activity of the heart.

Molecule A combination of two or more atoms forming a specific chemical substance. Thus a small molecule like water has two atoms of hydrogen and one of oxygen. Macromolecules may consist of many hundreds of thousands of atoms in fixed combination and taking up specific shapes, which, in living organisms, determine their function.

Morbidity Referring to disease. The morbidity rate is the ratio of sick to healthy persons in a population.

Mucosa The soft lining of most of the sacs and absorptive surfaces of the body. Mucosal structure and function are regionally adapted to local needs. For example, the intestinal mucosa has many fine, finger-like projections which greatly increase its absorptive efficiency and its surface area (*see* Villus).

Myelography A procedure in which a radio-opaque dye is injected into the space surrounding the spinal cord and radiographs are taken.

Neoplasm Literally, 'new growth'. Any lump or tumor derived from a single class of cells of the body may properly be termed a neoplasm. If these cells grow in an orderly way and remain under the control of body mechanisms, this would be classified as a benign neoplasm. Malignant neoplasms, or cancers, differ in their unruly and unregulated growth which spreads from one to another part of the body. *See* Carcinoma.

Nephropathy Chronic disease of the kidney.

Neuritis This term, which strictly means inflammation of nerves, is applied to many nerve disorders which are not actually inflammatory. It is accurately applied to the nerve disorder of leprosy. The term 'Alcoholic neuritis', though frequently used, does not describe a strictly inflammatory process. The term neuropathy is more often applied to non-inflammatory nerve disorders.

Neurology The study of nervous diseases. Neurology encompasses disorders of the brain, spinal cord, peripheral nerves and muscles.

Neuron A nerve cell with its processes. One of the structural units of the nervous system.

Neurophysiology The study of the function of nervous tissue.

Neurosensory Relating to a sensory nerve.

Nosology The study of disease classification.

Obstetrics The speciality dealing with the management of pregnancy, labor and the period immediately after it, the puerperium. Originally the province of the midwife and tribal matriarchs, the orderly development of this discipline has preserved the lives of countless mothers and babies.

Ocular Pertaining to the eye.

Oscilloscope An instrument which provides a visual display of electrical currents. Its familiar form is the cathode ray oscilloscope of the television screen. Most commonly used in intensive care situations to monitor the electrical impulses from the heart in the electrocardiogram.

Palpation Examination by touch, using the fingertips, the palm or the whole hand. The medical student learns the arts of inspection, palpation, percussion (tapping) and auscultation (listening).

Pancreas Gland lying across the posterior wall of the abdomen. Most of its substance produces digestive enzymes and juices which are discharged into the duodenum (i.e. it has an exocrine gland function). Scattered throughout are the small islets of Langerhans which make insulin and glucagon, hormones which pass directly into the bloodstream (i.e. they have an endocrine function). (*See* Insulin.)

Parasite A creature which lives on and draws sustenance from another, not seriously affecting its capacity to survive, or even enhancing it. The commonest troublesome parasite of humans is the head louse. Microorganisms living parasitically in the human bowel may manufacture and provide vitamin B_{12} necessary for blood formation.

Pathogenic Disease-producing.

Pathology The branch of medicine which deals with structural changes in the tissues brought about by disease. Its interests extend from examination of the whole body at autopsy to the detailed microscopic study of tissue samples, often removed diagnostically in life. Chemical pathology has come to describe the biochemical study of disease processes due to chemical disturbance in the tissues.

Pharmacopoeia A book containing lists of drugs and their uses. Official pharmacopoeias also describe chemical tests for purity and identity and contain recommendations about dosage.

Pituitary Endocrine (q.v.) gland lying in the skull, beneath the mid-brain and attached to the hypothalamus (q.v.). Anatomically and functionally divided into anterior and posterior parts, the anterior pituitary produces several hormones which regulate the activity of other endocrine glands to which it responds by sensitive feedback mechanisms.

Placebo The 'placebo' effect of a drug or treatment is one which arises from the mind of the patient, rather than from a specific effect of the treatment. In order to measure the strength of this placebo effect when evaluating a new drug, it may be necessary to give a preparation identical in appearance with the genuine preparation, but lacking any specific effect. Ideally, comparison of drug and placebo should be carried out 'double blind', with neither patient nor observer aware which preparation is which. Placebos are never used as such in ordinary medical treatment.

Plasma The fluid, non-cellular part of the blood. It is a rich soup containing fats, proteins and sugars which it supplies for tissue nutrition as well as carrying away soluble breakdown products.

Platelet The smallest formed cellular element in the circulating blood. The platelet performs an important function in arresting blood loss after injury. It plugs openings in small blood vessels and releases substances from its surface which cause constriction of blood vessels and which contribute to the formation of the insoluble fibrin clot. Like many other cells platelets are formed in the bone marrow.

Polymorph Literally, many-shaped. Refers to the predominant circulating white blood cell, whose main function is to engulf foreign organisms and particles, and which, when killed, forms pus.

Portal system Usually refers to the vessels which collect blood from the intestines and related glands and transport it to the liver. A minor but important portal system collects blood from the hypothalamus and transports it to the anterior lobe of the pituitary gland.

Pneumothorax Collapse of the lung caused by air passing into the pleural space between the lung and the lining of the chest cavity. It may be introduced by traumatic injury of the chest wall or by the rupture of a small air-filled cavity on the surface of the lung itself. For many years artificial pneumothorax was used therapeutically in the treatment of pulmonary tuberculosis to relax and so rest the diseased lung.

Prophylactic Substance given or procedure undertaken to prevent illness. Thus chloroquine is taken prophylactically to guard against malaria.

Prosthesis An artificial replacement. Thus a plastic or metal replacement heart valve or an artificial limb is generally known as a prosthesis. Even false teeth qualify.

Protozoa Primitive, single-cell organism. Some, like amoebae, cause disease in man.

Psychosis A term used to describe the more severe forms of mental disorder, especially those involving delusions and hallucinations, and including schizophrenia, manic-depressive psychosis, and endogenous depression. Although the term used to be used to distinguish these disorders from the lesser neuroses, the distinction is not absolute.

Psychosomatic Psychosomatic symptoms are bodily symptoms produced by emotional or mental disorders. It was fashionable to ascribe many disorders to psychosomatic causes—peptic ulceration, high blood pressure, diabetes, migraine have all been called psychosomatic diseases. Though emotional upsets may certainly influence the course of these diseases, it now seems very unlikely that they are ever the cause of them.

Psychotherapy Treatment designed to produce a response by non-physical means. Techniques include reassurance, suggestion, hypnosis, abreaction and group therapy, as well as Freudian or other techniques of psychoanalysis.

Psychotropic Refers to drugs which have their main effect upon the emotions. They may calm anxiety or relieve depression and often act by changing the concentration of amines (q.v.) in certain areas of brain.

Puerperal fever Happily now a thing of the past in civilized countries, this infection of the raw surface of the maternal womb following the recent delivery of a child used to claim a high proportion of recently delivered mothers. It is mainly due to streptococcal infection. The disease was virtually eradicated when simple measures of hygiene such as hand washing and isolation helped by the use of antiseptics was introduced. It was finally defeated by the introduction of antibiotics.

Pulmonary Pertaining to the lung. Pulmonary tuberculosis, for example, is infection of the tissues of the lung with the tubercle bacillus. In a pulmonary embolus one of the main blood vessels to the lung becomes blocked by a clot brought to it from elsewhere in the circulation.

Purine Nucleic acids, the constituents of DNA (see Chromosome) and RNA, contain two kinds of bases—purines and pyrimidines. Gout is a disorder of the metabolism of purines, resulting in the accumulation of uric acid, the main breakdown product, in the body. Crystals of urate in the joints provoke an acutely painful inflammatory arthritis. Deposits in the kidney may cause renal failure.

Radiation Used non-specifically for various kinds of electromagnetic rays—X, gamma, beta, alpha—as well as for light.

Radiography The production of an image on a film or a television screen by means of X-rays. The photographic image results from the contrast between structures or tissues through which X-rays pass easily (radiolucent) and those, like bones, which hinder the passage of the rays (radio-opaque).

Radio immuno-assay An elegant technique for detecting and measuring substances present in body fluids at very low concentration, based upon the use of antibodies to the substance to be measured. The antibody, raised in another species, e.g. the guinea pig, is saturated with a radioactively labelled form of the substance to be measured. The saturated antibody is then exposed to the fluid containing the unknown quantity of the substance. The higher the unknown quantity, the more radioactivity it will displace from the antibody, and the residual radioactivity can be measured. The use of this simple technique which has revolutionized our understanding of endocrinology and has found widespread medical and biological applications is attributed to the American workers the late Solomon Berson and Rosalyn Yalow.

Renal dialysis (hemodialysis) A procedure in which substances in the blood normally secreted by the kidneys are removed by exchange across an artificial membrane in a machine called a dialyser.

Rheumatic fever An allergic illness affecting the joints and the valves of the heart which may occur after infection with certain streptococcal bacteria. Progressive changes in the heart valves may lead to heart disease later in life.

Schizophrenia An abnormality of mind with many definitions. Its characteristic features are a withdrawal from reality into a fantasy existence, a loss of drive and interest in the real world, and sometimes inexplicable hallucinations and delusions. The schizophrenic state has been likened to the condition between sleeping and waking experienced by many normal people.

Sclerosis Hardening of a tissue (see Arteriosclerosis, Atherosclerosis).

Sepsis A general term indicating infection of the surface or interior of the body, often as the result of some other happening, e.g. childbirth, or during the course of surgery or other therapeutic activities. Antiseptic measures combat infection, while aseptic conditions are achieved when sources of infection have been excluded.

Serum Blood minus the corpuscles, platelets and fibrinogen. Obtained from blood which has clotted, this blood fraction contains all the antibodies against disease, and these may be used for diagnostic or therapeutic purposes.

Septicemia Widespread infection including the blood itself.

Spasticity Impaired movements with stiffness and resistance to passive movement, usually due to brain damage. (See Cerebral palsy.)

Spina bifida Congenital malformation of variable severity due to incomplete closure of the spinal canal during fetal development. The damage to the nerves in the spinal cord may be associated with paralysis of the bladder and lower limbs.

Spirochete Spiral bacterium, progressing by corkscrew rotatory movements. One variety (*Treponema pallidum*) is the cause of syphilis. Another causes Weil's disease, an infection of liver and kidneys.

Spleen Thought by the ancients to be one of the seats of the emotion, the spleen is actually a large lymph glandular organ situated in the left upper abdomen. Its role is essentially that of a filter, removing abnormal particles and effete cells from the circulation. It is not essential to life.

Sputum Mucoid material secreted by bronchial glands and coughed up from the lungs.

Staphylococci Cocci are small ball-like microorganisms (unlike bacilli, which are rod-shaped). Staphylococci are bunched together like grapes. Streptococci are grouped in chains. Cocci of both groups are responsible for many of the infective diseases of man.

Steroids A term which refers to a class of chemical compounds with a strong family resemblance to each other, and all very similar to cholesterol, from which may be derived. The characteristic feature is the 4-carbon-ring structure, and the specific hormonal properties depend upon the nature of the side chains tacked on onto the 4-ring nucleus. Adrenal steroids or corticoisteroids are formed by the cortex of the adrenal gland. The sex hormones, testosterone in the male and estrogens in the female, are also steroid hormones.

Streptococci *See* Staphylococci.

Sulfonamide A family of antibacterial drugs which interfere with bacterial metabolism and prevent multiplication of organisms. The sulfonamides were introduced before the antibiotics, but still have useful roles in certain infections.

Suture A stitch. Although much surgical suturing is done with a threaded needle, many machines have been developed to insert sutures into delicate, intricate or inaccessible structures. The end to end, watertight suturing of small arteries is an example of this.

Syndrome Collection of symptoms or signs which are repeatedly found occurring together and so are characteristic of a disease or disorder.

Systemic Affecting the whole body.

Thrombosis Clotting of blood within a vein or artery. A valuable property of blood following trauma, when thrombosis occurs in an uninjured artery or vein the result may be disastrous. Anticoagulant drugs are used to prevent this.

Thymus The thymus gland is located high up in the chest, at the front. Long regarded as a vestigial area of lymphatic tissue, it has lately been recognized as a most important organ controlling the immune processes of the body. Lymphocytes discharged from it are 'programmed' to recognize a number of foreign substances and to attack them. It becomes progressively smaller with age and can hardly be found in elderly people.

Thyroid The endocrine gland lying in the neck in front of the trachea. The thyroid produces a hormone, thyroxine, which regulates the activity of every cell and tissue in the body.

Toxin Toxins are poisonous substances produced by bacteria. Tetanus, for example, is caused by a toxin. A toxoid is a modified, non-poisonous toxin injected to produce antibodies in the host which neutralize the toxin itself and so confer protection.

Trachea The main air-conducting pathway leading from the

189

pharynx or throat and terminating by dividing into the two main bronchi carrying air to the right and left lung. Obstruction to the trachea causes asphyxia which may sometimes be relieved by tracheotomy—the making of an opening into the trachea through the throat.

Transducer An instrument which converts one kind of energy to another, in medicine often into electrical impulses; used for measuring, for example, the pressures within body cavities or temperatures at inaccessible sites.

Trauma An injury or a disturbing experience.

Trivalent vaccine A single vaccine protecting against diphtheria, tetanus and whooping cough.

Tuberculosis An infective disease caused by the mycobacterium tuberculosis. Different strains affect man, cattle, birds and rodents. In man, it most commonly affects the lungs, but may spread from there to other parts of the body.

Tumor Literally, a swelling. A general term which refers to any growth, whether benign or malignant.

Typhoid Literally, 'clouding'. The word describes a severe infective disease due to the most virulent of the food poisoning organisms, *Salmonella typhi*. Spread in milk, water and food, it ravaged unprotected populations but in addition to its control by public health measures the organisms can now be killed with appropriate antibiotics. The only resemblance that it has to typhus fever, a quite different serious houseborne infection, is the 'clouding' of consciousness due to the severity of the infection.

Vaccine A preparation of organisms (bacteria or viruses) of low virulence which, when injected, nevertheless stimulates the production of antibodies which are also effective against the virulent strains of the organisms, and thus provide protection against that particular infection.

Vagus nerve The tenth cranial nerve, which arises from the brain and pursues a long, wandering route to supply the heart, the stomach and the intestines.

Ventricle Literally, 'a little stomach'. This term is applied to the blood-filled muscular chambers of the heart (right and left ventricles) and to the fluid-filled spaces deep within the brain (the cerebral ventricles) through which the cerebrospinal fluid circulates.

Vertebra An individual component of the backbone. Essentially composed of a solid body and a bony arch. The backbone forms a flexible but strong support for the body structure and conducts the spinal cord under protected conditions.

Vibrio The comma-shaped microorganisms first seen by Koch in cases of cholera are examples of the vibrio. Though they were recognized as the cause of cholera, it was not until comparatively late that its transmission in water supplies was understood. On the incorrect assumption that it was airborne, the British army was always forced to march at right angles to the wind during campaigns in cholera-ridden countries.

Villus A finger-like projection from the lining of the small intestine. The very large number of the villi increases the effective area for the absorption of foodstuffs.

Virus One of the simplest and most primitive living organisms, only able to multiply within the cells of other living things. Many human diseases are caused by viruses, including poliomyelitis, influenza and the common cold.

Vitamin Originally 'vitamine' or 'vital amine', because these substances were thought to be amines (q.v.). Now means a substance necessary to life (in quite small quantities), only obtainable from dietary sources and not capable of synthesis within the body from simpler precursors.

Index

Key to endpapers

1. **Hippocrates** (460–377 BC) Greek physician of antiquity who is traditionally regarded as the father of modern medicine.

2. **Aristotle** (384–322 BC) Greek philosopher, logician and scientist who, perhaps more than any other thinker, has characterized the orientation and content of all that is termed Western civilization.

3. **Asclepiades** (124–c. 40 BC) Established Greek medicine in Rome; opposed humoral doctrine of Hippocrates.

4. **Celsus, Aurelius Cornelius** (flourished AD 10–37) Known as Roman Hippocrates, gave first indication of how neuropsychiatric disorders were grouped relative to other medical problems.

5. **Galen** (AD 129–199) Greek physician who founded experimental physiology.

6. **Susruta** (5th century AD) Indian surgeon and author of a great medical treatise.

7. **Rhazes** (died c. 923) Persian alchemist and Muslim philosopher, considered to be the greatest physician of Islam.

8. **Avicenna** (980–1037) The most famous and influential of the philosopher-scientists of Islam.

9. **Paracelsus** (1493–1541) Swiss physician and alchemist who established the role of chemistry in medicine.

10. **Paré, Ambroise** (1510–1590) French surgeon regarded as the father of modern surgery.

11. **Harvey, William** (1578–1657) British physician and discoverer of the true nature of the circulation of the blood.

12. **Borelli, Giovanni Alfonso** (1608–1679) Italian physiologist and physicist who was the first to explain muscular movements and other bodily functions according to the laws of statics and dynamics.

13. **Sydenham, Thomas** (1624–1689) British physician, a founder of clinical medicine and epidemiology.

14. **Boyle, Robert** (1627–1691) Chemist and natural philosopher noted for his pioneer experiments on the properties of gases and espousal of a corpuscular view of matter that was a forerunner of the modern theory of chemical elements.

15. **Leeuwenhoek, Antony van** (1632–1723) Dutch microscopist, the first man to observe bacteria.

16. **Boerhaave, Hermann** (1668–1738) Dutch physician and professor of medicine who was the first great clinical or 'bedside' teacher.

17. **Lind, James** (1716–1794) Founder of naval hygiene in England; a physician whose recommendation that fresh citrus fruit and lemon juice be included in the diet of seamen resulted in the eradication of scurvy from the British Navy.

18. **Hunter, John** (1728–1793) Surgeon and founder of pathological anatomy in England, early advocate of investigation and experimentation.

19. **Pinel, Philippe** (1745–1826) French physician and a founder of psychiatry, who pioneered the humane treatment of the mentally ill.

20. **Jenner, Edward** (1749–1823) British physician and discoverer of vaccination against smallpox.

21. **Davy, Sir Humphrey** (1778–1829) Chemist and scientist who discovered several chemical elements.

22. **Laënnec, René-Théophile-Hyacinthe** (1781–1826) French physician who invented the stethoscope and is considered to be the father of chest medicine.

23. **Chadwick, Sir Edwin** (1800–1890) Social reformer who made achievement of sanitary reform in Britain his life work.

24. **Bernard, Claude** (1813–1878) French physiologist known chiefly for his discoveries concerning the role of the pancreas in digestion, the glycogenic function of the liver, and the regulation of the blood supply by the vasomotor nerves.

25. **Snow, John** (1813–1858) British physician who showed that the London cholera epidemic was caused by contaminated water.

26. **Ludwig, Carl Friedrich Wilhelm** (1816–1895) A founder of the physico-chemical school of physiology in Germany, best known for his study of the cardiovascular system.

27. **Morton, William Thomas Green** (1819–1868) American dental surgeon who in 1846 was the first to demonstrate the use of ether during surgery.

28. **Nightingale, Florence** (1820–1910) British nurse, founder of trained nursing as a profession for women.

29. **Helmholtz, Hermann von** (1821–1894) The greatest figure in the experimental study of vision. His *Physiological Optics* is still the most important work on the subject.

30. **Virchow, Rudolf** (1821–1902) German pathologist, anthropologist and statesman who pioneered new concepts of pathology by applying the cell doctrine to the concept of disease.

31. **Galton, Sir Francis** (1822–1911) British explorer, anthropologist and eugenicist, known for his pioneering studies of human intelligence.

32. **Pasteur, Louis** (1822–1895) French chemist and microbiologist who proved that microorganisms cause fermentation and disease.

33. **Charcot, Jean-Martin** (1825–1893) French medical teacher and clinician, a founder of modern neurology.

34. **Lister, Joseph** (Lord Lister) (1827–1912) Surgeon and medical scientist who pioneered the use of disinfectants for the prevention of surgical infection.

35. **Jackson, John Hughlings** (1835–1911) British pioneer neurologist whose studies of epilepsy, speech defects and nervous system disorders arising from injuries to the brain and spinal cord remain among the most useful and best documented.

36. **Koch, Robert** (1843–1910) German physician and one of the founders of the science of bacteriology.

37. **Metchnikoff, Elie** (1845–1916) Russian zoologist and microbiologist, discovered that amoeba-like cells in animals engulf foreign bodies such as bacteria – a phenomenon known as phagocytosis.

38. **Röntgen, Wilhelm Conrad** (1845–1923) German physicist who in 1895 discovered X-rays.

39. **Pavlov, Ivan Petrovich** (1849–1936) Russian physiologist known chiefly for his development of the concept of the conditioned reflex.

40. **Ehrlich, Paul** (1854–1915) German medical scientist known for his pioneering work in hematology, immunology and chemotherapy and for his discovery of the first successful treatment for syphilis.

41. **Freud, Sigmund** (1856–1939) Founder of psychoanalysis, published in 1899 his major work, *The Interpretation of Dreams*.

42. **Garrod, Sir Archibald Edward** (1857–1936) British physician who conducted important research on the biochemical genetics of inherited human metabolic diseases, especially the first direct study of alkaptonuria.

43. **Ross, Sir Ronald** (1857–1932) British bacteriologist who discovered that malaria was transmitted by the anopheles mosquito.

44. **Curie, Pierre** (1859–1906) French professor of physics who, with Marie Curie, isolated radium in uranium ore.

45. **Hopkins, Sir Frederick Gowland** (1861–1947) British biochemist who discovered essential nutrient factors now known as vitamins.

46. **Curie, Marie** (1867–1934) Physicist and first woman professor at the Sorbonne who, together with Pierre Curie, isolated radium in uranium ore.

47. **Landsteiner, Karl** (1868–1943) Born in Vienna, immunologist and pathologist who discovered the major blood groups and developed the ABO system of blood typing.

48. **Cushing, Harvey Williams** (1869–1939) American neurosurgeon whose work on the pituitary body gained international attention and who first described a type of obesity of the face and trunk known as Cushing's disease or syndrome.

49. **Fleming, Sir Alexander** (1881–1955) British bacteriologist whose discovery of penicillin in 1928 prepared the way for antibiotic therapy for infectious diseases.

50. **Anitchkow, Nikolay Nikolaevich** (born 1885) Russian pathologist who has done important research on blood vessels and correlation of medullary centers.

51. **Kendall, Edward Calvin** (1886–1972) American chemist who isolated, from the adrenal cortex, the steroid hormone cortisone and, with Philip S. Hench, applied the hormone in the treatment of rheumatoid arthritis.

52. **Waksman, Selman A.** (1888–1973) Biochemist who discovered the antibiotic streptomycin.

53. **Muller, Hermann Joseph** (1890–1967) American geneticist. Demonstrated that X-rays speed up the natural process of mutation and remembered for his theoretical idea of a 'sperm bank' to 'conserve genius'.

54. **Dam, Henrik** (born 1895) Danish biochemist who discovered vitamin K and did research on antihemorrhagic substances.

55. **Penfield, Wilder Graves** (1891–1976) Canadian neurosurgeon who located several functional areas of the human cerebral cortex in the development of surgical treatment of epilepsy, discovered that stimulation of interpretive cortex activated neuronal record of past experience, and developed centrocephalic hypothesis of memory control.

56. **Banting, Sir Frederick Grant** (1891–1941) Canadian physician who, with Charles H. Best, discovered insulin in 1921.

57. **Domagk, Gerhard** (1895–1964) German bacteriologist and pathologist who discovered the antibacterial effects of Prontosil, the first of the sulfonamide drugs.

58. **Hench, Philip Showalter** (1896–1965) American physician who made important discoveries concerning the hormones of the adrenal cortex, their structure and biological effects. In 1948 he successfully applied an adrenal hormone (later known as cortisone) clinically in the treatment of rheumatoid arthritis.

59. **Castle, William Bosworth** (born 1897) American physician. Major research has been in pathological physiology of nutritional and hemolytic anemias. Discovered intrinsic factor which, together with extrinsic factor (now known to be vitamin B_{12}), is required to prevent pernicious anemia.

60. **Enders, John Franklin** (born 1897) American microbiologist who cultivated poliomyelitis virus in tissue culture, a preliminary step to the development of the polio vaccine.

61. **Reichstein, Tadeus** (born 1897) Polish chemist who made important discoveries concerning hormones of the adrenal cortex, their structure and effects.

62. **Florey, Baron Howard Walter** (1898–1968) Born in Australia. Pathologist who, with Ernst Boris Chain, isolated and purified penicillin for general clinical use.

63. **Best, Charles Herbert** (born 1899) American physiologist who, in 1921, with Sir Frederick Grant Banting, was the first to obtain a pancreatic extract of insulin, the anti-diabetic hormone, in a form that controlled diabetes in dogs. Successful use of insulin in treating human patients followed.

64. **Burnet, Sir Frank MacFarlane** (born 1899) Australian physician and virologist; discovered acquired immunological tolerance to tissue transplants.

65. **Müller, Paul Hermann** (1899–1965) Swiss chemist who discovered the potent toxic effects on insects of DDT.

66. **Krebs, Sir Hans Adolf** (born 1900) Biochemist who discovered the series of chemical reactions in living organisms known as the Krebs cycle.

67. **Forssmann, Werner** (born 1904) German surgeon, a pioneer in heart research, particularly in the development of cardiac catheterization.

68. **Chain, Ernst Boris** (born 1906) German-born biochemist who, with Howard Walter Florey, isolated and purified penicillin and performed first clinical trials.

69. **Sabin, Albert Bruce** (born 1906) American virologist who developed an orally administered vaccine for the prevention of paralytic poliomyelitis.

70. **Hodgkin, Dorothy Mary Crowfoot** (born 1910) British chemist whose determination of the structure of vitamin B_{12} brought her the 1964 Nobel Prize for Chemistry. Has since elucidated the three-dimensional structure of insulin.

71. **Salk, Jonas Edward** (born 1914) American virologist who first developed a vaccine for the prevention of poliomyelitis.

72. **Medawar, Sir Peter Brian** (born 1915) British zoologist who discovered acquired immunological tolerance when he found that adult animals injected with foreign cells early in life accept skin grafts from the original cell donor.

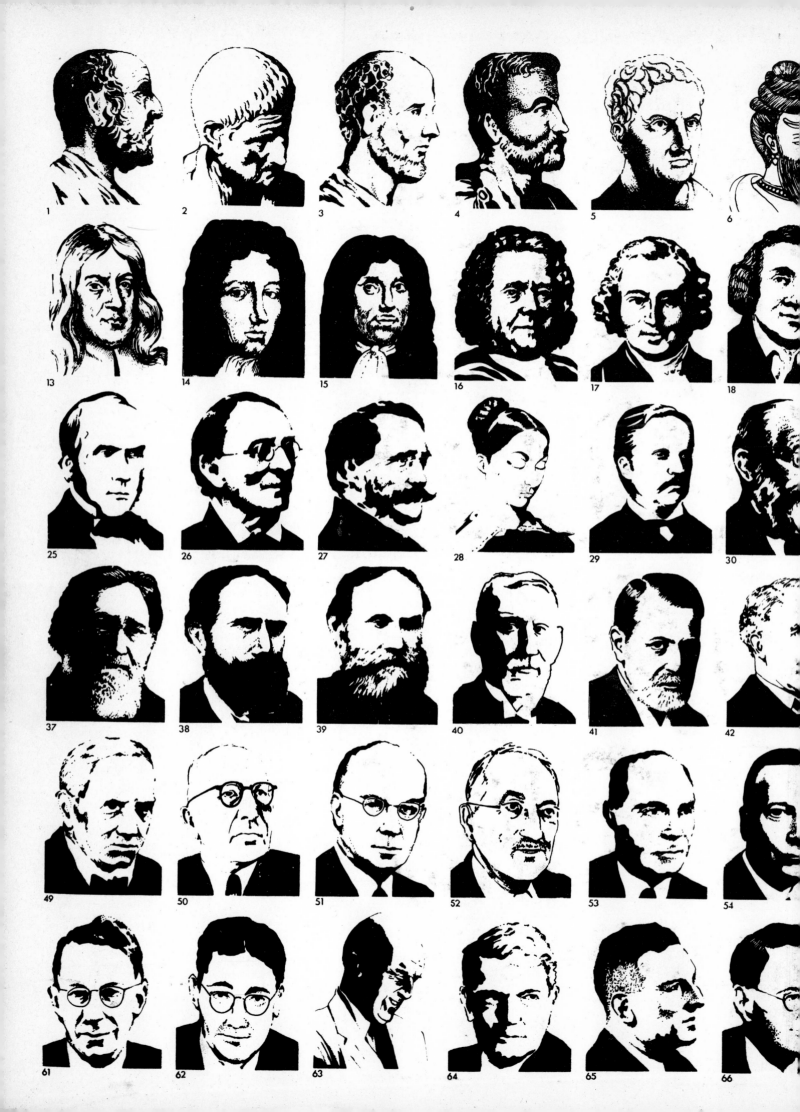